Diabetic Retinopathy for the Comprehensive Ophthalmologist

SECOND EDITION

Raj K. Maturi, M.D.

Associate Clinical Professor

Department of Ophthalmology

Indiana University School of Medicine, Indianapolis

Retina Service, Midwest Eye Institute

Jonathan D. Walker, M.D.

Clinical Assistant Professor

Indiana University School of Medicine

Fort Wayne

Robert B. Chambers, D.O., FAOCOO

Associate Clinical Professor

Havener Eye Institute

Department of Ophthalmology & Visual Sciences

The Ohio State University, Columbus, Ohio

Deluma Medical Publishers
7900 West Jefferson Blvd.
Suite 300
Fort Wayne, IN 46804
retinopathytext@gmail.com

Editor
Steve Lenier
editor@stevelenier.com

Layout and Design
Lauren Peacock
lauren@canalstreetwinona.com

Line Art
Roberta J. Sandy-Shadle
Publications
Indiana University-Purdue University, Fort Wayne

Financial Disclosures

None of the authors have any proprietary interests in either the book or its subject matter. Dr. Maturi serves as a consultant to Eli Lilly and the Jaeb Center for Health Research. He is on the advisory board for Allergan and Regeneron, and is a principal or sub-investigator for Alcon, Alimera, Quark, Allergan, Sanofi, Eyegate, GlaxoSmithKline, Jaeb Center, Parexel and Santen.

Legal Disclaimer

The author provides this material for educational purposes only. It is not intended to represent the only or best method or procedure in every case, nor to replace a physician's own judgment or give specific advice for case management. Including all indications, contraindications, side effects, and alternative agents for each drug or treatment is beyond the scope of this material. All information and recommendations should be verified, prior to use, with current information included in the manufacturers' package inserts or other independent sources, and considered in light of the patient's condition and history. Reference to certain drugs, instruments, and other products in this publication is made for illustrative purposes only and is not intended to constitute an endorsement of such. Some material may include information on applications that are not considered community standard, that reflect indications not included in approved FDA labeling, or that are approved for use only in restricted research settings. The FDA has stated that it is the responsibility of the physician to determine the FDA status of each drug or device he or she wishes to use, and to use them with appropriate patient consent in compliance with applicable law. The author specifically disclaims any and all liability for injury or other damages of any kind, from negligence or otherwise, for any and all claims that may arise from the use of, any recommendations or other information contained herein.

ISBN-13: 978-0-9821472-2-1

DEDICATED TO:

My wife Dheepa R. Maturi, for her years of steadfast support, love and kindness; my children, Vikas and Jay, for their incredible humor, good nature and love. Each of you has made this lifetime so much more joyful.

Raj K. Maturi

My wife Deborah, and my children Lucius and Maria. No soy nada sin ellos. The truth of that continually amazes me.

Jonathan Walker

To my wife DeAnne and my children Christopher and Megan with an equal measure of thanks for your support of me and pride in your own accomplishments.

Robert B. Chambers

ACKNOWLEDGEMENTS

There are many broad shoulders upon which this book stands. First of all, there are the pioneers of retinopathy treatment that have given us the tools that we have and the elegant studies that tell us how to use them. There are also the folks all around the world--like the members of the DRCR.net--that are trying to provide even better therapies. They intuitively grasp the infinity of things not covered in Chapter 2. On a more personal level, I owe a great debt to all the attending physicians and ancillary staff at the Ohio State University, the USC/Doheny Eye Institute, and the University of Iowa. They are not only busy performing all the tasks mentioned above; they also had to suffer through training me.

I want to thank Dr. Sandeep Nakhate, Dr. Robert Goulet III, Lucius Walker and Dr. Alan "Patience is Your Most Valuable Surgical Tool" Kimura, who were willing to spend their time reviewing the first edition. And this book has been brought to a new level by my co-authors, Bob Chambers and Raj Maturi, who took on the thankless task of making right the things I wrote. They also have been invaluable friends and colleagues over decades of retinal practice. Of note, I was responsible for the final version, so anything that is wayward is totally my doing.

Thanks also to Drs. Giorgio Dorin, David Sorg, Valerie Purvin, James Schmidt, Dale Fath, Donald Reed, Thomas Wheeler, Taniya de Silva, Krishna Murthy, Lik Thai Lim and John Pajka, who contributed to individual chapters in various ways. Everyone's advice has been invaluable and is reflected in anything in the book that is actually useful.

Thanks to Lauren Fath and M. Walt Keys; they made the first edition happen. And the second edition now exists thanks to the editing skills of Steve Lenier and the artistic skills of Lauren Peacock; their contact info is in the front matter if you have a book in you that is hankering to come out. The marvey line art was provided by Roberta Sandy-Shadle and the photos in Chapter 7 were done by James Whitcraft—both at Indiana-Purdue University, Fort Wayne. Mike Neeson helped out by confirming my memories of lasers of old, and Larry Hubbard of the Wisconsin Reading Center generously shared his Zen Master knowledge of retinopathy grading. Thanks to my partner—Matt Farber—who actually saw the patients while I was locked in my office Photoshopping laser spots, and thanks to my exemplary office staff for keeping everything going when I wasn't. Of course, there are no words to thank my wife and kids for doing all the real work while I alternately napped and typed on the couch.

Finally, thanks to the referring doctors for entrusting me with their patients and especially thanks to the patients themselves, who extend the ultimate honor of entrusting us with their eyes.

Jonathan Walker

Contributors

Taniya de Silva, MD
Associate Professor of Clinical Medicine
Program Director, Endocrinology Fellowship
Section of Endocrinology, Diabetes & Metabolism
Louisiana State University School of Medicine
New Orleans, LA

Lik Thai Lim, MBBCh, BAO(UK), FRCOphth, FRCSEd, MFSTEd
Consultant Ophthalmologist
Malaysia

Krishna R. Murthy, MRCOphth
Prabha Eye Clinic & Research Centre
Vittala International Institute of Ophthalmology
Indira Gandhi Institute Of Child Health Sciences
Bangalore, India

James E. Schmidt, MD, FACC
Clinical Associate Professor of Internal Medicine
Boonshoft School of Medicine
Wright State University
Dayton, OH

TABLE OF CONTENTS

AN INTRODUCTION

This book is designed to transfer useful skills for the clinical management of diabetic patients. It does not start with the fundamentals; instead, it is assumed that the reader has basic examination skills and is at least partially familiar with various tests, such as fluorescein angiography and optical coherence tomography.

Nor does this text offer an in-depth discussion of basic science or an exhaustive review of the available literature. If you want an in-depth look at the literature behind treating retinopathy, you are encouraged to review the sections on diabetes in any of the major ophthalmology texts. Another excellent resource is the book **Diabetic Retinopathy: Evidence-Based Management** by David J. Browning—it is a must read for anyone who wants to really understand the disease.

The goal of this book is simply to make the trenches where most of us live a bit more comfortable.

The voice of this text is different from standard texts—something done in hopes of conveying useful information without too much tedium. However, as a wise person once said, "There is a fine line between clever and stupid." If anything offends or interferes with the smooth download of information, let us know.

Also, there are no absolutes here. Once you think you know the best way to do anything, you have lost the ability to learn. Try these suggestions and techniques, and if they don't work, throw them out. Run them by your mentors and your friendly neighborhood retinal specialists—get other opinions and synthesize a style of your own. We welcome any comments and/or complaints. If the gods of retina smile on this book, then perhaps there will be further editions with plenty of input from people way smarter than us. Our contact info is below.

Mostly, we hope that you can peruse these pages and find something that will help you to help patients who have one of the most prevalent and vicious causes of blindness on this planet.

Robert B. Chambers, D.O.

Raj K. Maturi, M.D.

Jonathan Walker, M.D.

Contact info:
Deluma Medical Publishers
7900 West Jefferson Blvd. #300
Fort Wayne, IN 46804
260 436-2181
retinopathytext@gmail.com
Drcobook.com

P.S. At various points in the text, there are unavoidable opportunities to harass our surgical colleagues who have mastered more refractively oriented procedures. Recognize that this is meant in good sport and, in truth, stems largely from professional jealousy— they can actually understand things like high order aberrations and apodized lenses *and* they have patients who hug them after surgery.

Retina specialists do not generally get hugged by their patients. Moreover, the only bit of optics we understand is The Retina Refraction: room lights on—better one; room lights off—better two.

Onward...

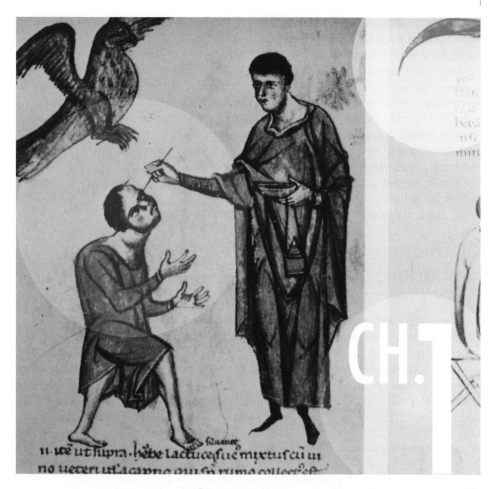

A Tiny Bit of Statistics and a Big Pep Talk

Whatever you do will be insignificant, but it is very important that you do it. Mahatma Gandhi

First, some really big numbers: An estimated 20.2 million Americans have diabetes mellitus, and the number is expected to grow to over 30 million cases by the year 2025. And, half of them may not even know that they have the disease! Thanks to exports like the Great Western Lifestyle, the number of worldwide cases is expected to increase by 72%—to 333 million—by the year 2025.[1] That is a lot of microaneurysms. By contrast, currently the number of patients blind from cataracts worldwide is estimated to be 18 million people. In other words, although a lot of ophthalmic effort is (correctly) directed towards decreasing the worldwide cataract burden, the number of patients at risk for vision loss from diabetes will soon be almost 20 times greater. Moreover, once a cataract is popped out, the job is done. Treating diabetes goes on forever for both the patient and physician—it isn't one-stop shopping.

Diabetic blindness also tends to occur at a time when people are younger and more active in society; it is the leading cause of new blindness in patients under the age of 65.

The rate of onset is variable, but after 20 years, about 60% of Type 2 and essentially all Type 1 diabetics will have some sort of retinopathy. You will spend a great deal of time caring for these patients. It may seem that the treatment of diabetic retinopathy has been well defined thanks to the large clinical trials with which you are no doubt familiar. However, the reality is that each patient you see presents an incredibly complex array of variables—social, emotional, physical and retinal. Addressing all of these variables requires a lot more than the ability to memorize the definition of clinically significant macular edema. It is axiomatic that we all went into ophthalmology to avoid dealing with the morass of an entire patient. Unfortunately, when it comes to treating diabetic retinopathy, your results are going to suck if you don't start by understanding the entire patient. At the very least, recognize that by the time a diabetic needs your help, they are usually facing the risk of irreversible vision loss—real, life-changing vision loss—not Nerf vision loss that can be fixed with Lasik.

Dharma Break: *Each diabetic patient whose vision you save probably represents more quality-of-life units than a whole surgery schedule full of 20/30 glare cataracts. Think about it...*

And the battle is bigger than just honing your clinical skills and trying to deal with the entire patient. At the risk of sounding hyperbolic, you also have to look at the society in which you function. It has been said that if patients are examined in a timely fashion and the standard treatment guidelines are followed, less than 5% of diabetics will develop severe vision loss.[2] A huge part of your job lies in recognizing the importance of the first clause of that sentence: if patients are examined in a timely fashion. Not only do you need to develop the ability to treat these people, but you also have to be aggressive about getting them in to be evaluated. Far too many diabetics show up only when they start having symptoms, and this is not the best way to keep people seeing.

Educate the patient and the patient's physicians at every visit. Educate the patient's family about the importance of getting everyone in the family routinely checked for diabetes and getting anyone who is diabetic in for an annual exam.

Educate society. Give talks to local diabetes support groups. Offer to provide information for the health desk editors at local newspapers, magazines or TV stations. Do the free clinic thing—or more ambitiously, get them a camera so they can send photos of all their diabetics and you can treat the ones with disease well before they fall apart. Make general information slides for the local cinema multiplex so they can be interspersed with all of those fascinating questions about which actor said what in which movie. Whatever. Just get these people in.

(All this may not only help prevent blindness; it can also help build your reputation and your practice—a twofer! Watch the ethical ramifications, though. It is one thing to generate public service messages that help patients and their doctors. It is quite another thing to plant your smiling face on an ad that says you are the bronzed god or goddess of retinopathy. This is a test.)

Unfortunately, you will still see plenty of cases that don't show up in time. Helping a pair of eyes—and the patient attached to them—by slowing their descent into severe vision loss is still a good thing, but it is way better to stop the retinopathy before it can get to the fovea or up into the vitreous. You can only do this if you see the patient long before the real trouble begins. Aggressive monitoring and treatment can easily keep someone seeing until they leave the planet. Hopefully this is something you will be able to do many times and for many people before you hop off the globe, too.

References

1.   Wild S, Roglic G, Green A, Sicree R, King H. Global prevalence of diabetes: estimates for the year 2000 and projections for 2030. *Diabetes care.* May 2004;27(5):1047-1053.

2.   Rosenblatt B, , Benson W. Diabetic Retinopathy in: Yanoff M, Duker J, et al., eds. *Ophthalmology.* Second Edition ed. USA: Elsevier; 2004:877-886.

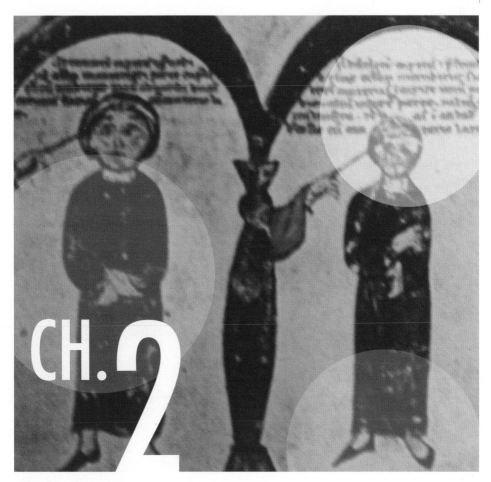

Basic Science

Didn't you read the intro? This is not a basic science text. If you want basic science, get a real textbook. Or go to ARVO. Sheesh...

moving on >>

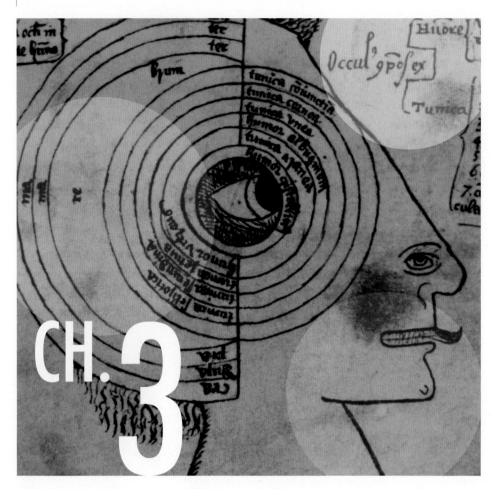

Diabetic Macular Edema—the Basics

Instead of seeking new landscapes, develop new eyes. Marcel Proust

DOING THE EXAM IN 2-D

This chapter discusses macular edema resulting from microvascular leakage around the posterior pole. Basically, diabetes turns the retinal capillaries into the vascular equivalent of leaky old garden hoses. The result is that patients develop microaneurysms, hard exudates, and hemorrhages in varying amounts. If there is a lot of leakage from the damaged vessels, then the retina will swell up like a sponge. If this swelling builds up in and around the center of vision, then permanent damage can occur, so the goal is to identify swelling and treat it well before this happens.

Besides causing leaky blood vessels, diabetes can also just kill off blood vessels. Most of the time, there is a combination of both problems—vascular leakage and capillary death. In some patients, the destruction of blood vessels is the predominant problem, and this is referred to as capillary dropout or macular ischemia. This is always bad and it can cause marked vision loss; so far there is no treatment other than prevention with good systemic control and by trying to address any treatable leakage. Although capillary dropout can cause retinal edema at first as a result of ischemia, the end result is a thinned-out retina. It usually requires a fluorescein angiogram to identify this problem, although it can be inferred if patients have marked vision loss and an atrophic-appearing fovea. (Figure 10 is an example of capillary dropout around the fovea.)

Unless the patient is truly unlucky, ischemia is usually not a predominant feature in the early stages of diabetic macular edema. Instead, vascular leakage tends to be the initial finding. Because this leakage is very treatable, it is crucial to be able to identify the clinical signs that indicate the beginnings of damage. At the very start of your career it is exciting to simply be able to see these findings—your first direct glimpse of a disease hard at work. However, once you master the mechanics of examining the fundus it is easy to become jaded about spotting the signs of retinopathy. Try not to let this happen. You can get a lot of clues about a patient's situation just by looking carefully at each of the various manifestations. For instance, you are no doubt aware that most intraretinal hemorrhages in diabetic retinopathy are blot-shaped because they stem from broken capillaries in the outer retinal layers, where the neurons are all jumbled together. As a result, the hemorrhage seeps out radially like a drop of food coloring on a paper towel. Flame-shaped hemorrhages occur when capillaries break in the more superficial nerve fiber layer, where the linear arrangement of the axons spreads the blood lengthwise rather than in all directions.

You may think that you are too cool to care about this second-year medical student stuff. You aren't. If a patient has an excessive number of flame-shaped hemorrhages and/or dot-blot hemorrhages, you should worry about superimposed problems like leukemia or thrombocytopenia (Chapter 27 goes into this much deeper). If there are no other diseases, you need to find out if the patient has other vascular risk factors that are not well controlled. The most likely culprit would be superimposed hypertension, but you might also see this with progressive renal failure or anemia. Many such patients also have poor compliance—usually due to a combination of lack of motivation, lack of insurance or lack of a motivated primary-care doctor. Based on a few red smears it is possible to make massive inferences about everything from a patient's creatinine to their socioeconomic status—and your deductions and consequent actions can have a dramatic impact on how the patient responds to your ministrations.

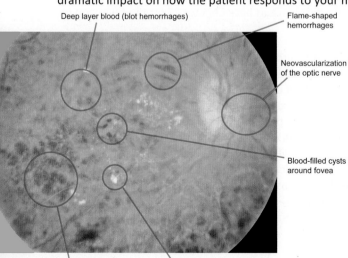

Deep layer blood (blot hemorrhages)

Flame-shaped hemorrhages

Neovascularization of the optic nerve

Blood-filled cysts around fovea

Confluent blot hemorrhages

Exudates

Figure 1: A patient with macular edema and multiple ugly looking hemorrhages. You can also see the tiny dots of heme around the fovea that suggest cysts filled with blood—even in the 2-D photo you can get a sense that those little dots are floating above the other damage. This patient had severe hypertension, early renal failure with secondary anemia and had been uninsured and unable to afford an eye exam until he could no longer function. You can infer a lot from a retina. (By the way, this book is produced without the benefit of corporate or drug company sponsorship, and a digital version is provided for free at the book's website so that anyone can access it. Some of the printed images have subtle findings and don't reproduce well in print—you may want to look at the digital version if you want a higher rez view of any given figure.)

In Chapter 1, it was pointed out that we all went into ophthalmology because taking care of an entire patient is not our bag, man. If we could get the eye mailed to us—without the attached patient—that would be fine. However, if you see worrisome hemorrhages, it is definitely time to dust off those atrophied clinical skills and check a blood pressure. Right there in the lane. While you are at it, you should also order a CBC, hemoglobin A1c and renal studies if no one has done them lately. These tests will identify significant problems much faster than a referral letter will, and the results will jumpstart the patient's care. Oh yeah, you might also help save their life (which is a nice break from a day full of "better one, better two"). Try to take advantage of all the information the fundus is willing to give you. If you look, but do not see, you will be failing to treat the patient's eye properly (and also be very un-Zen).

Another hemorrhagic nuance occurs in patients who are taking Coumadin. These patients will often have many more hemorrhages in the retina relative to their overall degree of retinopathy (in other words, they have more hemorrhages than you would expect, given the number of microaneurysms and non-hemorrhagic vascular changes that you see). All these hemorrhages may have varying sizes and unusual shapes. Make sure that your patients that are on this rat poison are really getting their levels checked; you will find occasional patients that are not being monitored properly. A more complete discussion of this drug and other anticoagulants in the setting of diabetic retinopathy is found in Chapter 26.

Cotton wool spots are another fundus finding that can tell you a lot about the patient. These used to be considered very important in terms of predicting future proliferative disease, but this has been disproven (which makes one wonder what other "facts" will be disproven in the future, which, in turn, makes one glad this book is produced with software and not woodcuts). A few scattered cotton wool spots are to be expected, and individual spots may last for several months. However, if there are a lot of cotton wool spots or if crops of new lesions appear rather quickly, it may signal problems with hypertension, renal failure, or hematologic abnormalities. Never forget that patients are also allowed to get completely unrelated problems, and it is always possible that a patient with lots of cotton wool spots may have an additional disease such as AIDS, retinal vasculitis or radiation retinopathy. Given the overall sturm and drang of diabetic retinopathy, it may be difficult to dissect out the presence of these other diseases unless you remember to think of them in the first place. (Check Chapter 27 for the full scoop on this.)

When actively studying hemorrhages and cotton wool spots, the Renaissance Retina Observer also inspects the hard exudate situation. Hard exudates begin to appear as more and more leakage occurs. You can think of them as high-water marks—the serum bathtub rings that outline where the retina is desperately trying to suck the abnormal fluid back into the capillaries and the leftover protein and lipid congeal into little yellow lumps. These lumps may be all over, but often they show up on the border between the healthy and damaged retina. Large amounts of hard exudates should always suggest the possibility of hyperlipidemia, so be sure to inform their medical doctor. Patients should be taught to consider their lipid profile to be as important as their blood pressure and hemoglobin A1c. Tight lipid control is a little-recognized aspect of total diabetic care, at least in the ophthalmic community, and pointing out to the patient that you can see "all those little fatty deposits" in their retina may be more of a motivator for healthy living than weeks of diabetic education classes.

There is always *something a bit mysterious, even to sophisticated patients, bout having someone look into their eye and state that damage is visible. Sometimes this can be a very effective tool for encouraging patients to take better care of themselves. Sometimes, however, it can be very depressing for patients to hear this—and you need to be sensitive to this as well. This is a good reason why it really is better that we don't get the eyes mailed to us. Chapter 22 will elaborate on issues like this a bit more.*

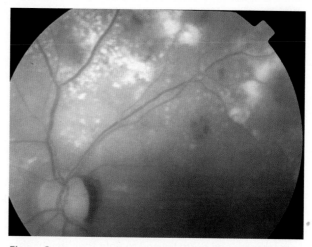

Figure 2: This kind of extensive hard exudate formation, especially along peripheral vessels, is very suggestive of hyperlipidemia.

DOING THE EXAM IN 3-D

Having developed some familiarity with the two-dimensional findings of background diabetic retinopathy, it is now time to go 3-D by looking for macular edema. Macular edema may be focal, which means that small, localized areas of microaneurysms create circumscribed areas of thickening, often surrounded by rings of hard exudates. Macular edema may also be diffuse, involving larger areas of the posterior pole and arising not only from microaneurysms, but also from diffuse capillary leakage throughout the vascular bed. Usually, there is a combination of both types of leakage. It has been argued that making a distinction between focal and diffuse leakage is irrelevant, especially in the era of intravitreal injections. Nevertheless, this is a good way to begin understanding the disease, and it can definitely help with planning laser treatment if you identify discrete areas of leakage to treat (more on this later).

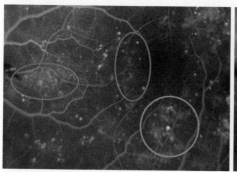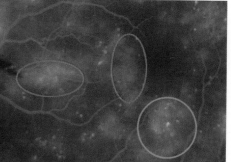

Figure 3: An example of different types of leakage. The green circles show areas where focal leakage from several microaneurysms predominates. The red ovals show areas where diffuse leakage from capillary beds predominates. Most areas are a mix of both.

Occasionally, diffuse macular edema may be difficult to diagnose because the whole retina is uniformly thickened, and unless you have a sense of "normal" thickening on clinical examination, the diagnosis may not be obvious. Most of the time the associated vision loss will point you in the right direction. Of course, your optical coherence tomography machine (OCT) is perfect in this situation, but not everyone reading this will have access to one. Plus, you really can't do a good laser without being able to readily identify retinal swelling on clinical exam, so do try to perfect your clinical exam. (More on OCT coming up.)

Perfecting Your Clinical Exam

It is crucial that you take the time to put a diagnostic contact lens on these patients, especially in the early stages of your diabetic retinopathy treatment career. Seriously. If you find yourself rationalizing a way to avoid using a contact lens, then you should go be a physiatrist or something. There is not enough axial magnification with the indirect slit lamp lenses (such as a 90- or 78-diopter lens) to really allow you to get a sense of how succulent the retina can become. It helps to visualize individual microaneurysms, hemorrhages and exudates and to note their height above the pigment epithelium at various places in the posterior pole. You can get a very definite feel for how thick the retina is by going back and forth between flatter, more peripheral areas and more swollen central areas. A thin off-axis slit beam helps somewhat in bringing out the three-dimensional structure, but nothing helps as much as just getting the contact lens on patients and doing the exam multiple times.

By the way, there are some other options to try to get a nice stereoscopic view without resorting to a contact lens—but like most things in life, the easier way is usually not the best way. You can get a 60-diopter lens (or something close to that number). The lower dioptric power will give you more axial magnification—you will get an enhanced stereoscopic view that can be almost as good as a contact lens. However, it is harder to line up both of your eyes through a 60-diopter; the patient has to be very well dilated and cooperative. If you can easily get the info you need from such a lens, then more power to you, but it is better to just put on the contact lens, especially at first. Another non-contact option is the Hruby lens. This is a plano-concave gizmo that may already be attached to the front of your slit lamp. It works by neutralizing the corneal curvature from a distance, and you usually click it down or lift it into a slot so that it is directly in your line of sight, and then you can study a non-inverted image of the macula. There is only a small field of view, and you are very dependent on patient cooperation, but the stereo is pretty good. Most folks find that the Hruby is too tricky to use, but you should at least try it if you have one on your slit lamp.

It is also very instructive to look at a recent fluorescein angiogram as you are examining the patient (and definitely when you are performing laser treatment). Carefully study each little lesion in the fundus and compare it to the angiographic appearance. You will note that many of the tiny red dots that you assume to be microaneurysms on clinical examination actually do not light up at all on the angiogram. These are simply dot hemorrhages and you may be wasting laser spots (and the patient's non-expendable RPE) if you shoot at them. Worse, these dot hemorrhages may readily take up laser energy and change color very easily—one of the criteria for successful treatment—and you may feel like you have done a great job, but you may simply have toasted valuable portions of the patient's nerve fiber layer. On the other hand, there will be many real microaneurysms that are invisible on your initial clinical exam but will then become apparent when you trace their location on the angiogram and track them down in the patient's fundus. These represent your true targets. Chapter 9 will cover all of this at length, but you have to know what you are looking for by doing the drills discussed here.

After tracing all of these lesions out on the angiogram and then finding them in the fundus on several patients, you will find that you are better and better at identifying these tiny lesions without an angiogram. Even if you try this only two or three times, you will be amazed at how your clinical skills will improve (and how your lasers will be more effective and less damaging). The result is better patient care and more efficient use of your valuable time—everybody wins!

The point is that you really need to get a feel for how "unobvious" diabetic retinopathy can be in order to fine-tune your ability to treat it properly, and the only way to develop your skills is to take the time to compare the fluorescein to the patient on a microscopic level, ideally using a contact lens, before you take on the responsibility of treating the disease with laser.

Stereo Photographs   *In the days when retinal photographers used film, it was common to obtain stereo photos of fundus pathology. You should ask around, because even the most digital photography departments may have some old stereo slides of diabetic retinopathy in the files. Another good source of stereo photos can be some of the older, beat-up textbooks in the back of your departmental library—especially the ones that have the little discs and 3-D viewer inside the back cover. For instance, old editions of Gass's Stereoscopic Atlas of Macular Diseases are so fantastic they can induce Ecstasy flashbacks.*

Stereo photos and fluoresceins are a beautiful way to get a sense of what is meant by the term "retinal thickening". If you are having a hard time figuring out just what you are supposed to see, it will take a few seconds of browsing stereo pics and you will understand. Note that stereo imaging with the fundus camera is more exaggerated than on clinical examination, and do not expect your patients to have the kind of dramatic elevation that is seen on good stereo photographs. It will, however, give you a very good idea of what to train your eye to look for, and it is way better than trying to hallucinate swelling based on what your OCT is telling you.

BUT ENOUGH ON THE EXAM. ON TO THE DISEASE...

All of the above is about being able to identify macular edema in general, but the real goal is to identify edema that is vision threatening, i.e., edema that needs to be treated. For decades, the primary enemy was defined by the Early Treatment of Diabetic Retinopathy Study (ETDRS) as "clinically significant diabetic macular edema" (CSDME). This term is reserved for findings that indicate a very high risk of progressive visual loss. The exact criteria for CSDME should be burned into your brain at this point in your career, but here it is for reference:

Criteria for Clinically Significant Diabetic Macular Edema

1. Retinal thickening within 500 microns of the center of the fovea.

2. Hard exudates within 500 microns of the center of the fovea that are associated with some degree of surrounding retinal thickening. (You should take a moment to ponder this second criterion. Both hard exudates and microaneurysms may be present without retinal thickening and, if there isn't any thickening, there definitely isn't any CSDME.)

3. One disc area of thickening, part of which is within one disc diameter of the center (or, to paraphrase Edgar Allan Poe, a disc within a disc).

The whole reason for defining CSDME this way is because the ETDRS showed that unless a patient actually has CSDME, the rate of vision loss was so low that there was hardly any treatment effect. (It is a tribute to the genius of the pioneers of diabetic treatment that they could define the disease in absolutely the most useful way—and do it before they even started the study!)

I stand amid the roar
Of a surf-tormented shore,
And I hold within my hand
Grains of the golden sand—
How few! yet how they creep
Through my fingers to the deep,
While I weep—while I weep!
O God! can I not grasp
Them with a tighter clasp?
O God! can I not save
One from the pitiless wave?
Is all that we see or seem
But a dream within a dream?

(This is just the second stanza. That guy could write...)

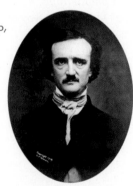

On the other hand, if patients did have CSDME, then laser treatment resulted in about a 50% decrease in the incidence of moderate visual loss at the three-year mark (Figure 4). Moderate vision loss was defined as doubling at the visual angle (i.e., 20/30 going to 20/60). Preventing this much vision loss is truly a Good Thing, and should rev you up for reading the chapters that follow.

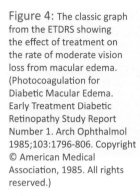 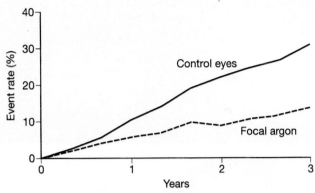

Figure 4: The classic graph from the ETDRS showing the effect of treatment on the rate of moderate vision loss from macular edema. (Photocoagulation for Diabetic Macular Edema. Early Treatment Diabetic Retinopathy Study Report Number 1. Arch Ophthalmol 1985;103:1796-806. Copyright © American Medical Association, 1985. All rights reserved.)

Now, CSDME is a bit of an Eighties construct, and it is a clinical definition—it is only there if you think you see it, and that means that there can be notable differences between examiners. Still, it is a useful definition, because laser is the best treatment when you are dealing with disease that is largely eccentric to the center of the macula. Knowing the definition of CSDME helps you decide which patients need laser treatment. (No worries. The next chapter will go over the nuances of DME treatment in detail—this section is just about definitions.)

But two things have combined to revolutionize the categorization of DME: optical coherence tomography (OCT) and intravitreal injections. OCT allows very precise measurement of retinal thickening—we are no longer dependent on subjective decisions about whether a macula is swollen or not. And intravitreal treatment allows treatment of foveal edema—something that is verboten with traditional laser. The combination of those two things has created the need for another DME definition: center-involved diabetic macular edema (CIDME). This is defined as central subfield thickness ≥250 μm (and vision impairment defined as Snellen equivalent of 20/32 to 20/320).[1]

To understand what that means, though, we need to bail out and talk about OCT. So hold that thought on CIDME for just a beat.

OPTICAL COHERENCE TOMOGRAPHY OCT

OCT has revolutionized our ability to visualize the architecture of the retina, and it can be extremely valuable for evaluating and following patients with diabetic retinopathy. As with fluorescein angiography, this review will assume that the reader has some familiarity with OCT testing already and will not cover finer points of how the test works or interpretation. If this is all new to you, there are lots of online resources, for instance, at oct.zeiss.com/blog.

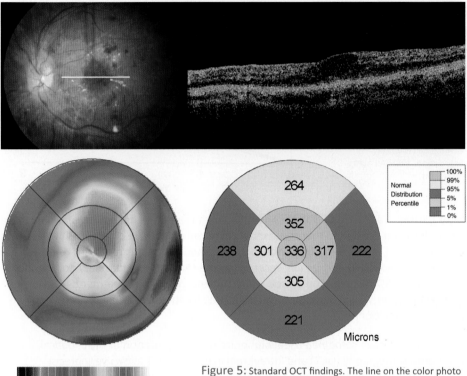

Figure 5: Standard OCT findings. The line on the color photo indicates the cut of the B-scan (upper left). The B-scan shows retinal thickening centrally (upper right). The lower left is the topographic retinal thickness map generated by averaging the different B-scans; it shows a focus of retinal swelling in and above the fovea. The color coding below the thickness map helps—they use "stoplight" colors: red is thickest, yellow intermediate and green normal, with white being the thickest (snow on top of the peak) and dark blue to black for the thinnest (the deepest ocean depths—this usually denotes pathologic atrophy). The middle right figure gives the average numeric thickness of nine sections of the scan—the "average retinal thickness map". Note that the average retinal thickness map uses a different color scale compared to the topographic retinal thickness map—for instance, dark red is used for the thinnest and pink for the thickest. The number in the central circle is the "central subfield thickness"—this is the number used to determine whether the patient has center-involved diabetic macular edema.

There are a few things to be aware of, however. OCT results come in two flavors: the individual B-scans that give you cross-sectional anatomy of the retina, and the various macular thickness protocols that give you a topographic map and 3-D cube of an entire region of the retina. One of the problems with the older Zeiss Stratus OCT machine—the machine used for most studies—is that it only obtains six individual B-scans and then "smears" those scans together in order to extrapolate the retinal surface. This means that a lot of the Stratus thickness map represents a digital extrapolation rather than real data—you definitely need to look at the individual B-scans in order to know what is truly going on. Plus, all OCT machines try to recognize specific retinal layers in order to calculate the overall retinal volume. It is possible for the computer to misinterpret the different retinal layers and give you information that is misleading—this is known as a boundary line error. Boundary line errors are especially common if the signal is weak due to a poorly done study or media opacity. Figure 6 shows the characteristic appearance of the effect of boundary errors on the Stratus topographic map.

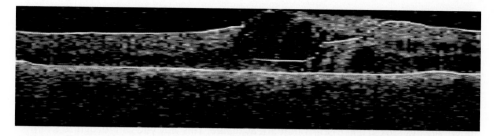

Figure 6: OCT boundary error. Note that the white lines do not follow the actual retinal architecture (above). This usually happens with very abnormal morphology and low signal strength (in this case the signal was attenuated by a vitreous hemorrhage). If you don't look at what the algorithm is doing, you can be very much misled, although you can usually get an idea that something is wrong when you study the retinal thickness map (right). When it looks like something you made at the spin-art booth at your elementary school fair, with weird hourglass colors and everything, you can bet that the computer misread the image. Note that this applies primarily to the Zeiss Stratus, which tries to average the retinal thickness from a small number of radial B-scans. Modern machines generate a large number of horizontal B-scans, but they can still generate boundary line errors. The errors look different on the thickness map—they tend to be more localized or linear because there is less extrapolation. The main point is never to rely on the thickness map alone to make a treatment decision. Be sure you know exactly what is going on with the retinal anatomy by looking at your B-scans.

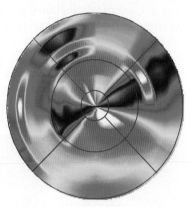

Whatever machine you have, you should always study all your B-scans to get a sense of whether the boundary lines are screwed up and to get an idea of the retinal microarchitecture. If you are only looking at one horizontal B-scan, you are missing a lot of useful data. For instance, Figure 7 shows a situation where one cut has a little bit of retinal thickening and an epiretinal membrane, but does not appear particularly ominous. A cut 90 degrees away shows a traction retinal detachment encroaching on the fovea.

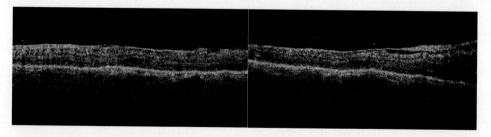

Figure 7: This is why you need to look at more than one cut of the OCT results. The left shows some retinal thickening and an epiretinal membrane—no big deal. The right is 90 degrees away, showing a much more ominous tractional detachment extending toward the fovea. Yes, you should have seen this on your clinical exam, but sometimes the clinical exam is subtle; you never want to be reassured by only one or a few cuts from the OCT—in the same way that you would never treat a routine glaucoma patient based on one pressure measurement.

The Zeiss Stratus is a "time domain" machine (TD-OCT), whereas most new machines, like the Zeiss Cirrus or Heidelberg Spectralis, are "spectral domain" (SD-OCT). A real textbook might actually explain those terms. Suffice it to say that spectral domain machines can obtain much more information in much less time, so there are a lot more B-scan cuts to provide more accurate measurements of thickness and volume. These machines can still have boundary errors, though, but they tend to show up as linear defects in the thickness map rather than as the crescents in the Stratus map above. *Always* look at the B-scans that are available. This way you can recognize when the machine has made a boundary line mistake, but more importantly there is a huge amount of information you can get from the B-scans that won't show up on the thickness map. Indeed, if you are using a time domain machine, recognize that you may be missing useful information and if a patient is not doing as well as you would think, you may want to refer the patient to someone with a spectral domain machine in order to get a better look at the anatomy. For instance, Figure 8 shows a patient with a normal looking thickness map yet worrisome cystic changes near the fovea. You might miss a finding like this if you are only looking at the thickness map or a few low-resolution cuts on a time domain machine.

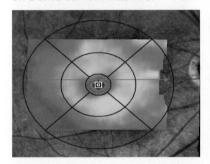 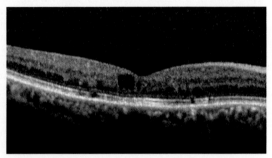

Figure 8: The image on the left shows a fairly unremarkable thickness map (although the yellow is a bit irregular compared to a truly normal OCT, which should make you suspicious). However, the patient had symptomatic vision loss and the B-scan shows why. You have to look at the cuts, not just the thickness map.

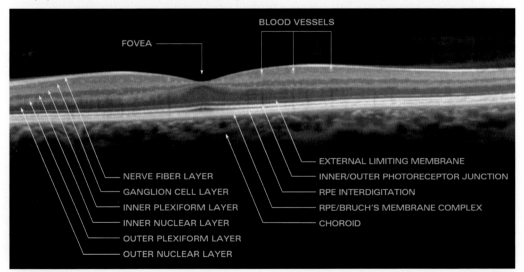

Figure 9: The anatomic detail available with a good scan using spectral domain OCT. Of particular importance is the inner/outer photoreceptor junction, also known as the inner segment/outer segment line. The patency of this line seems to be correlated with visual prognosis. Of note, there is controversy about whether this line really represents the inner and outer segment junction—it is more accurate to refer to it as the ellipsoid zone and the lucency above it as the myoid zone.[2] This book will use both terms together so everyone is on the same page. *(Image courtesy of Heidelberg Engineering, Heidelberg, Germany)*

There are other nuances of retinal microanatomy that the newer machines can provide—Figure 9 shows what kind of detail you can get. For instance, it is increasingly recognized that the continuity of the ellipsoid zone (inner/outer photoreceptor segment junction) is crucial in terms of a patient's visual potential.[3] This is true in diabetic retinopathy as well as almost any other disease state, such as macular pucker or macular degeneration. Figure 10 shows an example of damage to this line, which tells you that even if you eliminate the edema the patient's vision will likely be limited. The detail provided by spectral domain machines also allows DME to be classified into different anatomic subtypes, for instance, patients with diffuse retinal thickening versus cystoid changes versus subretinal fluid versus traction. Research is being done to determine whether these morphologies have prognostic significance—for instance, it appears that diffuse retinal thickening may respond better to anti-VEGF drugs whereas macular edema associated with subfoveal fluid may do better with intravitreal steroids.[4, 10]

Newer OCT techniques provide enhanced imaging, especially of the choroid. Enhanced depth imaging (EDI) OCT moves the focal point of spectral-domain OCT more posteriorly, resulting in a more detailed view of the choroid. Swept-source (SS)-OCT employs a tunable laser that can do over 100,000 A-scans/sec, providing for greater tissue penetration compared to standard SD-OCT and EDI-OCT. Since diabetes can also affect the choroid, the ability to better study choroidal architecture with these approaches may help our understanding of the overlying diabetic retinopathy. And it is now possible to use OCT to create images of vascular networks within the retina and choroid, a process known as OCT angiography. This allows visualization of the retinal capillaries without the need for injecting dye--a very promising technology, but not in wide use yet.

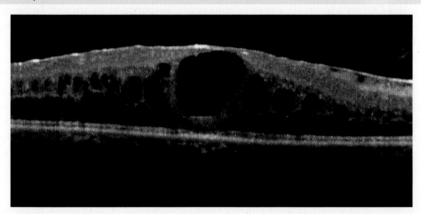

Figure 10: You can see that the ellipsoid zone (inner/outer segment line) breaks down below the big cyst in the fovea (as does the external limiting membrane, the RPE and the outer segments—basically everything that one needs to see). Don't give up, though—if you leave the retina this swollen things will only get worse. With treatment the patient was able to go from 20/400 to 20/100; you just have to be sure they understand the potentially guarded prognosis. By the way, you get 50 points for recognizing the thing on top of the retina. As we will see in subsequent chapters, an epiretinal membrane usually makes things harder to control and a patient like this may eventually need a vitrectomy. For now, one would simply try to deturgess the retina and then determine if removing the epiretinal membrane would help further.

As part of this, an extremely important use of OCT is the ability to identify problems with the vitreoretinal interface that can contribute to persistent edema. Although a careful clinical exam can usually suggest the presence of a subtle epiretinal membrane or taut cortical vitreous, abnormalities like this tend to become immediately obvious with OCT testing. This is useful when you have a patient with persistent edema and decreasing vision in spite of treatment. If you identify subtle traction, then you know that such a patient should be referred to your friendly neighborhood retina specialist, rather than given 300 more laser spots or 20 injections in a fruitless attempt to seal leaks in a retina that is slowly being pulled apart by the vitreous. There will be much more on this in subsequent chapters.

By the way, as you familiarize yourself with OCT results, you should also look at some of the options available for performing a scan. And maybe even get your retina scanned so you can fully grok the patient's experience. You should understand what the technicians are doing and be aware of the different fixation parameters, line cuts, and image processing techniques that are available. You can even—gasp—scan a patient yourself so you have a really good idea about what can be done to optimize the data you get. For instance, you may want to have the tech do some very high resolution scans in a patient that has visual symptoms but no definite findings on the standard scan—you can pick up subtle changes in retinal morphology that the standard scan misses. Or you may want to do a large number of closely spaced raster lines right at the fovea in a patient that may have vitreofoveal traction; sometimes the more widely spaced raster lines in a standard scan can miss very localized traction. If you don't know about these things you will not be able to get all the information that your very expensive device is capable of giving you.

Whatever machine you use, one of the great research advances created by the OCT is the ability to obtain numeric data describing the thickness of individual points and specific subfields of the macula. We no longer depend on subjective interpretation of fundus exams or stereo photographs, instead, studies looking at diabetic macular edema use OCT data to assess patient eligibility and response to treatment. Remember a few pages ago when we were talking about the definition of center-involved diabetic macular edema (CIDME)? Well, the Stratus got the whole ball rolling by handily providing the central subfield measurement (also known as the central subfield mean thickness measurement). This is the average thickness of the central millimeter of the retina. (It is the central circle in figure 5; in that example the thickness is 336 microns.) OCT can also determine the center point thickness, which is, duh, the thickness of the central point of fixation. However, the center point thickness is not very reproducible, especially if the retina is swollen and the patient has poor fixation. The central subfield thickness is felt to be more reliable, and most studies consider a central subfield thickness of greater than or equal to 250 microns to indicate center-involved edema.

Note *that the definition of CIDME also includes the visual criteria of 20/32 to 20/320. This refers to an ETDRS visual acuity, a very specific process using standardized charts, lighting and refraction techniques in order to obtain a vision that is accurate and reproducible. Because the process is designed to get the best possible vision, the ETDRS vision for a given patient tends to be better than the standard Snellen vision, but in practice everyone just uses the Snellen vision because ETDRS refractions are very labor intensive. Plus, it is likely that you will be trying to decide about how to treat patients whose vision falls outside this range. An example would be trying to decide whether to treat a patient with 20/20 Snellen vision and early cystic changes, or a patient with severe DME and count fingers vision—such patients would not have been enrolled in a trial. Be aware that the results of the studies really only apply to patients* *with the allowed level of vision, but—right or wrong—the tendency is to extrapolate those results to all patients. We won't be rigorous about including the visual acuity definition when talking about CIDME in this book, because most doctors worry about what to do with patients when their fovea starts to swell regardless of the vision. By the way, the DRCR.net is already on this with studies looking at how to treat patients with early edema who haven't lost vision yet—that will help define the best approach for patients with normal vision.[5]*

This number—250 microns—is much easier to remember than all the criteria for CSDME, and it is very important because it helps you decide which patients might benefit from intravitreal injections. However, identifying center-involved diabetic macular edema does not necessarily mean that a patient has to be treated—sometimes you will treat someone who does not meet the criteria and sometimes you won't need to treat a patient that does. Plus, sometimes the disease might be better treated with laser versus injections depending on where the leakage is. There is a whole chapter coming up that will help you with those kinds of decisions—for now it is good enough to know how to define your two big enemies: CSDME and CIDME.

Except for one thing. Sometimes that 250 number doesn't work.

As mentioned above, newer spectral domain OCTs can obtain a much more accurate measure of retinal anatomy. The older time domain Stratus defines retinal thickness as the distance between the internal limiting membrane and the junction of the photoreceptor outer segments and inner segments. This is because the whole region between the inner segments and Bruch's membrane is mashed together into a fuzzy line—there is little detail. In contrast, spectral domain machines can separate out all the different layers (Figure 9). The boundary lines can then be set for very specific layers—for instance, the Zeiss Cirrus defines retinal thickness as the distance between the internal limiting membrane and the retinal pigment epithelium. This adds between 30-70 microns compared to the thickness obtained by a Stratus. It is therefore very important to know a given machine's correction factor relative to the Stratus (as an example, Heidelberg recommends subtracting 50 from thickness measurements obtained by their Spectralis OCT to get a "Stratus equivalent"). Unfortunately, this conversion factor is itself only an approximation—studies looking at different machines find that the difference measured between those machines and a Stratus can vary quite a bit from patient to patient, and this is why researchers can't easily use different machines interchangeably.[6] However, the conversion factor is a good place to start as you try to decide what to do with slightly swollen maculae.

When you have a hammer...

Not everything needs to look like a nail. The decision to treat a patient is usually more complex than deciding that someone has "crossed the line" into CSDME or CIDME and then attacking them with lasers and needles. Here is a brief preview of things to consider as you build up your diagnostic skills:

> 1. What is the patient's systemic status? A well-controlled patient, with mild or eccentric disease, may do very well with just observation. Such patients may actually heal themselves and end up not needing treatment. Follow them closely, though, to be sure they don't progress.

> 2. Conversely, a poorly controlled patient may need more aggressive treatment to keep them out of trouble. Be aware that these patients tend to go downhill even if the treatment works well, and this creates nuances that need to be addressed with the informed consent.

> 3. Be careful with disease close to the fovea if you are considering laser treatment. If you think you have to drop spots into a patient's perifoveal vision, think again. It may be better to treat with injections, eye drops or even just browbeat them about their control. Mild disease in this location can be very indolent, and some patients may actually be better off in the long run without intervention.

> 4. Is there a reversible factor that is contributing to the edema? For instance, some patients with renal failure and fluid retention will lose their edema once they are on dialysis. Or, edema in pregnant patients may resolve without treatment after they deliver.

The above issues, as well as others, will be discussed at length in the upcoming chapters. For now, just concentrate on doing the best exam you can and becoming familiar with how to call CSDME and CIDME. Oh, and one other thing...

DIPLOMACY FOR DUMMIES
Something to Not Do as You Begin to Study Diabetic Fundi

If you are examining a diabetic that has already had macular laser—especially old-school treatment that tended to be heavy—you may be surprised by the number of visible laser spots. You have to be very careful about how you refer to these previous laser spots.

For instance, early in your career you may be excited that you have managed to identify spots in the first place and you may gleefully carry on about all the scars that you can see with your newly acquired 90-diopter skills. Or you may develop the tendency we all have: to try to make oneself look good by pointing out how others have done poorly, for instance by commenting about "all those spots back there"—vaguely implying that you are way too chill to drop that many hits into someone's macula.

Avoid doing these things.

First of all, if you are seeing a patient years after a treatment, it is very hard to comment wisely because you did not see what the fundus looked like at the time and you don't have any idea how bad the patient might have been without the laser. Also, remember that if you refer uncharitably to previous laser treatment, it may just be a matter of time before what goes around comes around and your treatments are being disrespected.

More importantly, patients can be very frightened to learn about "laser scars" in the back of their eye because at some level they may imagine crazed doctors trying to carve up their vision in order to pay for BMWs. They also will assume that any vision problems they have are due to the scars; they usually do not understand that the lasers have, in fact, managed to save what vision they have.

The problem is that when patients draw incorrect conclusions about the effect of laser on their vision, they can become very reluctant to undergo any treatment by anyone—including your own bad self—when they desperately need it. As subsequent chapters will discuss, it can be hard enough to get a patient to return for follow up, and you don't want to contribute to the problem by carrying on about oodles and scads of spots.

This warning also applies to any primary-eye-care practitioners who may be reading this. It is not uncommon for patients to return from their optometrist somewhat upset because, with the best of intentions, the OD has referred to 'all those scars everywhere'. A casual remark like that can really interfere with appropriate follow up. If you are going to talk about laser scars, be sure to remind the patient why they are there in the first place—and where their vision would have ended up without intervention. Perhaps it is better to use the term "treatment" rather than "laser scars" in order to describe the findings.

In fact, carefully placed laser spots usually have nothing to do with a patient's symptoms. For instance, many diabetic patients will complain of microscotomas around the center of their vision as they age—often manifesting as missing parts of words or letters. It is very easy for them (and you) to assume that these scotomas are from laser scars. However, most of the time laser spots are well outside the area where they could interfere with reading. Instead, the "spots" they are seeing are actually caused by capillary dropout around the fovea (Figure 11). If you casually blame the symptoms on the laser, you will have unjustly maligned one of your colleagues and you will be risking the patient's compliance forever.

You are managing to do two really bad things at once without even trying.

Of course, there is no question that previous scars can enlarge over time, and you will see patients that were treated years ago with very heavy treatment and who have undergone scar expansion that can look rather frightening (Figure 10.1 in Chapter 14 is an example). Although many times these patients are surprisingly asymptomatic for such scars, some patients will clearly have vision loss due to this process. If you feel that this is indeed the case, then you have to call it as you see it, but it still helps to remind the patient that without treatment, their vision would likely be far worse. By the way, a large part of this book is designed to help you avoid creating such problems.

Here is something else to be aware of. When hard exudates build up in the fovea, they can sometimes leave a focal depigmented scar when they fade away. This scar can look for all the world like someone placed a laser spot right in the fovea. A classic tyro move is to tell the patient that their fovea was lasered when this was not the case at all. This results in a whole bunch of needless grief and once again manages to unjustly malign a colleague and alienate a patient in one fell swoop. Just be careful what you say.

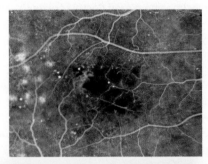

Figure 11: A patient complaining of difficulty seeing parts of words when reading. The laser scars are far away from areas involved in reading. The paracentral scotomas are from the capillary dropout and are not iatrogenic.

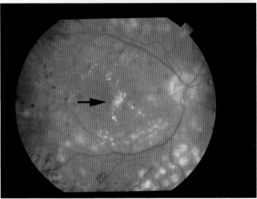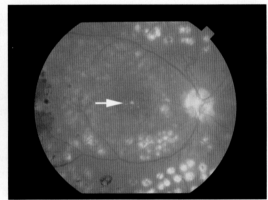

Figure 12: Hard exudates can build up in the fovea, as in the picture on the left (black arrow). When the exudates resolve, they can leave an area of focal depigmentation that can look just like a laser scar, as in the photo on the right (white arrow). No one lasered this fovea, so don't even think about freaking the patient out by calling this a laser spot. By the way, note how the real laser scars have expanded over time.[7]

OCT & DME That You Don't See

There is no doubt that one can sooner identify retinal thickening with OCT testing than with clinical examination. What is not clear is whether this has therapeutic implications. You have to remember that all of the early studies looking at the treatment of diabetic macular edema were based on how the retina appears clinically. If the OCT shows thickening that one cannot see on clinical exam, it is not known for sure whether such patients benefit from treatment, and the finding is referred to as subclinical edema.

If you do not see any obvious thickening, then it has been suggested that about one-half to two-thirds of the time the subclinical edema will not progress to clinically significant disease.[8,9] This can become hard to call, though, because once the OCT brings something to your attention, you can easily start to hallucinate some thickening. You have to be intellectually honest and promise not to manufacture clinically significant disease in your head just because you want to treat a retina.

Ultimately, deciding whether to treat such patients is an art-of-medicine thing—there are a lot of variables that may play into the decision. If the process appears to be progressive, then it may be reasonable to get in some early treatment to head off trouble. This is especially true if the thickening appears to be due to a few small microaneurysms that are away from the fovea and can be safely treated. On the other hand, if the patient does not have any symptoms and is systemically well controlled, very early edema will often resolve without the need for treatment (i.e., without the need for putting permanent spots in and around the patient's fovea or harpooning their eye with a 30 gauge needle). On the third hand, there is newer data suggesting that the anti-VEGF drugs can actually reverse retinopathy in general, so a patient with mild edema but who has worrisome nonproliferative retinopathy may benefit from earlier treatment (more on this in the next chapter).

It is also important to remember that, in general, the treatment of diabetic macular edema that is not fovea-threatening is never an emergency. It is reasonable to simply re-examine the patient in six to eight weeks and monitor the changes (this interval may vary depending on their disease and your level of concern). If nothing else, being able to use the pretty OCT colors to show asymptomatic patients how they are developing evidence of their diabetes can sometimes serve to motivate them better than a ton of handouts. It gets trickier if the fovea is involved and the patient is asymptomatic and you don't see anything on clinical exam—the concern is that microarchitectural damage is occurring and something needs to be done. Even in these cases, though, there is usually time to let the eye tell you what to do, but you may want to bring the patient back sooner as well as bug them to tighten their systemic control—sometimes even a topical non-steroidal can help out (much more on this later).

But I Don't Have an OCT...

Are you going to go to Retina Hell if you try to manage diabetics without an OCT? There are plenty of places around the world where it is simply not possible to generate the capital to obtain an OCT machine. Fortunately, most of the groundbreaking studies about treating diabetic retinopathy are totally based on clinical examination. Moreover, a careful observer can usually identify—or at least suspect—the kinds of problems that an OCT machine can find. The only difference is that the OCT makes detecting such findings effortless.

On the other hand, most retinal specialists would say that having an OCT is the standard of care when it comes to managing complex diabetic patients, especially if you will be doing injections. OCT is really useful for guiding therapy, and all the latest studies include OCT findings. As a result, if you think you can get an OCT it is a good idea to obtain one. The machine will likely keep you from doing the wrong thing to diabetics, and there are lots of other good things it can do. (Perhaps the most useful is the ability to identify subtle macular problems prior to cataract surgery, such as a diaphanous epiretinal membrane. You do not want a patient that is paying you the big bucks for a multifocal implant to be surprised by post-op pucker.)

If you can't get an OCT, do not worry. Just keep on improving your exam and keep watching for the kinds of things discussed in this book that can mess you up—almost always, a high index of suspicion and a careful contact lens exam will keep you reasonably informed about the retina. However, even if you are working in a totally impoverished region, don't forget that there are service organizations like the Lion's Club or Rotary International that may be able to help you. You will feel a lot better, and be a better doctor, if you can be the first on your block to have an OCT. See Appendix 2 for more details.

Of course, things start to get complicated if you might be able to obtain an OCT machine but you really need something more important, like a faster car. Only you and the Great Ophthalmic Court in the Sky can decide the answer to that one...

References and Suggested Reading

1.   Aiello LP, Beck RW, Bressler NM, et al. Rationale for the diabetic retinopathy clinical research network treatment protocol for center-involved diabetic macular edema. *Ophthalmology*. Dec 2011;118(12):e5-14.

2.   Staurenghi G, Sadda S, Chakravarthy U, Spaide RF. Proposed Lexicon for Anatomic Landmarks in Normal Posterior Segment Spectral-Domain Optical Coherence Tomography: The IN*OCT Consensus. *Ophthalmology*. Aug 2014;121(8):1572-1578.

3.   Maheshwary AS, Oster SF, Yuson RM, Cheng L, Mojana F, Freeman WR. The association between percent disruption of the photoreceptor inner segment-outer segment junction and visual acuity in diabetic macular edema. *American journal of ophthalmology*. Jul 2010;150(1):63-67 e61.

4.   Shimura M, Yasuda K, Yasuda M, Nakazawa T. Visual outcome after intravitreal bevacizumab depends on the optical coherence tomographic patterns of patients with diffuse diabetic macular edema. *Retina*. Apr 2013;33(4):740-747.

5.   Jampol LM, Bressler NM, Glassman AR. Revolution to a new standard treatment of diabetic macular edema. *JAMA : the journal of the American Medical Association*. Jun 11 2014;311(22):2269-2270.

6.   Bressler SB, Edwards AR, Chalam KV, et al. Reproducibility of Spectral-Domain Optical Coherence Tomography Retinal Thickness Measurements and Conversion to Equivalent Time-Domain Metrics in Diabetic Macular Edema. *JAMA ophthalmology*. Jul 24 2014.

7.   Schatz H, Madeira D, McDonald HR, Johnson RN. Progressive enlargement of laser scars following grid laser photocoagulation for diffuse diabetic macular edema. *Archives of ophthalmology*. Nov 1991;109(11):1549-1551.

8.   Browning DJ, Fraser CM. The predictive value of patient and eye characteristics on the course of subclinical diabetic macular edema. *American journal of ophthalmology*. Jan 2008;145(1):149-154.

9.   Bressler NM, Miller KM, Beck RW, et al. Observational study of subclinical diabetic macular edema. *Eye (Lond)*. Jun 2012 26(6):833-840.

10.   Liu Q, Hu Y, Yu H, et al. Comparison of intravitreal triamcinolone acetonide versus intravitreal bevacizumab as the primary treatment of clinically significant macular edema. Retina. 2015;35(2):272-279.

Basic and Clinical Science Course Section 12: Retina and Vitreous. San Francisco: American Academy of Ophthalmology, 2013: pp 89-112

Bressler NM, Ahmed IIK. Essential OCT. Dublin: Carl Zeiss Meditech, 2006.

Browning DJ (ed). Diabetic Retinopathy: Evidence-Based Management. Springer, 2010.

Wiley HE, Ferris FL III. Nonproliferative Diabetic Retinopathy and Diabetic Macular Edema. In Ryan SJ, Schachat AP (eds). Retina: Expert Consult Premium Edition. Saunders, 2012. pp 940-968.

Ding J, Wong TY. Current epidemiology of diabetic retinopathy and diabetic macular edema. Curr Diab Rep. Aug 2012;12(4):346-354.

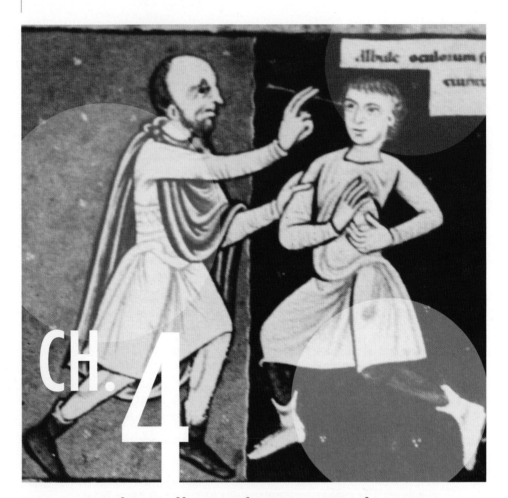

Lasers and Needles and Warm Woolen Mittens: an Approach to Treating DME

We are all apprentices in a craft where no one ever becomes a master. Ernest Hemingway

The approach to treating diabetic macular edema is evolving at a rapid pace. Coming up with a standardized protocol is almost impossible as new data keeps piling up--it is very much a moving target. Plus, the approach can differ from region to region, depending on local preferences and the resources available. Until we figure out a way to magically alter the words printed on this page, you really need to keep abreast of the field on your own. You also need to stay in touch with your neighborhood (or regional) retina specialists— they can not only give you lots of advice, but they can also keep you from doing things outside the local standard of care. In this chapter we are going to try to create a global approach to DME for you to start with, and then you can adjust it depending on the latest data, your results, and regional preferences. But first a couple of things:

Thing 1

It is easy to get totally absorbed in the tools at your disposal, especially when you are trying to understand things like OCT's, lasers and injections. But never forget the fundamental importance of the patient's systemic control. Your new found abilities to treat the retina will be far less effective if you are not also actively encouraging the patient to take proper care of themselves. There will be much more of this in The Chapter Whose Subject Must Not Be Named—but it bears repeating because you can't give your patient the outcome you both want if you ignore this aspect of their retinopathy.

Thing 2

Any discussion of modern treatment techniques has to include a shout out to recent collaborative trials. Carefully constructed large-scale clinical trials have always been instrumental in defining how diabetics are treated, and one of the latest and greatest innovations for this has been the Diabetic Retinopathy Clinical Research Network (DRCR. net). The DRCR.net consists of around 200 academic and private retina practices in the United States, and it functions as a collaborative network designed to facilitate multi-center research on various aspects of diabetic retinopathy. It allows the rapid initiation of trials looking at the latest fads to see if they really work, and it is funded by the National Eye Institute rather than by private corporations, which raises the credibility level. If you want to dig deeper into why you do what you do, their website is a must read (drcrnet. jaeb.org). And the DRCR.net is not alone—investigators around the globe have organized similar collaborative efforts, such as the Pan American Collaborative Retina Study Group. A lot of the latest treatment techniques discussed in this book will draw heavily on the trials performed by all these groups.

One caveat, though. The investigators in the DRCR.net and the other groups are the cream of the crop—they are true Retina Playuhs. Do you remember how your first few cataract surgeries looked like someone set off a small bomb in your patient's anterior chamber, and now your surgery is so slick you can't find one cell on post-op day one? Some of that is from doing a lot of cases, but some of it is due to subconscious learning—you automatically sense what micromove is best for reasons that you may not be able to describe, and your outcomes are way better as a result. Well, the same thing applies after doing thousands and thousands of lasers and injections—subconscious perceptions develop that make everything just go a tad bit smoother for the Major Dudes than it does for the rest of us mortals. Plus, the patients in the DRCR.net studies tend to be highly motivated, and that makes a big difference. Finally, the patients in these studies are subjected to a 15-minute, high contrast refraction at every visit – which ekes out the best vision possible.

All this means is that you should not be disappointed if your results don't seem to match the studies—and you should welcome the fact that the studies present a gold standard to strive for. Most importantly, you can't have your patients thinking that they will always do as well as the data suggests; Chapter 5 talks about this a lot. Also, remember that the results of any study apply primarily to patients with characteristics similar to those entered into the study in the first place. In other words, as you try to sort out how you will care for your personal patients, you will need to be flexible. Your patients may need a more custom approach that draws on the results of many studies.

But Back to the Subject of the Chapter

When trying to create a systematic approach to DME, the first concern is simply what tools are available to the treating ophthalmologist. If you are in a situation where you have diabetic patients but you do not have access to basic items such as laser and OCT, there is little that can be done. However, with motivation and persistence you can seek out organizations that can help you obtain equipment and training; check out Appendix 2 for suggestions. If you are one level up and have a laser but can't do intravitreal injections, you will find that each of the chapters on laser treatment includes advice about the approach to take when laser is your only option. The bulk of this chapter will assume that you have all the requisite toys and you can get your patients all the fancy drugs. Probably the one hang-up for most people around the world is that ranibizumab (Lucentis) and aflibercept (Eylea) are not options because of cost, and we'll cover that too. But on to the disease...

When treating macular edema, the first step is to be sure you are treating a diabetic problem. Chapter 27 is a whole discussion of the things that can look like DME but aren't— like vein occlusions or subtle intermediate uveitis. We will presume that you have ruled out all those other things.

The next step is to determine if you are dealing with an anatomic problem such as vitreomacular traction or macular pucker. Your clinical exam, and especially your OCT, will help with that. But it is not that simple. You also have to decide to what extent the anatomic problem is contributing to the leakage. If the edema is entirely due to the traction or pucker, then you can skip everything that follows and head straight to Chapter 19 on vitrectomy. On the other hand, if the patient has just a hint of surface wrinkling that doesn't seem to be contributing to the leakage, then you may be able to treat the retinopathy and ignore the surface wrinkling unless the edema proves refractory to your ministrations.

Unfortunately, nothing is simple, and many patients with a vitreoretinal interface abnormality and diabetic retinopathy end up with some degree of overlap, i.e., there is some leakage from microvascular damage within the retina from diabetes, and there is also some leakage caused directly by the traction or pucker. In fact, the two problems seem to synergize—a mild looking epiretinal membrane may accelerate the underlying retinovascular damage. It can be hard to know how much of the problem is due to trouble at the vitreoretinal interface versus pure diabetic retinopathy. Kind of like the distinction between art and pornography, though, if traction from any cause is the main problem it is usually fairly obvious. If it is not obvious, or if the patient is uninterested in addressing the problem surgically, it makes sense to start treating the macular edema with laser and/or injections and then reassess the role of surgery depending on how successful your treatments are. There may even be times when the effects of traction are masked by the swollen retina, and as the retina thins out with treatment the superimposed traction becomes apparent (Figure 1).

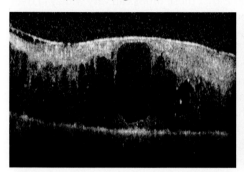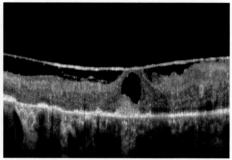

Figure 1: The OCT on the left shows a frighteningly swollen retina with an overlying epiretinal membrane (ERM). Successful treatment with laser and injections eliminated most of the edema, but on the right you can see a persistent cyst that is caused by traction from the ERM that became apparent as the retina deturgessed. By the way, you can also see that the ellipsoid zone (outer/inner segment line) is non-existent (as is most of the normal retinal anatomy). There is even some thickening of the subfoveal RPE, which suggests longstanding edema. When the retina is this slagged, it is unlikely that surgery to remove the traction would make any difference.

But wait. We need to discuss a side-topic that merits a change in font color.

There is one thing to think about in patients with edema from just about any cause, and it is something that you would automatically think of in one of your post-op cataract patients with CME.

It makes sense to consider the use of a topical nonsteroidal in patients with puffy diabetic retinas. This doesn't work for everyone—in fact, there was a DRCR.net study looking at this in patients with non-central DME who were largely phakic. There was a trend towards a response, but there was no statistically significant benefit.[1] There are other smaller studies that support the use of this medication, however.[2-5] The drops will not solve the problem in a poorly controlled patient with severe edema, and they don't work in everyone. And you should never postpone appropriate treatment in patients with progressive disease just to see if some topical ketorolac might solve the problem. However, it is an approach that can be very helpful for selected patients; it does seem to work better for pseudophakic rather than phakic patients.

For instance, in patients with a bit of swelling and a mild epiretinal membrane, the addition of a topical nonsteroidal drop may deturgess the retina enough that you may be able to avoid more aggressive treatment. Or in patients with diabetic macular edema alone--without any epiretinal membrane--the addition of a nonsteroidal can tip things in the direction of stability so they need fewer lasers and injections. Plus, patients who get a good anatomic response will often also notice subjective improvement in their vision, and it is always nice if there is a little positive reinforcement to help with compliance.

It is not clear if one nonsteroidal is better than another (although patients are more likely to adhere to the regimen if you use a medication that requires fewer drops a day). One thing to be aware of if you are going to try this is that these drops can vary widely in their cost--you might want to have someone in your office call the surrounding pharmacies to get some pricing. It seems to take at least a month or two of treatment to see if there is an effect, and often patients need to be treated for several months to stabilize things before tapering them. If one or two different drugs don't have any effect, then it is not worth trying others. But it may be worth retrying them again after several months if you get better control of the patient's disease with other modalities. Again, this is not something that works for everyone—and it has yet to be fully proven in a large trial--but it really seems to help decrease the overall treatment burden in selected patients. It is interesting that the addition of an NSAID has been shown to possibly be helpful in other retinovascular diseases like vein occlusions and macular degeneration.[4,53]

Remember, though, that there may be a risk of corneal melting with chronic use of a topical nonsteroidal, especially in patients with compromised corneas (i.e., exposure, neurotrophic problems or dry eyes--all things that can be more common in diabetics). The concern of a melt was more of a problem with older generic preparations, but it is still a risk so warn patients about this and instruct them to discontinue the drop and get checked if they are having problems. And don't act like a retina specialist—when you see them in follow up make sure you actually look at their cornea.

But back to the issue of combined epiretinal membranes and macular edema. There are no firm rules here; in patients with combined disease you simply need to reassess both the retinovascular status and the effect of any traction at each visit. These patients often take a lot of time as you go over the ups and downs of surgery versus treatment with lasers and injections. They need to understand that although there may be risks to vitrectomy, there are usually risks to observation in the form of permanent structural damage from chronic traction. Of course, the situation is complicated by the fact that vitrectomy by no means guarantees a favorable visual outcome--even if there are no complications. There are some foveas that just conk out even with successful surgical correction, and these patients can end up worse after vitrectomy even if their OCT is improved. There will be much more on the specific role of vitrectomy in Chapter 19; the point here is to look for problems with traction before you start skewering eyes with photons and needles. And don't spend years trying to figure out if an epiretinal membrane or traction is the main problem. There is a feeling that waiting a long time and then referring the patient for surgery when all else has failed results in less successful surgery. If you aren't sure, just send the patient to a retina specialist.

Most of the time mild *epiretinal membranes associated with mild diabetic retinopathy are annoying but not dangerous—especially the ones that keep the vision in the 20/25 to 20/50 range. If you are not a retinal specialist, you may think that such patients will automagically benefit from a vitrectomy, but if you are a retinal specialist you will have realized that operating on such patients can help, but often in a very underwhelming way. As a result, unless patients are bitterly symptomatic it is often better to just treat any identifiable leakage caused by the diabetes, but recognize that you won't get rid of all the edema so don't beat the proverbial dead horse with excessive lasers and/or injections. Adding a topical non-steroidal may also help, and you do need to always keep in mind the option of doing a vitrectomy if anatomic and visual problems get worse (for instance if the ellipsoid zone (outer/inner segment line) starts to disappear). Unless the patient is really type-A, most of these people--particularly older patients--are content to be monitored.*

But there is one situation where you can really get burned: cataract surgery. There is something about adding cataract surgery to the presence of a little bit of retinopathy and a little bit of an epiretinal membrane—the combination can really go south unexpectedly. This doesn't mean surgery is wrong. It just means that both you and your patient need to understand the risk. And putting in a multifocal lens in such a patient is not a good idea – very simply, diabetic retinopathy causes a huge loss in functional photoreceptor cells, even in patients with 20/20 vision. The reduced contrast sensitivity due to the multifocal lens, combined with reduced contrast in the diabetic retina, can leave a patient frustrated (more on this in Chapter 25 on cataract surgery in diabetics).

Okay. Presumably you have ruled out other diseases that mimic diabetes, and you are fairly certain that you are not dealing with some sort of vitreous traction or epiretinal membrane that is the main problem. Now we can actually start talking about treating DME.

Talking About Treating DME

The main branching point is whether or not the patient needs treatment with laser alone or whether injections will be required. This usually comes down to understanding the definition of center-involving edema. To review, the DRCR.net defines this as having an ETDRS visual acuity score between 20/32 to 20/320 with definite retinal thickening in the center of the macula on clinical exam and central subfield thickness ≥250 microns (using a Zeiss Stratus, which means that you might need to add 50-ish microns depending on how your spectral domain machine measures retinal thickness – see the OCT section in Chapter 3 for details).

Now this is where it gets tricky. Patients don't tend to come in with a binary degree of central involvement; they tend to have variable amounts of peripheral leakage and variable amounts of center involvement. If the patient does not have any center-involving disease and has clinically significant macular edema based on the "disc within a disc" rule, then things are pretty straightforward. Usually a gentle laser combined with not-so-gentle encouragement to improve their systemic control is all you need. There are two full chapters on how to do this located elsewhere in this book, so you should be all set.

It gets trickier if there is some peripheral leakage but also some swelling at the center, as defined above. This is more "art of medicine" stuff, and there are widely different approaches. Some docs think that laser is a waste of time (and RPE) and go solely with injections—we will see that there is a lot of data to support this. But there is also a sense that laser treatment is a good adjuvant to the injections; injections provide short-term control, whereas laser is for long-term control. In other words, you get the injections in to stabilize and protect the fovea and use laser to treat any leaks that are away from the center. Eventually the overall leakage will decrease and the need for chronic injections will also decrease, along with all the attendant risks and costs. Now, is there any randomized, controlled trial data that supports this? Nope. Nada. Still, it is an approach that seems really right to many retina folks, and we will spend more time discussing the issue of lasers versus injections later in the chapter. But first a slight digression.

It is important to understand where retina people are coming from when it comes to lasers--it will help you decide your personal approach. But you need to somehow absorb decades of experience with lasers, and the easiest way is to hop on the Wayback Machine.

Back in the Eighties, the Early Treatment of Diabetic Retinopathy Study (ETDRS) generated the graph in Chapter 3 that shows the results of treating macular edema with laser. Figure 2 is a refresher.

Figure 2.

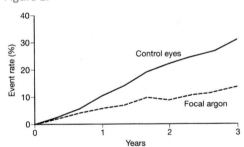

Those results were a breakthrough, but Figure 3 shows what it looks like if it is flipped around so you see it from the standpoint of a patient. Even with treatment, patients still deteriorated. It is just that their vision didn't suck as much as the controls.

Figure 3: A patient's-eye view of the graph from Chapter 3 showing the ETDRS results for treating macular edema. This graph made doctors happy, but patients still worsened on average, even with perfect treatment. Note the elegant symbolism suggested by the flipped labels: The doctor has to totally wrap his or her head around the patient's point of view to really be able to relate. This was not done because it is easier to flip the original image without changing the labels—it was done on purpose for art's sake.

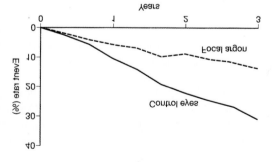

But ETDRS laser is old school, right? Absolutely. Over the years the original laser techniques were modified by making them gentler (upcoming chapters will review this at length). And although people were getting a sense that the newer techniques were working better, no one knew for sure. And then the DRCR.net published a study that dropped a real bass bomb on the house.[6] This study compared repeated use of laser versus repeated use of intravitreal steroids (albeit, short term off-label triamcinolone), and it was done before the big anti-VEGF studies (hence no anti-VEGF arm). Figure 4 shows the results—and this blew people away. Not only did laser smoke the steroids (and back then people thought for sure that steroids would be best), but look at that laser line—patients actually improved! So, for a brief time, laser was the gold standard, which made people feel really good about doing lasers.

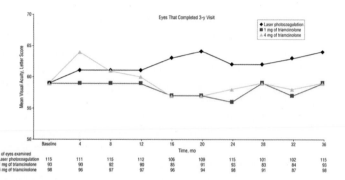

Figure 4: Mean visual acuity for the eyes that completed 3 years of follow-up comparing laser to two different doses of triamcinolone. Look at that laser line head north! (Courtesy of Archives of Ophthalmology.)

But remember, the DRCR.net results are from highly experienced doctors treating highly motivated patients—do not expect all your patients to do as well. For instance, Jyothi and Sivaprasad did an interesting study wherein they applied the DRCR.net laser protocol to a real world urban population—with poorer systemic control and more erratic follow up (Figure 5).[7] Suddenly the results of laser are not quite as stellar—in fact they start to look a lot like the boring old ETDRS results from 30 years ago. One can argue that maybe they just didn't have the same skill as the DRCR.net investigators, but it is far more likely that they were treating patients that couldn't or wouldn't take optimal care of themselves, and that makes a HUGE difference in terms of how well they respond to treatment.

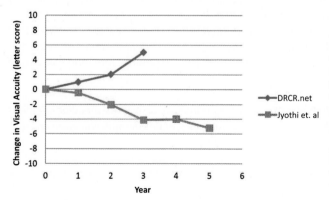

Figure 5: A graph of data from Jyothi and Sivaprasad.[7] The top line shows the 3-year results of the laser arm from the DRCR.net protocol that compared laser to triamcinolone. The lower line is what happened when the same laser protocol was used in a more diverse urban setting with patients with poorer systemic control and follow up. Do not let your laser patients think that the laser will automatically make them better.

What is the point of all this? It is that laser is a good thing—at the very least it will slow things down, and at best it can turn things around and actually get people better, albeit slowly. And all that explains why there is such a strong feeling that laser can help control macular edema and decrease the need for injections (assuming the laser is done parsimoniously and doesn't scar up the macula). It is just that no one knows for sure exactly how the laser fits in, especially in light of some of the anti-VEGF studies that suggest that laser may have little effect and in some cases may be deleterious. We will hit all this shortly; for now it is enough to understand that laser is a good adjuvant to include in your arsenal as long as you know how to use it wisely.

But speaking of quick fixes, now it is time to go from lasers to injections...

And when it comes to intravitreal treatments, the first thing to discuss is the use of triamcinolone acetonide (Chapter 11 talks about specific preparations). At first, people were shocked with the apparent efficacy of intravitreal triamcinolone for the treatment of diabetic macular edema. It was exciting to put a drug in the patient's eye and watch the edema completely disappear. It was also a lot of fun to have patients come back happy after a treatment for diabetic retinopathy—almost like a LASIK patient! All this created strong positive reinforcement to keep using steroids, but unfortunately, over time it became apparent that steroids didn't live up to their initial success. The efficacy seems to wear off with repeated injections, and of course there are always the potential side effects of cataract formation and glaucoma requiring surgical intervention. Perhaps the biggest indictment about the utility of steroids as a single treatment came from the DRCR.net study cited above where laser alone was more effective than triamcinolone.

As a comprehensive ophthalmologist, you may feel fairly comfortable with problems like cataracts and glaucoma. But remember, cataract surgery in diabetics, and especially diabetics with macular edema, can make things worse. And as for glaucoma, yes, you can treat with simple things like drops and even laser trabeculoplasty,[8] but some patients get a whopping pressure spike that just won't go away. And those patients need surgery to lower the pressure. If you are at an academic center where you can walk your patient with steroid-induced glaucoma down the hall to a world expert on glaucoma, your risk-benefit ratio may be very different than if you are practicing in a smaller town where the same patient may be operated on by someone who does only 10 filters a year. On top of that, diabetics tend to be more likely to have filters that fail.[9] And then there is bleb-related endophthalmitis. Bleb endophthalmitis scares retina docs, and it should scare you too. It can show up years down the road and can put an eye in a jar really fast.

Trading years of endophthalmitis risk for a few months of decreased macular edema is something that needs to be approached carefully as you decide how you want to treat these patients.

By the way, there is a suggestion in the literature that if the patients routinely have pressures lower than 15 they are less likely to get a significant pressure elevation with steroids.[10] Some doctors will take the extra step of putting patients on topical steroids to try to suss out a potential steroid response. Other risk factors for elevated pressure include the presence of actual glaucoma, suspect glaucoma and a family history of glaucoma. Younger patients may also be at higher risk.[11] There is also growing data that patients with a narrower angle recess as determined by anterior segment OCT may be at increased risk.[12] And just because nothing is simple, once you have put steroids in an eye, you really need to keep monitoring the pressure for a while. The pressure can rise insidiously, and this may show up well after the drug should have worn off.[13,52]

One final note—if you do end up with elevated pressure after intravitreal steroids, one option to keep in mind is that performing a vitrectomy and removing the residual drug may lower the pressure without the need for glaucoma surgery.[14]

However, the data from the above DRCR.net study does not mean that there is no role for steroids. First of all, there are doctors that feel you can get some of the benefit of intravitreal steroids with less risk by using a periocular injection instead. A few studies suggest that there is an effect, but others suggest it is not dramatic, including a different pilot study by the DRCR.net.[15] Still, there may be some situations where this "kinder, gentler" approach to using steroids can nudge an eye in the right direction. We do not regularly use this intervention, but you are welcome to take a look at the literature and decide for yourself.[16,17]

As for intravitreal treatment, although the laser versus steroid study suggested that steroids alone were not particularly useful on average, there are certainly a host of other studies that suggest that some patients will respond nicely to steroids--they can be a useful adjuvant. For instance, as we will see in the next section, Protocol I from the DRCR. net did include a steroid treatment arm. Although the steroids were not very helpful in phakic patients, they could provide some long-term help in pseudophakic patients.

And this gets to another main point in this chapter. In many ways, the treatment of patients with diabetic macular edema involves a search for whatever approach provides the least amount of risk and fewest interventions. There are definitely some patients for whom steroids work great and they need far fewer shots than if anti-VEGF drugs were used—you just have to figure out who those patients are.

Also, there are some patients whose edema just does not seem to go away no matter what you do. Many times the addition of a steroid injection to the other interventions may help control things. For instance, many docs will start treatment with anti-VEGF agents, and if the edema persists after, say, 4 to 6 monthly injections they will add a steroid injection. You may even have rare patients that are simply refractory to everything, and who need frighteningly frequent steroid injections just to hold onto their vision. These patients don't come along very often, but if you automatically write off the use of steroids you will have a lot of trouble controlling vision loss in such patients.

Which brings us to the subject of longer acting steroid implants such as Ozurdex, Iluvien and Retisert. The use of these modalities may be limited by cost, as well as the almost inevitable development of cataracts and high risk of glaucoma. However, in patients that do well with steroids, these longer-acting treatments can be useful. In fact, there is a sense that the sustained low-dose delivery that these modalities provide may actually be more effective than the intermittent pulsed dosing that occurs with periodic steroid injections. As more studies are performed using these long-acting implants, we will get a better sense of how they fit into the armamentarium. They will probably be most useful in patients that respond to steroids with few side effects, or for those patients that only partially respond to anti-VEGF agents and are willing to accept the risk of glaucoma and cataract to preserve their central vision.[18-20]

Quick review of the implants: Ozurdex has 0.7 mg of dexamethasone and is a small cylinder about .48 mm wide and 6 mm long. It is inserted via the pars plana using a special injector. It is biodegradable and lasts 3-4 months—patients may see a small telephone pole in their eye for a while and then it dissolves. One notable thing about Ozurdex is that there is a sense among clinicians that it is less likely to cause a big pressure spike compared to triamcinolone.[21] Iluvien is an even smaller cylinder and has .019 mg of fluocinolone acetonide. It is not biodegradable, but it lasts up to 3 years (Figure 6). Retisert has .59 mg of fluocinolone acetonide and is a small pellet that is inserted surgically via the pars plana and sewn in place. It lasts about 3 years also.

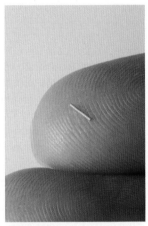

Figure 6:
Iluvien fluocinolone implant.
(Courtesy of Alimera Sciences)

Like triamcinolone, all these devices are effective for treating macular edema, but they all have the risks of glaucoma and cataract, plus they involve various degrees of leaving stuff inside the eye where it can cause trouble. For instance, Ozurdex and Iluvien can migrate into the anterior chamber in predisposed patients (such as those with a decentered IOL). Retisert requires surgery and a subconjunctival stitch that can erode; also, the medication pellet can become detached from the fixation plate and float around the eye. All of these devices are in various stages of being tested and approved (or turned down) around the world, so it is hard to say exactly how they will be used, but they will likely be a "last-resort" option for patients with refractory disease. One interesting fact that came out of the studies for the Iluvien implant is that it worked much better in patients that had had DME for over a year and a half—it didn't work as well for patients with fresh disease (although some question the statistics behind this conclusion).[22] This raises the possibility that different treatments may work better at different time points—something to keep in mind when you have a patient that doesn't seem to be responding—or stops responding—to any one therapy.

The next sentence is really important if you are just starting out using injections:

The key thing with intravitreal triamcinolone is to understand that it is not as good as you will think it is after the first time you put it in someone's eye.

Still, it does have a place, and for some doctors it is the go-to drug in patients that are pseudophakic with low pressures and no risk factors for glaucoma. It may also serve as an adjuvant to minimize the need for other injections, and for some patients it is the only thing that really works. We will get back to steroids in the end-of-chapter wrap up, so let's switch to the real stars of the show...

The Anti-VEGF Drugs: Bevacizumab and its expensive cousins

The anti-vascular endothelial growth factor (anti-VEGF) drugs have become the mainstay for treating center-involving diabetic macular edema. A real textbook could tell you why. Suffice it to say that blocking VEGF seems to seal leaky blood vessels. At first, everyone thought that they were just weak versions of triamcinolone, because it seemed that steroids gave a better immediate response. But as more studies have been done it is clear that regular anti-VEGF injections provide better control with fewer risks in general, and that explains why they are used so often.

You know this, but for completeness here is the gang: Bevacizumab (Avastin) is a humanized monoclonal antibody against VEGF. It is not approved for use in the eye—it is an anti-cancer drug that eye doctors have co-opted because it has effects similar to the approved drugs, but is way cheaper. The usual dose is 1.25 mg (.05 ml). Ranibizumab (Lucentis) was the first drug approved specifically for use in the eye; first for macular degeneration and then vein occlusions and most recently for diabetic macular edema. It is a specially modified fragment of the bevacizumab antibody. Note that the dose of ranibizumab is different for different diseases; the dose for vein occlusions and macular degeneration is 0.5 mg, whereas the dose for DME is 0.3 mg (the studies suggested that there was no reason to expose patients to the higher dose when treating DME). As of this writing, the 0.5 mg dose is about $1950 a vial and the 0.3 mg dose is about $1400. So be very careful about which vial you grab, because if you use the higher dose on a diabetic, you will lose several hundred dollars when the insurance company refuses to pay.

Aflibercept (Eylea) is a fusion protein that combines VEGF receptors with the Fc fragment of human IgG; it costs about $1850 a vial, it is the most recently approved drug for DME.[23]* Finally, there is pegaptanib (Macugen), the first anti-VEGF drug, but it is weaker and not used very often so we won't be discussing it much. Macugen's big claim to fame is that because it does not block all isoforms of VEGF, it may not have any of the systemic thromboembolic concerns that the other drugs have (to be discussed). Some doctors will therefore use it in patients that they perceive to be at risk for thromboembolic problems.

*In the same way that bevacizumab is used in place of ranibizumab, the drug ziv-aflibercept (Zaltrap) is the chemotherapeutic version of aflibercept. There has been some work looking at whether ziv-aflibercept can be used in the eye as a cheaper substitute, but it is too early to make any recommendations.[57] If it works well, it will be a great money saver.

Perhaps the sine qua non of anti-VEGF trials for diabetic macular edema is the Protocol I study by the DRCR.net.[24] Figure 7 shows the rather striking results, and if you are going to treat diabetic patients with these agents, you really need to take some time to study this trial—it was brilliant and it can serve as a nice template as you try to develop your own approach to the problem. Here is an overview of the whole thing.

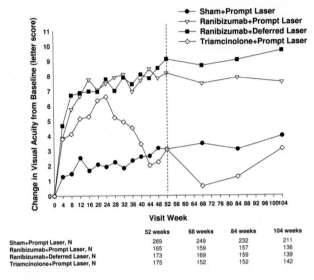

	52 weeks	68 weeks	84 weeks	104 weeks
Sham+Prompt Laser, N	269	249	232	211
Ranibizumab+Prompt Laser, N	165	159	157	136
Ranibizumab+Deferred Laser, N	173	169	159	139
Triamcinolone+Prompt Laser, N	175	152	152	142

Figure 7: The results of DRCR.net Protocol I comparing laser alone to ranibizumab with prompt and deferred laser and also to triamcinolone with prompt laser.

The protocol randomized patients into 4 groups. The first received standard laser (with sham injections). The second received laser along with intravitreal triamcinolone, and the triamcinolone could be repeated every 16 weeks. The final two groups were treated initially with monthly ranibizumab using the approach discussed below; of note, one of these groups received prompt laser at the start of treatment, whereas the other group received laser almost 6 months after starting ranibizumab if there was persistent edema. This last bit will become important as we try to figure out the role of laser in treating these patients. You can quickly see from Figure 7 that the ranibizumab groups did quite well, the laser alone and the laser and triamcinolone groups not so much.

It is important to understand the approach used for determining the need for a ranibizumab injection. The protocol required monthly visits through the first year and it used something called the "4-2-7" rule. Patients were given a monthly injection of ranibizumab for four consecutive months regardless of the functional or anatomic status of the retina at each visit. Once the patient received four monthly doses, therapy was based on how the retinal thickness and vision compared to the previous visit. If the central subfield thickness dropped to less than 250 microns or the vision improved to 20/20 then no injection was required—these were called the "success criteria". Otherwise, patients received two more monthly injections on the fifth and sixth visits. For months seven through twelve, if the treatment resulted in the success criteria, then treatment was deferred. However, if the success criteria were not met and patients were showing continued improvement then another injection was given at each visit. "Continued improvement" was defined by a five-letter (one EDTRS line) increase in vision or a 10% decrease in CSF thickening relative to the previous visit. If the findings stabilized—i.e., there was no study-defined continued improvement—then treatment could be deferred for that visit and injections were resumed if the retinal thickening returned or the vision deteriorated on subsequent visits.

During the second year of Protocol I, re-treatment once again continued as long as successive improvement occurred over each visit. However, once the eye either stabilized or reached success criteria, then the frequency of the visits could fall to every two months and then to every four months if the eye continued to do well. But if the vision decreased or the edema increased then the patient was treated and monthly followup was resumed. On average, patients required eight to nine injections in the first year and this decreased to two to three in the second year. However, patients in the DRCR.net had good hemoglobin A1c numbers (7.3 in the group finishing 3 years).[25] Your mileage may vary if you are dealing with a patient population that is less motivated. One also has to wonder about how much of the improvement—and the lower number of injections during the second year—was due to seeing patients on a monthly basis and beating them over the head about systemic control. (And having them realize, like Pavlov's dogs, that if they don't do their very best to take care of their diabetes someone in a white coat will stick a needle in their eye.) You need to remember about the excellent control of the patients in this study as you try to bring this approach to your real world—you may not get anywhere near the same results, and you are more likely to need other modalities to optimize your outcomes.

But getting back to the protocol, it is really important to get the concept of "continued improvement" down; it was very wise of the investigators to include this definition. In fact, in the DRCR studies, following the protocol injection frequency meant that after six injections monthly, you only treated edema if it was getting worse or getting much better with treatment – patients with edema and stable vision were just observed! It is easy to assume that when you are putting a $1400 medicine into an eye every month, the edema is going to go away. It often doesn't, and it is possible to beat a very expensive dead horse if you don't recognize this. In fact, if you look at the two-year data from this study, over 40% of the eyes in the ranibizumab groups still had a central subfield thickness of greater than 250 microns; they were still center-involved and still fairly boggy. And even at five years out, about one third of eyes still had edema.[26] You will find in some patients that no amount of continued intravitreal anti-VEGF drug will get rid of all of the edema. This is why the protocol included this out – you don't have to treat someone every month forever, you only have to treat them until you see things stabilize and then treat as needed if things worsen.

Now, this begs the question of whether you can get even better results if you add something else—and this is where the treatment of these patients turns into a mad scientist's laboratory with everyone having their favorite recipe (hence the serpentine nature of this chapter as it tries to cover all the different modalities). But understanding the DRCR.net Protocol I approach is a good platform upon which to build your particular anti-VEGF pyramid.

But yet another change in font color.

There are a couple of additional points to make based on the Protocol I results.

First, what about those steroids? The overall data shown in Figure 7 suggests that triamcinolone has an immediate effect similar to the anti-VEGF drugs, but that effect drops off and ultimately the drug doesn't work so well. But look at Figure 8—that shows the results with triamcinolone in patients that started out pseudophakic. That group did as well as the ranibizumab groups. This suggests that there is definitely a role for this drug, assuming that glaucoma is not a problem. It is also strange that this beneficial effect was not seen in phakic patients—and the lack of effect does not seem to be due to development of cataracts because patients were able to have visually significant cataracts removed (and many did—upwards of 70% by 2 years). It suggests that needing cataract surgery while treating DME may be more problematic in patients getting triamcinolone compared to using the drug in patients that have already had cataract surgery. This does not mean that triamcinolone should not be used in phakic patients—there may be patients who respond to nothing else. It simply means that, all things considered, triamcinolone may not be the best drug to start with in phakic patients. It is also a cautionary tale to remember when patients with diabetic retinopathy need cataract surgery; but we will save that for Chapter 25.

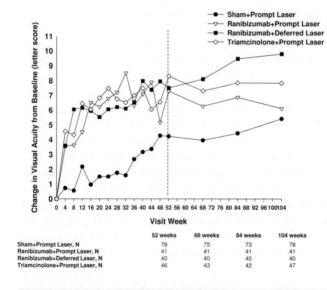

Figure 8: DRCR.net Protocol I results in pseudophakic patients. Note how the triamcinolone group did much better—it is up there with the ranibizumab group. (Figures 7 and 8 used with permission, Archives of Ophthalmology)

The second, and really important, point is the difference between the group that had prompt laser when the anti-VEGF treatment was started and the group that had deferred laser (remember—"deferred" meant waiting almost 6 months after starting injections before doing laser for persistent edema). In this study it looks like patients with deferred laser did better, suggesting that laser should be postponed—or avoided—rather than jumping in and treating with laser immediately. It so happens that the deferred laser group ended up needing a few more injections, and the investigators speculated that perhaps treating physicians were not as aggressive with the use of injections in patients that had received prompt laser (perhaps those investigators thought that the use of laser would decrease the need for injections, and with fewer injections patients did not do as well). Another explanation could be that doing prompt laser may have required more aggressive treatment that may have diminished vision over time—as we will see in Chapter 9, you need more power and can inadvertently create bigger burns when treating more swollen retina. Whatever the reason, it is important to understand that at least in this highly motivated group of patients there is good evidence to suggest that prompt laser is no better and possibly worse than waiting to do laser once the retina has been medically deturgessed.[25,26]

And Protocol I was not the only study that suggested that laser was either not useful or perhaps even deleterious. There are a host of company-sponsored studies--all beginning with the letter "R", strangely enough--that confirmed the DRCR.net results regarding the utility of ranibizumab for DME (READ, RISE, RIDE, RESOLVE, RESTORE). Each protocol was different, and none of them showed that laser alone or laser with ranibizumab provided better results than just injections alone, at least over the duration of the studies. There are also studies using bevacizumab showing the same thing, and all this raises questions about the utility of laser—so much so that at least one center has stopped using laser for DME.[27]

Wait. What?

Wasn't there a paragraph back there that said the opposite—that laser is really useful? Yep:

"There is also a sense that laser treatment is a good adjuvant to the injections; injections provide short-term control, whereas laser is for long-term control. In other words, you get the injections in to stabilize and protect the fovea and use laser to treat any leaks that are away from the center so that, over time, the overall leakage will decrease and the need for chronic injections will also decrease, along with all the attendant risks and costs."

How can that paragraph be reconciled with all the data from these trials suggesting laser is superfluous at best and maybe even deleterious?

To answer that, we have to take a brief trip to the Land of Abnormal Retinal Correspondence, where deeply held convictions are maintained in the face of, well, the data. There are several reasons why most retina specialists feel that laser has a definite role in spite of the results of these trials. A big reason gets back to the patient population—many patients simply don't have the inclination or wherewithal to take care of themselves like the patients in studies, and patients with poorer control seem to need more than just one type of treatment to treat their DME. You have to throw the book at them just to hold on to what they have.

A second reason comes from comparing the Protocol I results to the DRCR.net study that studied laser versus triamcinolone alone. Steroids alone did not do so well compared to laser, but steroids combined with prompt laser did much better in Protocol I, at least in pseudophakic patients (review Figures 4 and 8). Related to this is the consistent upward trend in vision for the groups in the other studies that had laser. Patients with laser tend to improve, but it takes a while (see Figure 4 again). The assumption is that over time the placement of careful laser will minimize the need for long-term injections, especially in patients with poor control. And as time goes by, it seems that more studies are suggesting this is actually the case.[28,29]

A third reason for embracing laser is based on the myriad ways that DME presents—there are some patients that have incredibly discrete leakage from microaneurysms that are away from the fovea, and treating those lesions will shut down the problem without the risk of injections. You just need to know when this approach is ideal, as well as to have skills to apply laser with minimal collateral damage. There are even newer laser techniques that use subthreshold treatments that don't seem to cause any damage, or that use highly accurate computer-guided treatment. These may be even safer and more effective than traditional laser, although definitive studies are pending (this will all be discussed in Chapter 6).

Finally, in many places around the world there are limited resources that make it impossible to follow the injection protocols perfectly—especially with the expensive drugs. In these situations, compromises have to be made and laser can be a low-budget vision saver. We will return to all this again at the end of the chapter.

> **Okay, okay.** Full disclosure here. *There is another factor that has the potential to encourage the use of lasers: Depending on the nature of your healthcare system, doing lots of lasers can be very remunerative. As mentioned at other points in this book, it is hoped you are well above such concerns. Plus, it is likely that if laser allows one to spread out visits and injections, one might make less money in the long run with appropriate laser. Still, just like you would want to know about which company is paying for a given study, you should know that this particular gorilla lurks around discussions regarding the utility of laser for DME, and you should salt folks' opinions accordingly.*

Back to those anti-VEGF agents.

You can be aware of all the protocols for using ranibizumab and aflibercept, but the real question is whether or not your patient and/or your healthcare system can afford to use the drugs. If not, you will probably need to substitute bevacizumab. There are a host of studies suggesting that bevacizumab works rather well for DME, an example being the BOLT study, which compared bevacizumab alone to laser alone (the main injection interval in the BOLT study was 6 weeks compared to the 4 week interval used in ranibizumab studies). The bevacizumab group gained 9 letters at two years, which is similar to the ranibizumab results above (the laser group gained 2.5 letters).[30] So bevacizumab for DME is not exactly uncharted territory. And when it comes to treating age-related macular degeneration, the

Comparison of AMD Treatment Trials (CATT) demonstrated equivalence, at least between ranibizumab and bevacizumab. But that is a very different disease, and even in that study bevacizumab did not dry out the retina quite like ranibizumab, and no one has compared aflibercept to the other two in AMD.[31]

But the three drugs have been compared for treating DME—a study the DRCR.net just finished known as Protocol T.[32] The results of that study are summarized in Figure 9. Basically, aflibercept seems to be a bit stronger than the other two. But before you become the first on your block to destroy your healthcare system by using Eylea on every single diabetic, let's take a closer look.

The investigators looked at whether the initial visual acuity made a difference when choosing a drug, and it did. For patients whose vision was 20/40 or better, all three drugs worked about the same. But for patients with vision worse than 20/50, aflibercept was better on average. Plus, patients receiving aflibercept required fewer laser treatments.

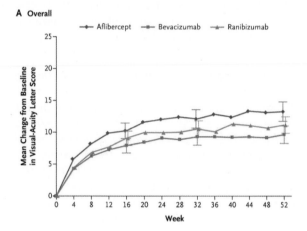

Figure 9a: The overall results for the Protocol T study showing that aflibercept is better, but not by a lot.

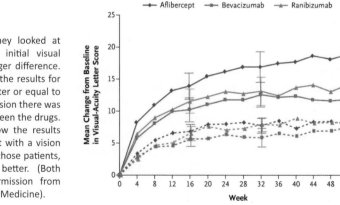

Figure 9b: When they looked at the results based on initial visual acuity, there was a bigger difference. The dashed lines show the results for patients with vision better or equal to 20/40. At that level of vision there was not any difference between the drugs. But the solid lines show the results for patients starting out with a vision of 20/50 or worse. For those patients, aflibercept is clearly better. (Both graphs used with permission from New England Journal of Medicine).

However, this does not mean that you are being a bad doctor if you don't start with aflibercept in every patient that is 20/50 or worse. First, remember that these are ETDRS visual acuities. There is no defined conversion factor between ETDRS visions and the acuities you get in your lane, but ETDRS visions tend to be at least a line or two better. So the efficacy of aflibercept may really kick in around 20/70-80 in the real world.

Also, in many places, those expensive drugs are simply not an option. And even if they are an option, patients may have huge copays with the pricier drugs. Most importantly, when you start treating patients you will learn that graphs can only show population averages; there are individual patients that do better with bevacizumab and there are also patients that just don't respond as well to aflibercept. Some patients actually need to use different drugs in rotation because of tachyphylaxis. And finally, the study didn't look at issues such as whether combination treatments including steroids and laser might change the results, or if patients with worse systemic control would respond differently (the average hemoglobin A1c in Protocol T was 7.7). As a result, it is not unreasonable to start with bevacizumab and see what happens. Of course, there are people that feel that it is profoundly wrong to do this, but until ranibizumab and aflibercept are available as a $25 generic injection, it is what it is.

In America, both Genentech and Regeneron (the manufacturers of ranibizumab and aflibercept, respectively) have patient access programs whereby they will provide the drug for patients who don't have the resources to pay for it. *They even have a copay assistance program so that patients making less than $100,000 a year may be able to get help covering the copay. (Basically, the companies make so much money off the drug that they developed a rather Byzantine set-up to help with the copay—they donate money to a separate charity that then sets aside money for the patient. This way the companies can still get most of the money from insurance when doctors give a dose.) All this can sometimes make ranibizumab and aflibercept even cheaper than bevacizumab, especially for indigent patients. It is a bit of a hassle for your staff, but it is well worth it to be able to have all options available for your patients. The policy in other countries varies on a geographic basis, and you may want to check with the regional representatives to see if any access programs are available.*

There are two big concerns, though. The first is that your bevacizumab will need to be compounded; and that adds some risk that patients need to know about (Chapter 11 talks about this more). The other problem is that doctors, governments and professional societies have wildly divergent views on the safety of bevacizumab. Unless you live in a cave, you know that the anti-VEGF drugs have potential systemic risks such as clots, strokes and heart attacks. Some people will be very dogmatic and insist that the only real data about how safe these drugs are comes from the controlled trials using the expensive anti-VEGF agents, and that it is wrong to use bevacizumab because the exact risk is not as well studied. Others don't think there is much difference, and don't distinguish between bevacizumab, ranibizumab or aflibercept as far as systemic risk.

Of course, the data about systemic safety is vague enough that you can find support for just about any opinion. For instance, one particular review suggests that bevacizumab has a greater systemic risk, but the company that makes ranibizumab paid for that paper.[33] Other population-based studies, and a Cochrane review, have not found a definite increased risk with either drug.[34-37] Yet another population study suggested that both bevacizumab and ranibizumab may slightly increase the risk of MI, but not stroke.[38] CATT suggested there was no big difference between the drugs, but the bevacizumab group did have more systemic problems that were not traditionally associated with bevacizumab—but the bevacizumab group was older and more likely to have problems anyway. Analyses of combined ranibizumab studies did suggest a possible association with strokes, which strongly suggests that there is at least a similar risk with bevacizumab.[39,40] And another study suggested that the risk might be greater with monthly ranibizumab compared to PRN dosing.[41] However, the Protocol T trial didn't find any definite safety concerns amongst the three.

Going deeper, bevacizumab does seem to affect plasma VEGF levels more than the other drugs, which is worrisome.[42] On the other hand, a recent editorial suggested that all the potential systemic issues—with all the drugs--may be spurious and are simply due to Type 1 statistical errors.[43] More recent studies concluded that there is probably some sort of small risk—especially in patients receiving monthly injections over a long period of time—and a large population study suggested the risk of a thrombotic event may be 1 in 127.[44,53,54] So there is likely a real risk, but you can almost pick your favorite results depending on your viewpoint.

However, the one thing everyone agrees on is that you can't ignore the issue.

Rather than becoming an epidemiologist, one thing to consider if you are going to give anti-VEGF drugs is to check with your regional experts regarding how they feel about these side effects. If they are really dogmatic about which drug to use, you might need to mirror their concerns because if your patients end up in their office for a second opinion you don't want your approach to be wildly different. They probably won't be so dogmatic, but their insights will still be valuable. And you for sure need to stay on top of the latest literature—if definitive studies ever do spell out the risk of one drug over another, you want to tell your patients before they read about it in the paper.

Then there is the question of whether you should use any of the meds in patients with known disease—for instance in patients with a history of stroke or cardiac disease (often an issue in diabetic patients). Many of the studies using these meds in diabetes specifically excluded patients with a recent history of an MI or CVA, so it is hard to extrapolate the safety data to the kind of trainwreck patients you see in your clinic.[41] There is data from some of the anti-VEGF studies that suggests that such patients may be more at risk for problems with treatment. At this point, many texts will add something about how you should consult the patient's internist before administering anti-VEGF agents. This seems like a reasonable thing to do—until you realize that there is no internist in the world who can predict the real risk of intravitreal anti-VEGF agents for any patient. It would even be impressive if the average internist were really familiar with the use of anti-VEGF agents for retinopathy.

This is one of those weenie things that we do as ophthalmologists in order to avoid any real responsibility. Basically, your level of "freaked-out-ness" over covering yourself will help you decide how far you want to pursue this—but you are ultimately the one doing the injection, and it is your job to stay on top of the data and the patient's systemic status in order to make the best decision you can. (Besides, getting some sort of vague clearance to do an injection is really only pretend protection. Plaintiff attorneys love it when doctors start blaming each other.)

Sample the opinions of the experts in your area; you don't want to be an outlier. Most will acknowledge the risk, but will still treat. You do want to be sure you have gone over this clearly with the patient and their family members, and that the discussion is well documented and repeated. If the patient ever does have a stroke or heart attack (which is pretty much guaranteed in this patient population), you don't want anyone saying you didn't tell them. This is also a situation where occasional doctors will suggest using the older drug pegaptanib (Macugen), which is weaker than the other drugs but seems to be free of systemic risk issues. Or you may want to default to steroids like triamcinolone or Ozurdex, depending on the clinical situation.

It would be awesome if we could just tell you what to do in a few paragraphs— but no one really knows so you have to do your homework and come up with a plan on your own. Chapter 5 focuses on doing a consent in this situation and has additional suggestions.

While we are talking about the risk of systemic thrombotic events due to the anti-VEGF drugs, it is worth noting that there are cases of intraocular occlusive events occurring shortly after using these agents as well. Patients have developed artery and vein occlusions, capillary nonperfusion, anterior ischemic optic neuropathy and ocular ischemic syndrome. It is not clear if these problems are due to the drug itself (for instance, anti-VEGF agents are known to have a vasoconstrictive effect on the retinal vessels). Or it could be due to other problems such as the post-injection pressure rise, acute hypertension from patient stress, and/or underlying poor ocular perfusion that predisposes to vascular occlusion. These problems do seem to be more common in diabetics and patients with pre-existing vascular disease. Fortunately, events like this are rare, but be aware that this is yet one more thing that can go wrong.[57]

Having discussed some if the potential problems with the anti-VEGF drugs, it is good to know that most patients require far fewer treatments over the years. But the really amazing thing is that patients in the studies were less likely to progress to more advanced types of retinopathy such as severe nonproliferative disease or proliferative disease (this trend was also seen in studies using triamcinolone).[45] Anti-VEGF drugs are not just changing the ocular milieu on a temporary basis; instead they are having a more fundamental effect on the basic mechanisms of diabetic retinopathy—it reverses diabetic retinopathy with frequent use![46,47] The FDA recently approved both aflibercept and ranibizumab for reversing retinopathy in patients with diabetic macular edema. It is encouraging to think that the injections are actually helping to cure the disease. Figure 9 is an example.

Figure 10: (facing page) This patient needed fairly constant anti-VEGF injections in the left eye to control DME. The right eye needed far fewer injections. Note how over time the background retinopathy progressed in the bottom image of the untreated right eye—there is even subtle proliferative disease at the nerve. The eye requiring regular treatment looks much healthier over time.

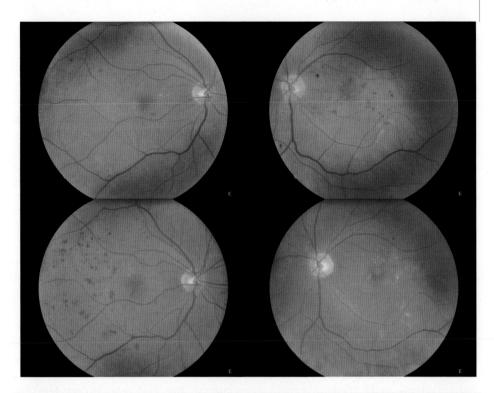

By the way, Figure 10 serves as a reminder for something else to keep in mind. If the DME goes away and the patient no longer needs anti-VEGF injections, you still need to watch them carefully. When the injections stop there may be a rebound-like effect and their background retinopathy may progress rapidly to proliferative disease, and the patient will have no symptoms until they start to hemorrhage. You want to catch that well before it starts—there will be more on this in Chapter 14.

What if nothing is working?

You missed something. How is the patient's body—any blood pressure problems, renal failure, etc.? Are they on any drugs that can perpetuate edema (prostaglandin analogs, Actos—see Chapter 12)? Go back and look for other problems like uveitis, a vein occlusion or all the other stuff in Chapter 27. And double check for traction. But this is also where people start to try everything—add a topical non-steroidal, use laser, combine steroids and anti-VEGF drugs, see if any of the long-acting steroid devices are available and might help.

Also, don't give up quickly, especially with the anti-VEGF drugs. Some patients don't seem to respond to the first few injections, but if you are persistent they will slowly improve. And look at the graphs for both Protocols I and T (as well as any of the other anti-VEGF studies). Note that the vision improves a lot at first, but then continues to slowly improve over time. This is different from what happens in age-related macular degeneration (AMD), where the vision also improves at first, but tends to level off or even backslide over time. If you are used to treating AMD, you need to reset your expectations with DME and be willing to continue treating to push for the best possible vision. Depending on your healthcare system, you may be able to switch drugs—there are always patients that seem to do much better with a specific drug (remember the enhanced efficacy for aflibercept in patients with worse vision in Protocol T). And finally, have a low threshold for referral.

Retina folks actually like this stuff, and they might have something up their sleeve that you don't (like a vitrector).

And sometimes you just can't get rid of the edema—remember the Protocol I data that about a third of patients still had swelling even after 5 years of treatment.[26] There are patients where the edema is there forever, or where the damage is permanent and the vision doesn't get better even if you can eliminate all the swelling. Under those circumstances you may end up just treating the patient palliatively—simply giving them a shot of something whenever it looks like they are about get a lot worse. But a retinal specialist should really make this call—as mentioned above, patients who are stuck with chronic edema should be referred.

What about PRP for DME?

If you jump ahead to the proliferative disease chapters, it will become obvious that a lot of diabetics have very ischemic peripheral retinas due to capillary dropout. Because VEGF comes from the ischemic peripheral retina, and because VEGF causes vascular leakage, it is thought that by doing mild panretinal photocoagulation in peripheral ischemic retina, one can help control leakage in the macula. Some doctors will use wide-field fluorescein angiography to identify areas of peripheral non-perfusion and then treat those areas with laser.[48-50] In fact, such an approach is not new—it was suggested years ago.[51] As we shall see in subsequent chapters, one is always worried that panretinal treatment will exacerbate macular edema, so this thinking seems a bit counterintuitive. Plus, other experts feel that there is data from the ETDRS that suggests peripheral treatment is unlikely to be effective in this way. Keep an open mind about this, though. As more studies are done, it may be another technique that can be useful in patients with refractory disease--what we know "for sure" can change with time.

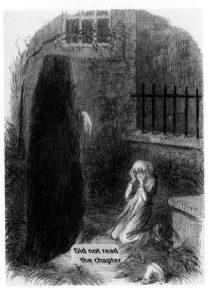

The End-of-Chapter Wrap-up.

If you are blowing off the rest of the chapter and just reading this section, you are really shortchanging yourself. We can't make you go back and read it all, but when you are visited by the Ghost of Christmas Future because you were a bad ophthalmologist, don't blame us.

So to review, first make sure you are actually treating diabetic edema and not one of the many things covered in Chapter 27. Second and third, beat on the patients to address their systemic control—that is the base of your therapeutic pyramid—and make sure that they don't have something else going on like renal failure, hypertension or pregnancy that is revving things up.

Then try to decide if there is any traction involved, and whether that traction is bad enough that a vitrectomy is warranted or if it is worth trying to treat the edema medically first. Then look at the areas of leakage. If it is peripheral to the fovea, and mild, you may not need to do anything—just watch it closely. If it is peripheral and worrisome (i.e., definite CSDME), your best bet is to do gentle laser and go back to the second and third steps above. If there is center-involving disease, you can still look at the areas of leakage. If you think that there are a few plump microaneurysms causing the trouble, and they are away from the fovea, you may still want to try laser. But if the leakage is more diffuse, or if there is a lot of central disease, you are going to need to go straight to injections (with or without laser depending on what the leakage looks like and where it is). If the patient is pseudophakic and does not have pressure problems, you may want to start with triamcinolone. If they are phakic, you will likely go with the anti-VEGF drugs, but your healthcare system and the patient's insurance company may be the ones that tell you which drug you will be using. Don't forget company sponsored access programs that may make it cheaper to use an expensive drug compared to having the patient pay for bevacizumab.

Also, if you are going in with anti-VEGF agents, remember the Protocol I results that suggested that it might be better to defer laser for a few months to see how things go—and then add laser if the disease is refractory. On the other hand, if there is a lot of disease and the patient has poor control, you may want to consider earlier laser because in these patients you may need to treat with everything you've got to stop their disease. As an aside, never forget about the potential utility of something simple like a topical nonsteroidal. They can be useful in some patients—and this can range from decreasing the number of injections to actually eliminating edema without the need for other treatments. Upcoming studies will better determine how these eye drops fit in.

One other thought on when to do the laser. If you think laser is the right thing to add to a patient's treatment--but if the retina is really swollen--you might want to get rid of some of the swelling with injections first. It is a lot harder to laser through thick retina, and your spot is more likely to spread out, resulting in a larger scar. Chapter 9 will go into this in greater detail, but it is worth mentioning here.

Mostly, remember to be flexible—you may need to combine treatments in difficult patients or switch back and forth between treatments depending on the disease or external issues such as insurance or problems with follow-up. For instance, some patients may need an occasional steroid shot to bolster the effect of chronic anti-VEGF therapy, or a little anti-VEGF can be added to extend the effectiveness of steroid shots. They may also need laser touch-ups if new areas of eccentric leakage develop that don't merit the risk of intravitreal treatment.

Recognize that you are in uncharted territory as you do these things. So far there are no big studies that really define how to mix and match therapies, so keep up with the literature and check with your colleagues to make sure you are not missing anything.

And don't keep repeating ineffective treatments if you aren't making progress. Sometimes you can't get the swelling to go away no matter what you do. In that case, share the love and get a second opinion with a specialist—there may be something you missed or there may be a role for a vitrectomy (more on this in Chapter 19). But don't wait a long time to do that—if you are going nowhere, refer the patient somewhere before too much chronic damage occurs.

Finally, recognize that sometimes patients have refractory disease and that nothing is going to completely control the process. If neither you nor your local specialist can solve the problem, then consider backing off and simply using palliative treatment on a PRN basis to keep things from getting worse. Fortunately this doesn't happen too often, but it is good to know when to give up.

References

1. Friedman SM, Almukhtar TH, Baker CW, et al. Topical Nepafenec in Eyes with Noncentral Diabetic Macular Edema. *Retina.* Jan 19 2015.
2. Callanan D, Williams P. Topical nepafenac in the treatment of diabetic macular edema. *Clin Ophthalmol.* Dec 2008;2(4):689-692.
3. Hariprasad SM, Callanan D, Gainey S, He YG, Warren K. Cystoid and diabetic macular edema treated with nepafenac 0.1%. *J Ocul Pharmacol Ther.* Dec 2007;23(6):585-590.
4. Shimura M, Yasuda K. Topical bromfenac reduces the frequency of intravitreal bevacizumab in patients with branch retinal vein occlusion. *The British journal of ophthalmology.* Sep 2 2014.
5. Singh R, Alpern L, Jaffe GJ, et al. Evaluation of nepafenac in prevention of macular edema following cataract surgery in patients with diabetic retinopathy. *Clin Ophthalmol.* 2012;6:1259-1269.
6. Beck RW, Edwards AR, Aiello LP, et al. Three-year follow-up of a randomized trial comparing focal/grid photocoagulation and intravitreal triamcinolone for diabetic macular edema. *Archives of ophthalmology.* Mar 2009;127(3):245-251.
7. Jyothi S, Sivaprasad S. Five-year visual outcome following laser photocoagulation of diabetic macular oedema. *Eye (Lond).* Jul 2011;25(7):851-858; quiz 859.
8. Rubin B, Taglienti A, Rothman RF, Marcus CH, Serle JB. The effect of selective laser trabeculoplasty on intraocular pressure in patients with intravitreal steroid-induced elevated intraocular pressure. *Journal of glaucoma.* Jun-Jul 2008;17(4):287-292.
9. Law SK, Hosseini H, Saidi E, et al. Long-term outcomes of primary trabeculectomy in diabetic patients with primary open angle glaucoma. *The British journal of ophthalmology.* May 2013;97(5):561-566.
10. Smithen LM, Ober MD, Maranan L, Spaide RF. Intravitreal triamcinolone acetonide and intraocular pressure. *American journal of ophthalmology.* Nov 2004;138(5):740-743.
11. Jones R, 3rd, Rhee DJ. Corticosteroid-induced ocular hypertension and glaucoma: a brief review and update of the literature. *Current opinion in ophthalmology.* Apr 2006;17(2):163-167.
12. Singer MA, Groth SL, Sponsel WE, et al. Association of OCT angle recess width with IOP response after intravitreal triamcinolone injection. *Retina.* Feb 2013;33(2):282-286.
13. Williams CP, Konstantopoulos A, Rowley SA, Luff AJ. Late intraocular pressure rise following intravitreal triamcinolone injection. *Clin Experiment Ophthalmol.* May-Jun 2007;35(4):385-386.

14. Agrawal S, Agrawal J, Agrawal TP. Vitrectomy as a treatment for elevated intraocular pressure following intravitreal injection of triamcinolone acetonide. *American journal of ophthalmology.* Oct 2004;138(4):679-680.

15. Chew E, Strauber S, Beck R, et al. Randomized trial of peribulbar triamcinolone acetonide with and without focal photocoagulation for mild diabetic macular edema: a pilot study. *Ophthalmology.* Jun 2007;114(6):1190-1196.

16. Tunc M, Onder HI, Kaya M. Posterior sub-Tenon's capsule triamcinolone injection combined with focal laser photocoagulation for diabetic macular edema. *Ophthalmology.* Jun 2005;112(6):1086-1091.

17. Sato H, Naito T, Matsushita S, Takebayashi M, Shiota H. Efficacy of sub-Tenon's capsule injection of triamcinolone acetonide for refractory diabetic macular edema after vitrectomy. *The journal of medical investigation : JMI.* Aug 2008;55(3-4):279-282.

18. Lazic R, Lukic M, Boras I, et al. Treatment of anti-vascular endothelial growth factor-resistant diabetic macular edema with dexamethasone intravitreal implant. *Retina.* Apr 2014;34(4):719-724.

19. Comyn O, Lightman SL, Hykin PG. Corticosteroid intravitreal implants vs. ranibizumab for the treatment of vitreoretinal disease. *Current opinion in ophthalmology.* May 2013;24(3):248-254.

20. Cabrera M, Yeh S, Albini TA. Sustained-release corticosteroid options. *Journal of ophthalmology.* 2014;2014:164692.

21. Scaramuzzi M, Querques G, Spina C, Lattanzio R, Bandello F. Repeated Intravitreal Dexamethasone Implant (Ozurdex) for Diabetic Macular Edema. *Retina.* Jan 8 2015.

22. Cunha-Vaz J, Ashton P, Iezzi R, et al. Sustained delivery fluocinolone acetonide vitreous implants: long-term benefit in patients with chronic diabetic macular edema. *Ophthalmology.* Oct 2014;121(10):1892-1903.

23. Korobelnik JF, Do DV, Schmidt-Erfurth U, et al. Intravitreal Aflibercept for Diabetic Macular Edema. *Ophthalmology.* Jul 8 2014.

24. Elman MJ, Bressler NM, Qin H, et al. Expanded 2-year follow-up of ranibizumab plus prompt or deferred laser or triamcinolone plus prompt laser for diabetic macular edema. *Ophthalmology.* Apr 2011;118(4):609-614.

25. Elman MJ, Qin H, Aiello LP, et al. Intravitreal ranibizumab for diabetic macular edema with prompt versus deferred laser treatment: three-year randomized trial results. *Ophthalmology.* Nov 2012;119(11):2312-2318.

26. Elman MJ, Ayala A, Bressler NM, et al. Intravitreal Ranibizumab for Diabetic Macular Edema with Prompt versus Deferred Laser Treatment: 5-Year Randomized Trial Results. *Ophthalmology.* Oct 28 2014.

27. Jusufbegovic D, Mugavin MO, Schaal S. EVOLUTION OF CONTROLLING DIABETIC RETINOPATHY: Changing Trends in the Management of Diabetic Macular Edema at a Single Institution Over the Past Decade. *Retina.* Jan 14 2015.

28. Do DV, Nguyen QD, Khwaja AA, et al. Ranibizumab for edema of the macula in diabetes study: 3-year outcomes and the need for prolonged frequent treatment. *JAMA ophthalmology.* Feb 2013;131(2):139-145.

29. Solaiman KA, Diab MM, Dabour SA. Repeated intravitreal bevacizumab injection with and without macular grid photocoagulation for treatment of diffuse diabetic macular edema. *Retina.* Sep 2013;33(8):1623-1629.

30. Rajendram R, Fraser-Bell S, Kaines A, et al. A 2-year prospective randomized controlled trial of intravitreal bevacizumab or laser therapy (BOLT) in the management of diabetic macular edema: 24-month data: report 3. *Archives of ophthalmology.* Aug 2012;130(8):972-979.

31. Martin DF, Maguire MG, Fine SL, et al. Ranibizumab and bevacizumab for treatment of neovascular age-related macular degeneration: two-year results. *Ophthalmology.* Jul 2012;119(7):1388-1398.

32. The Diabetic Retinopathy Clinical Research N. Aflibercept, Bevacizumab, or Ranibizumab for Diabetic Macular Edema. *The New England journal of medicine.* Feb 18 2015.

33. Kaiser PK, Cruess AF, Bogaert P, Khunti K, Kelly SP. Balancing risk in ophthalmic prescribing: assessing the safety of anti-VEGF therapies and the risks associated with unlicensed medicines. *Graefes Arch Clin Exp Ophthalmol.* Nov 2012;250(11):1563-1571.

34. Campbell RJ, Bell CM, Paterson JM, et al. Stroke rates after introduction of vascular endothelial growth factor inhibitors for macular degeneration: a time series analysis. *Ophthalmology.* Aug 2012;119(8):1604-1608.

35. Curtis LH, Hammill BG, Schulman KA, Cousins SW. Risks of mortality, myocardial infarction, bleeding, and stroke associated with therapies for age-related macular degeneration. *Archives of ophthalmology.* Oct 2010;128(10):1273-1279.

36. Moja L, Lucenteforte E, Kwag KH, et al. Systemic safety of bevacizumab versus ranibizumab for neovascular age-related macular degeneration. *The Cochrane database of systematic reviews.* Sep 15 2014;9:CD011230.

37. Ng WY, Tan GS, Ong PG, et al. Incidence of myocardial infarction, stroke and death in patients with age-related macular degeneration treated with intra-vitreal anti vascular endothelial growth factor therapy. *American journal of ophthalmology.* Dec 9 2014.

38. Kemp A, Preen DB, Morlet N, et al. Myocardial infarction after intravitreal vascular endothelial growth factor inhibitors: a whole population study. *Retina.* May 2013;33(5):920-927.

39. Bressler NM, Boyer DS, Williams DF, et al. Cerebrovascular accidents in patients treated for choroidal neovascularization with ranibizumab in randomized controlled trials. *Retina.* Oct 2012;32(9):1821-1828.

40. Ueta T, Noda Y, Toyama T, Yamaguchi T, Amano S. Systemic Vascular Safety of Ranibizumab for Age-related Macular Degeneration: Systematic Review and Meta-analysis of Randomized Trials. *Ophthalmology.* Jul 12 2014.

41. Yanagida Y, Ueta T. Systemic safety of ranibizumab for diabetic macular edema: meta-analysis of randomized trials. *Retina.* Apr 2014;34(4):629-635.

42. Zehetner C, Kirchmair R, Huber S, Kralinger MT, Kieselbach GF. Plasma levels of vascular endothelial growth factor before and after intravitreal injection of bevacizumab, ranibizumab and pegaptanib in patients with age-related macular degeneration, and in patients with diabetic macular oedema. *The British journal of ophthalmology.* Apr 2013;97(4):454-459.

43. Ahfat FG, Zaidi FH. Bevacizumab vs ranibizumab-an appraisal of the evidence from CATT and IVAN. *Eye (Lond).* Mar 2013;27(3):289-290.

44. Thulliez M, Angoulvant D, Le Lez ML, et al. Cardiovascular Events and Bleeding Risk Associated With Intravitreal Antivascular Endothelial Growth Factor Monoclonal Antibodies: Systematic Review and Meta-analysis. *JAMA ophthalmology.* Jul 24 2014.

45. Bressler SB, Qin H, Melia M, et al. Exploratory analysis of the effect of intravitreal ranibizumab or triamcinolone on worsening of diabetic retinopathy in a randomized clinical trial. *JAMA ophthalmology.* Aug 1 2013;131(8):1033-1040.

46. Campochiaro PA, Wykoff CC, Shapiro H, Rubio RG, Ehrlich JS. Neutralization of vascular endothelial growth factor slows progression of retinal nonperfusion in patients with diabetic macular edema. *Ophthalmology.* Sep 2014;121(9):1783-1789.

47. Ip MS, Domalpally A, Sun JK, Ehrlich JS. Long-term Effects of Therapy with Ranibizumab on Diabetic Retinopathy Severity and Baseline Risk Factors for Worsening Retinopathy. *Ophthalmology.* Feb 2015;122(2):367-374.

48. Takamura Y, Tomomatsu T, Matsumura T, et al. The effect of photocoagulation in ischemic areas to prevent recurrence of diabetic macular edema after intravitreal bevacizumab injection. *Investigative ophthalmology & visual science.* Aug 2014;55(8):4741-4746.

49. Patel RD, Messner LV, Teitelbaum B, Michel KA, Hariprasad SM. Characterization of ischemic index using ultra-widefield fluorescein angiography in patients with focal and diffuse recalcitrant diabetic macular edema. *American journal of ophthalmology.* Jun 2013;155(6):1038-1044 e1032.

50. Suner IJ, Peden MC, Hammer ME, Grizzard WS, Traynom J, Cousins SW. RaScaL: A Pilot Study to Assess the Efficacy, Durability, and Safety of a Single Intervention with Ranibizumab plus Peripheral Laser for Diabetic Macular Edema Associated with Peripheral Nonperfusion on Ultrawide-Field Fluorescein Angiography. *Ophthalmologica. Journal international d'ophtalmologie. International journal of ophthalmology. Zeitschrift fur Augenheilkunde.* Nov 26 2014.

51. Gardner TW, Eller AW, Friberg TR. Reduction of severe macular edema in eyes with poor vision after panretinal photocoagulation for proliferative diabetic retinopathy. *Graefes Arch Clin Exp Ophthalmol.* 1991;229(4):323-328

52. Aref AA, Scott IU, Oden NL, et al. Incidence, Risk Factors, and Timing of Elevated Intraocular Pressure After Intravitreal Triamcinolone Acetonide Injection for Macular Edema Secondary to Retinal Vein Occlusion: SCORE Study Report 15. JAMA ophthalmology. 2015;133(9):1022-1029.

53. Semeraro F, Russo A, Delcassi L, et al. Treatment of Exudative Age-Related Macular Degeneration with Ranibizumab Combined with Ketorolac Eyedrops or Photodynamic Therapy. Retina. 2015;35(8):1547-1554.

54. Avery RL, Gordon GM. Systemic Safety of Prolonged Monthly Anti-Vascular Endothelial Growth Factor Therapy for Diabetic Macular Edema: A Systematic Review and Meta-analysis. JAMA ophthalmology. 2015:1-9.

55.   Schlenker MB, Thiruchelvam D, Redelmeier DA. Intravitreal Anti-Vascular Endothelial Growth Factor Treatment and the Risk of Thromboembolism. American journal of ophthalmology. 2015;160(3):569-580 e565.
56.   Mansour AM, Al-Ghadban SI, Yunis MH, El-Sabban ME. Ziv-aflibercept in macular disease. The British journal of ophthalmology. 2015;99(8):1055-1059.
57.   Mansour AM, Shahin M, Kofoed PK, et al. Insight into 144 patients with ocular vascular events during VEGF antagonist injections. Clin Ophthalmol. 2012;6:343-363.

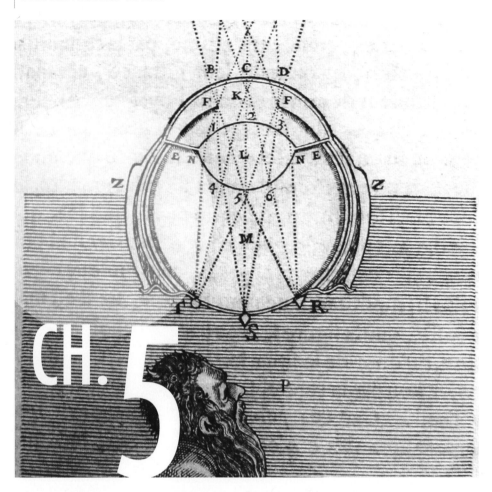

Trust Me, I'm a Doctor / PART ONE: The Informed Consent for Treating Diabetic Macular Edema

We are what we pretend to be, so we must be careful about what we pretend to be.
Kurt Vonnegut, *Mother Night*

The informed consent for treating DME will vary depending on whether you are using laser, injections, or both. It also depends on the level of disease, the comprehension of the patient and the patient's systemic control. We'll start with general principles, then focus on the consent for laser and finally talk about the specifics of the informed consent with injections. And don't blow this chapter off just because it's not hard science. This is where you learn to walk in your patient's moccasins, and that can make you more effective than a whole case of Avastin.

Communication with the patient is extremely important when one uses anything to treat diabetic retinopathy. You must remember that in spite of your best efforts to relate the concepts involved, there is a strong tendency for the patient's expectations to be very different from reality. It is certainly reasonable to provide the patient with ancillary information, such as discussions with office staff, videos and handouts. But don't depend on such things to replace you. (Besides, when was the last time you read that handout your dentist gave you about proper flossing?) Ultimately, it is the relationship that you foster with the patient that will—hopefully—keep them motivated to persist with the generally distasteful and often lifelong pursuit of having you fiddle with their retinas.

You should, first of all, take a deep breath and try not to display the overwhelming sense of near-drowning that one feels on a busy clinic day. You don't necessarily need to light your corncob pipe and put your feet up on the cracker barrel, but you should remember that your patient will not be impressed by how many treatments you can cram into an hour. They will be impressed if you take the time to carefully explain things, answer questions and skillfully anticipate unvoiced concerns. Make sure there is a family member or friend in the room, too. Having another person in the room will give the patient someone to share the experience with, and the second set of ears will be more functional than those of a stressed-out patient. It is simply a given that the average patient will be unlikely to remember much of what you say. Priluck, et al., wrote a fascinating paper on the ability of patients to recall an informed consent discussion concerning retinal detachment surgery.[1] On average, patients could only remember about 57% of what they had been told, and only 23% remembered the discussion of surgical risks.* Furthermore, patients would commonly state that anything that they did not remember had not been discussed. This is why you have to hyper-document anything you say—because in the polemic world of legal medicine, the paperwork becomes the reality, which is kind of absurd.

What all this really means, though, is that if you truly care more about your patients than about how your paperwork might look to a trial lawyer, you should realize that the data you provide may not be as important as the way in which you deliver it. A machine gun burst of risks will get the job done fast and will meet the "letter of the law" in your chart, but it is unlikely that the patient will remember much of it. A slow, careful discussion, with attention to the patient's concerns, will create a far better memory of the mood of the process in the patient's mind, even if the actual facts can't be remembered. Simply knowing that the doctor is interested in trying to transmit the information may be as important as how much is retained. In other words, you can probably deliver the informed consent in a completely unintelligible language, like maybe Klingon, but if you do it in a way that conveys that you will take all the time in the world to be sure the patient understands the situation, you will have accomplished a lot more than if you blast through the complications and then have them sign on the dotted line.

*And only 3% remembered that they could have a hemorrhage or infection that could destroy the eye. Think about *that* the next time you give some wired boomer attorney your best clear-lens-extraction-multifocal-IOL spiel.

On a darker note, remember that although you know you are a good person, people are constantly reading articles about maniac doctors cutting off the wrong leg or defrauding Medicare. In addition to having trouble understanding the nature of diabetic retinopathy, patients may also have an imperceptible lack of trust that can blossom into something really bad if a complication occurs. You have to anticipate this and recognize that careful communication from the start is the best way to avoid trouble.

In any event, here are the concepts to convey, regardless of how you choose to convey them (preferably not in Klingon)...

THE DISEASE

You have to make sure the patient has at least a rudimentary understanding of the pathophysiology involved by using your favorite analogy. For diabetic macular edema, this usually involves something like, "the diabetes has changed the blood vessels in your eye from nice new pipes into old rusty pipes, and they are leaking the clear fluid that is in blood. This makes the retina swell up like a tiny sponge in the same way the old veins in people's legs can leak and let their ankles swell up." Or anything similar to that—you can adjust it to the patient's level of interest and sophistication.

It is important to point out that, with macular edema, the vessels are not hemorrhaging actively. Many times patients will have been told that they have "burst blood vessels" or "hemorrhages in their eyes" and they visualize some horrible Niagara Falls of blood exploding out of their head. Terms like this generate unnecessary stress, and patients will wonder why you aren't treating the whole thing as a dire emergency and immediately lasering their gushing blood vessels into submission. You really want to dwell on the fact that you are dealing with interstitial fluid leakage and that any microscopic blood spots are really just old bruising and not any sort of active hemorrhage. Incidentally, using the word "bruising" to refer to intraretinal hemorrhages of any sort seems to be a much less inflammatory term than "blood" or "hemorrhage." It tends to avoid the whole Quentin Tarantino Kill Bill connotation and gives you a fighting chance that the patient's mind will not seize up completely.

It is extremely useful to have the patient's photographs, fluorescein angiogram and/or OCT available to show them during this discussion. If you can demonstrate a normal-looking fundus and then show them their own hard exudates and blot hemorrhages moving into the fovea, it is a lot easier for them to understand the gravity of this situation, especially if they do not have a lot of symptoms. This also allows you to point out the fact that, if you are going to use laser, you will be treating well away from the center of the vision. You would be surprised at how many patients have an unvoiced concern that your main goal is to simply chop away at their vision like a Civil War barber-surgeon and that they might be better off going blind slowly without treatment, rather than letting you hurry things along with your foolish laser and injections.

THE GOALS OF TREATMENT

The patient must also understand the goals of the treatment, especially if you are starting with laser. They strongly assume that your laser will improve things. This is partly because any time they have gone to a doctor in the past, the doctor usually does something that makes their life better, such as fix a sore throat or stitch a cut. They also know lots of people who have had lasers (YAG and LASIK) and who saw much better immediately after the laser. The distinction between your laser and those lasers can be quite, uh, blurry.

Welcome to the world of retina—a place where patients may get worse no matter what you do, and where you will spend a ton of time trying to convince your patients (and perhaps yourself) that going bad slowly is the greatest thing on the planet.

To review this, Figure 1 shows the graph from Chapter 4 comparing DRCR.net laser results to laser results in a less motivated patient population. Patients can definitely improve with laser, but there are still many patients for whom it can only slow things down.

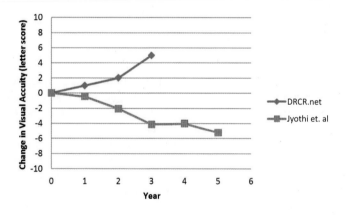

Figure 1: The graph from chapter 4 showing the point spread of modern lasers for DME. The top line shows the 3-year results of the laser arm from the DRCR.net protocol that compared laser to triamcinolone. The lower line is the result when the same laser protocol was used in a setting with patients who had poorer systemic control and follow up. Do not let your laser patients think that the laser will automatically make them better.

Careful laser is going to help your patients a lot, but they need to understand that it won't be Hollywood. Don't forget that you devoted a large chunk of your life to understanding the statistics that make your treatment logical, but these concepts are very new and counterintuitive to your patients who expect LASIK-like outcomes.

But wait. With intravitreal treatment, patients for sure do better, right? We saw that in the last chapter, and Figure 2 shows it again. But like the laser results, you can't expect all your real world patients to do as well as those in the study. And even if they do well, they may not share your enthusiasm for the results, because even great results won't be as good as the vision they had before they developed retinopathy. Figure 2 gives you a taste of this.

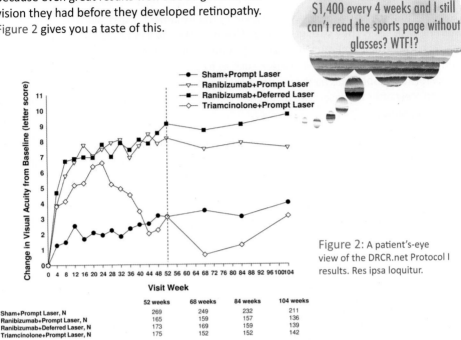

$1,400 every 4 weeks and I still can't read the sports page without glasses? WTF!?

Figure 2: A patient's-eye view of the DRCR.net Protocol I results. Res ipsa loquitur.

The point is, that thanks to the hard work of many people, we have made dramatic improvements when it comes to treating diabetic macular edema, and most conscientious patients won't get the downhill slide that most ETDRS patients experienced in the olden days. But not all patients will do so well, and if you dwell too much on the possibility of stability or improvement, it may be all the patient remembers of your discussion. And then they can become very frustrated when the reality of even successful treatment sets in, and that can lead to a very bad thing—they become disappointed and stop coming back for follow-up.

This is by far the worst thing you can let happen, because they usually return only when they have severe symptoms and awful disease that may be impossible to control. You must anticipate and address this type of frustration with treatment upfront. Here is one of the most important points in the book:

When it comes to treating diabetic retinopathy, anything that interferes with patient compliance will result in far more vision loss than complications from your treatments. Unfortunately, the patients that are most likely to be unhappy are the ones who are most likely to be less sophisticated, and they are also the ones that are likely to do poorly because of poor compliance and control. And if they wander off with no follow-up it is guaranteed that they will do terribly—you don't want this to happen as a result of your failure to make sure they had the right expectations.

The real art is to titrate what you say so that it is customized for each patient. But that discussion depends on a multivariate analysis that you have to perform in your head. Those variables include the interventions you have available to you, how bad their disease is, how good their systemic control is, and your sense of how able they are to process the info you give them. A knowledgeable, well-controlled patient with good insurance will likely do well; they need to know the risks, but they will "get it" and be on your side. A less sophisticated patient with poor control may need a complete review of the goals of treatment at every visit—especially if you can't offer them all the various treatments because of limited resources. Depending on your assessment of their prognosis, they may need to be reminded that getting worse slowly will be a good result; if they happen to stabilize or even improve, then that is gravy. (This is also a good time to remind them that their systemic control has a lot to do with what will happen.)

Even if you are sure they will do well, you need to avoid painting too much of a rosy picture. Patients tend to develop a really overblown idea of what "doing well" may mean, and their expectations will leave them disappointed. You even need to be careful if you use terms that suggest stabilization, because most diabetics don't remain the same over the long-term.

Here is why: Even if your treatment works superbly, diabetics can still have gradual deterioration of their visual quality—the fine print is harder to read, going from light to dark is trickier, it is harder to see traffic signs, etc. And this gradual deterioration occurs whether they have treatable retinopathy or not—even normal looking diabetic retinas usually don't function normally. [2] In addition, diabetic eyes just don't work as well starting from the front—subclinical changes in the tear film, cornea and lens all contribute to image degradation on top of retinal changes.[3] Although you can very effectively overcome large-scale damage like macular edema, you cannot as easily overcome the gradual deterioration of optical and retinal function that occur at the cellular level with diabetes.

This is especially true if you are primarily using laser, either because you don't have access to intravitreal treatments or if you are treating eccentric leakage in a patient with minimal symptoms. Intravitreal therapy tends to get the patient on your side because patients will often notice some degree of improvement and keep coming back for more. Laser is less likely to provide that kind of immediate gratification. Plus, the perception that diabetics have of the laser can change over time. Initially there is a strong tendency for patients to assume that laser will make them better, and you have to address such expectations so they aren't too disappointed. Later on there is a tendency to assume that any visual problems they have must be from the laser and not from progression of their disease, and you have to routinely address this as well. (Of course, sometimes older laser techniques would mess up their vision. However, more often patients think that the laser is causing vision loss because some doctor that doesn't know squat about treating retinopathy looked in and said as much. Chapter 3 covered this, so don't be that doctor.)

There is another big reason why a patient may want to blame your treatment if it doesn't magically make them normal again: It is easier to blame you than to accept responsibility for years of poor control. The only way you can work around this is with continual education—and sometimes you have to accept the fact that you will always be the bad guy, even if you have snatched such a patient from the jaws of blindness.

Here is another thing that is really important:

There is a problem with trying to convey the fickle nature of diabetic retinopathy. If patients understand that they may not get as good as they want, or that you may only be able to slow the rate of decay, then they may draw a very erroneous conclusion—that they will go downhill forever and you will only delay their inevitable descent into total blindness.

Anticipate this type of conclusion, and try to head it off. Remind them that although you can never guarantee anything, it is very unlikely that they will go totally blind from diabetic macular edema, especially if they are good about their control and follow up. Explain that, over time, they may be irritated by their vision, but they are unlikely to ever become helpless, which is what they really fear. Again, throw in plenty of "no guarantees" so their conclusion pendulum doesn't swing to the other side and have them thinking they are off scot-free—but by giving them this reasonable assurance you can save them lots of unnecessary anxiety. And then you can pull out all stops and try to actually get them better with whatever methods you have.

Have you ever had a patient tell you that some doctor told them that they were going blind when they weren't even close to going blind? You may get a sense of superiority from such a comment—you can reassure the patient (and yourself) that there is no way you would ever be so stupid as to say such a thing. Well, it is hard to imagine that any doctor would be so stupid as to say such a thing, but now you can see how a patient could come to such a conclusion after a thorough informed consent.

If you think you are a great communicator and that no patient would ever think that you would say that they are going to go blind, try this simple experiment: After you explain the potential for disappointment with even successfully treated diabetic retinopathy, ask the patient if this means that they will inevitably go blind. You will be surprised at the answers you get. And get ready to take a deep breath and start over— patience is your most valuable surgical tool.

COMPLICATIONS

But back to the specifics of the informed consent. For all patients, you need to clearly point out that without treatment there is a very good chance the patient will be losing vision over the next one to two years. Patients tend to focus on the complications of treatment, and you have to remind them of the far greater risk of doing nothing.

This is tricky. Never underestimate a patient's ability to mentally assign a huge significance to a tiny risk of complications while ignoring the vastly greater risk of vision loss if they do not get treated. Patients are very likely to remember your discussion of complications if their vision isn't as perfect as they want, and then they will assume the treatment is the problem. This puts them on the path to the Dark Side of Noncompliance. The point is that you have to cover the bad things but think carefully about how you do it.

You will be a sucky doctor if you do not make sure patients clearly hear the words "There is a small chance that the treatment can make you worse." Even if you become a retinal sensei, it is a sad medical fact that bad things can happen, and you never know when both you and the patient will get an unpleasant surprise. You do not want any patient coming back at you claiming that you never said such a thing—no matter how bullet-proof your malpractice carrier says your written informed consent is. And remember, this is where it is really important to have a family member or friend in the room.

However, you should not leave this (or any other negative concept) hanging at the end of a conversational paragraph. You need to remind them in the next sentence that the risk of treatment is very tiny, but the risk of permanent loss of vision is extremely large without treatment.

Another important warning should be mentioned if you are using laser, especially for Astute Patients (i.e., engineering types): Sometimes, a good observer may forever-after identify the laser spots that you placed in their macula. This is surprisingly unlikely—most patients are oblivious of careful, gentle laser for macular edema. However, some patients will notice this, and you get lots of style points for mentioning it before they come to you to complain about it. If you are seeing such a patient for a second opinion, it is charitable to point out that it is a heck of a lot better to have a few spots on one's peripheral vision than to lose chunks of central vision from untreated disease. But hopefully you will be able to protect your patient's central vision with injections that offer short term stabilization combined with parsimonious laser that helps minimize the need for multiple injections, all in a way that avoids having to trade peripheral laser spots for central vision.

And speaking of injections—the informed consent for shots is a whole nuther can of worms. You have to mention all the immediate risks of injection like intraocular hemorrhage, retinal detachment and endophthalmitis (Chapter 11 covers all the complications). You also have to discuss the possible complications related to each type of drug—cataract and glaucoma for steroids and all that weird stuff about thromboembolic events for the anti-VEGF drugs. And then you have to talk about how the injections usually need to be repeated multiple times and—yet again—make sure patients have the appropriate expectations. Finally, even though the above issues are really, really important, you also have to mention things that patients will consider far more important than you do. Like how their eye may be scratchy and irritated for a day after the injection or how they can get a subconjunctival hemorrhage or corneal abrasion—things that you consider a nuisance, but when the patient and their family act like they have PTSD from a scratched eye, you will be glad you mentioned it first.

Dealing with the potential thrombotic complications of the anti-VEGF drugs is complicated by the fact that different experts have very different takes on the issue. Plus, there is conflicting data about whether there is a difference between the risk of bevacizumab versus ranibizumab and aflibercept. There are experts that think it is immoral to use bevacizumab because it was never studied like the latter two drugs, and there are experts that think it is immoral to use the latter two drugs because of lack of difference and cost. And all those experts tend to say fairly irrelevant things like "inform the patient and let them decide", which is a joke because the patient will respond to all the nuances you generate in the consent based on your personal feelings. The paragraph from Chapter 4 where all this was discussed is worth repeating here:

"One thing to consider if you are going to give anti-VEGF drugs is to check with your regional experts regarding how they feel about these side effects. If they are really dogmatic about which drug to use, you might need to mirror their concerns because if your patients end up in their office for a second opinion you don't want your approach to be wildly different. They probably won't be so dogmatic, but their insights will still be valuable. And you for sure need to stay on top of the latest literature—if definitive studies ever do spell out the risk of one drug over another, you want to tell your patients before they read about it in the paper."

You may live in a place where the decision has already been made for you; for instance, if a governing body has decided that you can't use bevacizumab. For the rest of us, it is a bit more complicated. But regardless of the drug you favor, there are some things you need to cover: 1) When bevacizumab is used systemically at much larger doses in people with cancer, they can get some bad side effects such as blood clots, strokes and heart attacks. 2) There is a possibility that patients who get any of these drugs in their eye may get the same side effects, but the risk, if real, seems to be small. It helps to point out that diabetics are at increased risk for strokes and clots and heart attacks anyway, and even if the patient gets such a problem it will never be clear if the drug caused it.

And this is really the crux of the matter. The one thing everyone agrees on is that no one can say that the drugs are 100% free of this risk, so the patient has to decide if this scares them more than inevitably losing their vision without treatment. And you should repeat this every so often—it is guaranteed that if you are treating someone for years and they have a TIA or heart attack, they will NOT remember your discussion and they will be convinced that your stupid injections caused the problem because you never mentioned it.

If you are using bevacizumab, you need to add some additional stuff. First, there are some people who think the risk of thrombotic or other side effects is greater with bevacizumab, but others do not. Second—and this is a biggie—bevacizumab will never be FDA approved for ocular use (you can substitute the appropriate governing body for your region). You can tell them why (the drug company that makes both bevacizumab and ranibizumab would never go through the hassle of approving bevacizumab and lose billions of dollars in revenue). You can then point out that doctors are always using drugs off-label—once a drug is approved we can use it for other reasons when there is good evidence that it works, and you can point out that there are lots of drugs that we use that have never been FDA approved. Like aspirin and Tylenol.

Finally, you do need to discuss the fact that bevacizumab needs to be compounded, with all the associated risks discussed in Chapter 11—but you can avoid those risks by following the guidelines discussed in that chapter. (Of course, it may well be safer to use properly compounded bevacizumab compared to you drawing up ranibizumab or aflibercept in your grubby lane—but hopefully you are careful even though no one is looking over your shoulder.)

Once you work through the medical stuff, you also need to discuss the cost (if that is an issue—it may not be depending on your healthcare system). And patients need to understand that you aren't getting all that cash yourself—otherwise they will worry about your motives if you recommend the expensive drugs. But you might as well be honest about the money you do get so they have the whole picture—for instance Medicare pays docs about $60 when using ranibizumab or aflibercept, but much less when using bevacizumab (it has to do with how Medicare reimburses in-office drugs— ask your business manager if you don't know about this stuff, because you should). And then you really need to know what the patient-assistance options are—it is crucial to protect them from whopping copays. Doing the paperwork can be a real hassle for your staff, however many doctors won't even consider a more expensive drug until patients are signed up for such programs in order to protect both the patient and the practice from a big financial hit if the insurance company denies payment.

Then there is the question of whether you should use any of the meds in patients with known disease—for instance in patients with a history of stroke. There is data that suggests that such patients may be more at risk for problems with anti-VEGF treatment. Plus, most of the big studies using anti-VEGF agents in diabetes excluded such patients, so we can only make inferences about how the drugs affect a more vasculopathic population. Again, you are wise to sample the opinions of the experts in your area; you don't want to be an outlier. Some will ignore this concern and just treat. Others acknowledge the risk, but still lean towards treating. Others are reluctant to treat or may even suggest using the old drug pegaptanib (Macugen), which is weaker than the other drugs but also seems to be free of systemic risk issues. Just make sure the patient understands why you are doing what you are doing.

Phew. This is a lot of stuff to cover. Are you sure you still want to use these drugs? And you need to get all this written down so that the patient has something to sign. There is a handy resource provided by the Ophthalmic Mutual Insurance Company (http:// www.omic.com); you can go to their site and download various informed consents. Be warned—they are written by people who are trying to protect doctors from the free-for-all known as the American tort system. As a result, they are written in a way that may leave your patients feeling that they will be lucky if they get out of your office alive—let alone seeing. And you want to make sure they are upgraded to reflect the latest data.

Of course, if you are using steroids you don't have to deal with all the systemic anti-VEGF issues. But you do have to talk about cataracts and elevated pressure that may require surgery—which means you have to at least briefly talk about those types of surgical risks.

But back to the consent process in general...

Okay. Once you have gotten the part about complications out of the way, it is now even more important to dwell on the biggest problem with treatment: that it may not completely control the disease. Patients must be prepared for the possibility of multiple treatments and worsening of vision from progressive disease in spite of treatment. Even very intelligent patients have a tendency to assume that your intervention will be like Walmart: one-stop shopping. You may need to constantly reiterate how the treatment will need to be repeated, especially if you are using injections. This is also a good time to reemphasize the importance of good systemic control so the patient understands that your treatment alone is not going to solve their problem—the patient needs to be an active participant in this process. (Much more on this in The Chapter with a Tantalizing Name.)

You may even need to add that, unfortunately, there are times when the treatment simply does not work very well at all. This is particularly true in patients with longstanding poor control, bad disease, and who present late in their disease course. Still, with all the cool stuff we can do the odds are we can make them way better than they would be without treatment.

As you read this, it may seem like a lot of information to convey when time is limited. However, it really just takes about five minutes to go through this if you are only doing laser; plan on more time if you are doing injections. Making sure the patient understands is perhaps the most important part—and you cannot assume that they really get everything (even though you know you are the world's best communicator). The best way to assess their comprehension is to ask patients in a non-judgmental way to repeat the gist of what you have talked about. And when they respond with something way off base, just take a deep breath and start over. The actual treatment will soon become the least of your worries; making sure that patients understand what you are doing is a job that never stops.

SPECIAL PROBLEMS WITH INFORMED CONSENT IN DEVELOPING COUNTRIES
(and uniquely American institutions such as free clinics, county hospitals, and other examples of how our healthcare system can bring developing world medicine to your backyard)

The bulk of this chapter deals with patients who have a reasonable chance of getting access to the care they need. But many readers of this book will be in situations where patients have less of an opportunity to obtain state of-the-art healthcare. And the extended section title will hopefully encourage readers in a certain developed country to keep on reading, because there are problems that arise when resources are limited, no matter how big the gross domestic product is.

Developing regions are cursed with a combination of limited healthcare resources and a limited desire on the part of the diabetic population to access healthcare until their disease is far advanced. The reasons for the latter are numerous and include the cost, the difficulty of obtaining an exam, and the lack of symptoms until things are really bad. One big problem is the perennial dilemma inherent in treating diabetic retinopathy: the perception, on the part of patients, that treatment causes blindness.

This dilemma deserves further elaboration. Cataract surgery in developing countries (or any country, for that matter) is met with enthusiasm because the patients experience immediate benefit, and once a cataract is popped out, the problem tends to be over. This sets a level of expectation that is never met by treating diabetic retinopathy in the same setting. Treating diabetic retinopathy usually involves recurring, unpleasant treatments, and there is usually not much benefit that the patient can perceive.

This is because diabetics in this situation tend to seek evaluation only when they are forced to by progressive symptoms, at which point their disease is very advanced. Lasers and injections are then attempted, and although the treatment usually helps to some degree, the patients can still develop severe vision loss. Although one can explain this course of events to patients and their families, there is an inevitable tendency for patients to assume that the treatments caused their disease progression rather than to understand that their disease was so hopelessly advanced that the treatment could only slow things down. The problem is exacerbated by the fact that the affected population tends to be unsophisticated and to have a hard time understanding the nuances discussed in this chapter. The problem is even further exacerbated by the fact that the healthcare workers have limited time and resources to convey such nuances—let alone have time or equipment to perform the treatments in the first place.

A vicious circle is created as patients receive treatment and then go out and tell their friends and family that "it didn't work". The word spreads, and more diabetics become afraid to come in for early screening and treatment, and then eventually show up with advanced disease that treatment can't stop. They think the treatment made them worse, they tell their friends, and so on and so forth. The problem is compounded by extremely poor systemic control, which makes even timely treatment much less effective, and it is more likely to occur in places where the only treatment option is laser rather than injections. Lasers don't have the "wow" factor that injections do.

Dealing with this type of situation—whether it is in a developing country or a local free clinic—can change how the informed consent is presented to the patient. When these patients come crashing into the system with horrible disease, you have to be a bit more blunt and you have to try to offset the whole "treatment is bad" thing right from the start. The patient needs to understand that your goal is to try to hold on to any vision whatsoever and that they cannot expect to get better or even remain stable. You don't need to be the death of hope—they may do well with all your treatments, but make sure they aren't expecting perfect results. Emphasize that you are going to do everything you can to help them, and it will be a heck of a lot better than doing nothing, but things would have been a lot better if you had seen them well before this point.

You can also beat on them about control, but there may not be much they can do about it in their circumstances. What is really important is that you beat on them to be sure their relatives get checked for diabetes regularly, and if they are found to have diabetes, then they have to get an eye exam once a year. Also, if the patient knows anyone with diabetes, they should tell that person to get in for regular eye exams—no matter what— because if that person doesn't, they may end up in the same mess that the patient is facing.

All this sounds harsh, but you really have to go after the tendency for folks to expect that lasers and injections will solve their visual problems in this situation and you have to try to break the vicious cycle of having patients being unwilling or afraid to get an exam and then showing up too late. Finally, you have to try to do all this in a setting where your time and resources are likely very limited.

If you are in such a situation—ask for help. As stated before, there are international organizations that may be able to lend a hand. The American Academy of Ophthalmology maintains a list of such organizations on their web site. There may also be local religious or service-group organizations that can help you, like the Rotary or Lions clubs. You may be very surprised at what a difference you can make for your practice and your patients if you are persistent. You are also welcome to contact us. Just try not to get frustrated and give up. Appendix 2 has more insights and info.

Finally, there will be sections in the upcoming chapters that address how one needs to alter the treatment approach in locations where resources are limited and patients with awful disease are plentiful. It turns out that the focus of the informed consent is not the only thing that may be very different in these situations.

References

1.   Priluck IA, Robertson DM, Buettner H. What patients recall of the preoperative discussion after retinal detachment surgery. *American journal of ophthalmology*. May 1979;87(5):620-623.

2.   De Benedetto U, Querques G, Lattanzio R, et al. Macular Dysfunction Is Common in Both Type 1 and Type 2 Diabetic Patients without Macular Edema. *Retina*. Jun 23 2014.

3.   Calvo-Maroto AM, Perez-Cambrodi RJ, Albaran-Diego C, Pons A, Cervino A. Optical quality of the diabetic eye: a review. *Eye (Lond)*. Nov 2014;28(11):1271-1280.

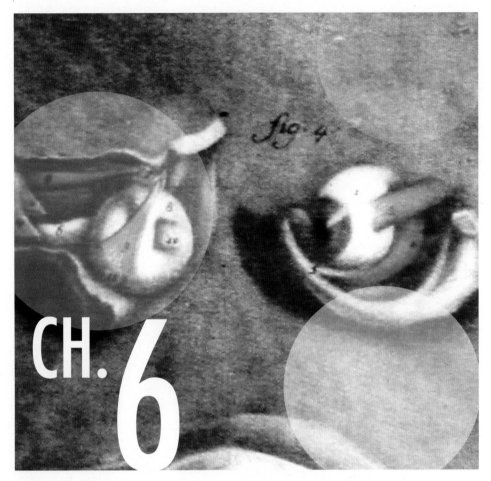

Know Your Weapons—Lasers and Their Ilk

God grant me a good sword and no use for it. Polish proverb

PART A. LASER PHYSICS FOR WIMPS

This section really does not have a heck of a lot to do with patient care issues, but it is useful to have some idea about how the little demons inside the laser box do their thing. It so happens that the acronym says it all: Light Amplification by Stimulated Emission of Radiation. But what does that mean?

It starts with the fundamental fact that electrons orbiting an atomic nucleus want to ditch their extra energy and get to lower levels. This process results in the emission of photons.

It turns out that electrons can release photons of only certain wavelengths because electrons can only live in certain orbitals, which are determined by the atom in which the electron resides. If the electron falls to a lower orbit, the electron releases a photon whose energy corresponds exactly to the difference in energy between the two orbitals—no in-betweenies allowed. The electron can also be bumped up to a higher orbital if it happens to absorb a photon of the exact energy that matches the energy difference between the lower and upper orbitals. If you can bump a bunch of electrons up to a given orbital and then get them to drop back down to a lower level at the same time, you can—for instance—stop diabetic retinopathy.

Getting the electrons to do this involves a weird and mysterious variation of the whole bumping up and dropping down process (this is where the Stimulated Emission part comes from). It turns out that if a photon happens to have the same energy as the difference between the pumped-up orbit where an electron is and the next-lowest orbit, and if said photon happens to pass by one of these electrons—without hitting it—the photon will stimulate the electron to drop into the lower orbit and produce a second photon that is coherent (meaning the peaks and troughs of the waves of both photons occur at the same time). It is this rather amazing property that allows the production of laser light from a host of stimulated electrons. Furthermore, a given photon can stimulate a whole bunch of electrons as it whizzes by, and each photon released will go out and stimulate the release of even more photons (the Light Amplification part of LASER).

In 1917, Albert discovered that the oscillating field of the stimulating photon perturbs the electron's field, which causes it drop to the lower energy level sooner than it otherwise would. It took several decades, however, to turn this theoretical knowledge into something that even an ophthalmologist could use.

Older lasers use some type of gas to provide a population of high-energy electrons for this process to occur. You can usually identify a gas ion laser because it tends to be large with big black cables running from the laser to the wall; many such lasers are also water cooled, which adds a gurgling-broken-toilet ambience to the treatment experience. The gas molecules are "pumped" by either an electric discharge or a powerful light source, which creates a large population of high-energy electrons. There is also a fully reflective mirror at one end of the gas tube and a partially reflective mirror at the other. This makes the photons bounce back and forth a bit, which ensures that as many electrons as possible are stimulated to drop to a lower orbit and release a photon. Only a small number of photons escape through the partially reflective mirror and this, in turn, produces the laser light that you then put into a patient's eye.

Nowadays, most lasers generate coherent light from a light emitting diode; such lasers tend to be much smaller and look not unlike a home theatre amp, but with fewer buttons. These diode, or solid-state, lasers are a bit more complicated to explain. They involve things such as electrons moving from high-energy conduction bands to low-energy valence bands, skipping altogether the delightfully named "forbidden region" of energy. This sets up a situation where stimulated emission can occur in a chunk of matter that is much smaller than the gas tube of an older laser. Electrical energy is used to shove electrons into the higher valence levels and the release of photons is stimulated at the junction of the diode. The diode itself is still sandwiched between mirrors, just like in a gas tube laser. The whole process is far more efficient than in a gas laser, hence the lack of big cables and pipes that made gas ion lasers unsuitable for use as laser pointers.

Lasers used to treat retinal diseases are known as continuous wave lasers because the laser beam can be generated, well, continuously. The user sets the actual duration of the beam, and the power output is relatively low, which allows a gradual, controlled response in the target tissue. This is in contrast to the "pulse lasers" that are used in ophthalmology—the neodymium: yttrium-aluminum-garnet laser (Nd: YAG) and the excited dimer laser (excimer). This type of laser puts all of its energy output into a very brief period of time. Because the energy is the power per unit of time, a laser pulse released in a very short time can have a very high peak power, which, if focused in a small spot, can reach an extremely high power density (irradiance) and can essentially be explosive.

The frequency of light generated by a laser depends on the substance being used to generate the light. If the frequency produced is not ideal for the chosen application, it can be changed by using either harmonic generation or organic dyes. An organic dye laser can produce a spectrum of wavelengths, but such lasers are inefficient—a lot of energy is lost when the primary laser is fired into the dye to excite and lase its fluorescence spectrum in the dye laser cavity. Dye lasers tend to be expensive and difficult to maintain, and you are not likely to see such a laser nowadays.

Harmonic generation is a far more common technique for changing a laser's frequency. In this case, the laser light is passed through a special crystal that will vibrate at the laser's frequency and generate harmonics that are multiples of the laser's frequency. Such crystals are commonly used to double the frequency of the output of a YAG laser in order to produce a wavelength in the green spectrum (i.e., from 1064 to 532 nm). A typical diode green laser generates light in this fashion.

All of this is a horribly oversimplified explanation of one of the mainstays of retinal therapy. If you ever want to feel overwhelmed, pick up a bona fide textbook on lasers to get an idea of how complex they really are. We all have to be very grateful for the fact that there are plenty of good folks out there that actually understand this stuff on a fundamental level and are always working to give us better and better tools. This way we can concentrate on part B.

PART B. FROM ACRONYM TO VERB: LASERING PEOPLE

Once you manage to get your hands on a laser and point it at a patient, you can expect three types of tissue interactions, depending on the nature of the laser: photocoagulation, photodisruption and photoablation. These categories are a bit arbitrary because they are really part of a spectrum of how tissues respond to laser energy. It is convenient, though, to use these terms to distinguish the tissue effects of the different types of ophthalmic lasers. For instance, if you devote your life to fighting the demon scourge known as spectacles, you will depend on photoablation to provide your worldly needs. In this case, an excimer laser generates a wavelength of 193 nm (in the ultraviolet range), which can break chemical bonds. This allows very precise removal of tissue with only minimal damage to the surrounding structures. Photoablation is definitely a "now you see it, now you don't" kind of thing.

When you perform a YAG peripheral iridectomy or capsulotomy, you will be depending on photodisruption. This is more of a mechanical effect that results from tightly focused, high-power laser light, which produces an explosively expanding vapor bubble of ionized plasma. This bubble then quickly collapses, producing acoustic shockwaves that happily blow apart the structure you are treating. This is very satisfying from a single-player-shooter point of view, but it is not particularly user-friendly when you want to treat something delicate and squishy like the retina. A variation of the standard YAG laser is the femtosecond Nd:YAG laser, which uses a much shorter time interval to deliver the laser energy. This allows the photodisruption to be extremely precise—hence its growing use in corneal and cataract surgery.

Retinal laser treatment depends on the far more gentlemanly tissue effect known as photocoagulation. In this case, the laser light is absorbed by chromophores—usually the melanin in the RPE and choroid. That induces an elevation in the temperature of the tissue that spreads out from the pigment and literally cooks the surrounding tissue at a microscopic level. The resulting coagulation of proteins causes the desired effect—hopefully without any photoablative or photodisruptive pyrotechnics.

There is a fourth tissue interaction—photochemical—but you are unlikely to use it. In this case, a very low-power laser is used to activate a specific chemical to obtain the desired effect in the tissue. The use of a red laser to activate verteporfin (Visudyne) in order to treat neovascular age-related macular degeneration is the best example of this.

PART C. THE MOST IMPORTANT STUFF

Regardless of how the laser is produced, there are certain variables that you need to intuitively understand if you are going to treat patients safely and effectively. The first one is the wavelength of the laser you use. Figure 1 is the classic display of how each laser color is absorbed in various ocular tissues. For a long time, people hoped that different colors would allow one to customize the treatment depending on the indication. For instance, you can see that yellow really nails one of the peaks of oxyhemoglobin relative to green, and if you ever have occasion to use a yellow laser, you can detect a significant difference in how, for instance, microaneurysms respond to a different wavelength (they tend to be very easy to pick off with the yellow—often with very little disruption of the retinal pigment epithelium and outer retina). Perhaps more clinically significant is both the marked drop-off in hemoglobin absorption and the gradual drop-off in melanin uptake as you move into the red end of the spectrum. This explains in part why red and infrared burns require more power and tend to penetrate deeper into the more pigmented choroid. It also helps explain why the infrared diode laser in particular is so different to use relative to a green laser.

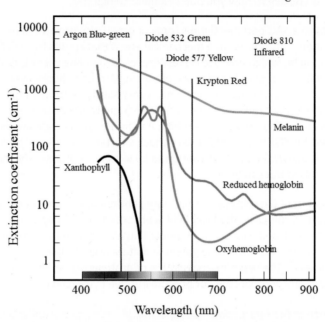

Figure 1: The absorption of different laser wavelengths by different substances in the retina, RPE and choroid. Note that, in general, the further you go toward red, the less the absorption—hence the need for more power and a resultant deeper burn with longer wavelengths. You can also see how yellow hits a peak of oxyhemoglobin absorption relative to green, which accounts for the difference in how microaneurysms are affected by each wavelength. Finally, you can see why it is a very bad idea to use blue light anywhere near the fovea, where xanthophyll pigment is found. (Data from Mainster MA. Wavelength selection in macular photocoagulation. Tissue optics, thermal effects, and laser systems. *Ophthalmology* 1986;93:952-8.)

However, although one does get different tissue responses depending on the wavelength, no one has proven that there is a huge difference in the ultimate treatment effect. Besides, you will basically be using whatever laser has been plopped in your clinic because there is no way you can go out and shop and compare with these enormously expensive devices. Fortunately, most of the studies on diabetic retinopathy were performed using some sort of green wavelength—usually argon green or its kissin' cousin diode green—and that is pretty much the standard color of laser found anywhere.

Some places do have the fancy lasers that can generate different colors, and you should experiment with these colors for yourself. Modern solid state lasers can generate green, yellow and red wavelengths, and some retinal specialists enjoy using a yellow laser because it seems to allow more selective treatment of retinovascular lesions and they feel there is less long term scar formation. A red laser can be useful when there are media opacities because the longer wavelength can get through better than green. An infrared laser can penetrate even better, but that wavelength is so different to use that it gets its own chapter at the end of the book.

However, no large study has proven that there is a definite difference between wavelengths in terms of clinical outcome. In fact, the Diabetic Retinopathy Clinical Research Network allows interchangeable use of yellow and green lasers for focal treatment of macular edema. For simplicity, the rest of this book will assume you have some sort of green laser to work with because that is the most common. Go Irish.

The one thing to remember with any wavelength is what you learned in second-grade science class: Black absorbs everything and white reflects everything. In other words, if you are treating happily in an area of the retina and you come upon a dark area like a nevus or a previous laser scar, you need to watch out, because you can get an explosive burn as the pigment sucks in the laser (higher absorption translates into higher photothermal elevation). Remember to Turn It Down When You Hit Brown (and Cut Way Back When You Hit Black). Alternatively, if you need to treat a very pale area, you will need to crank it up—but be super careful when you hit pigment again.

FLUENCE

Although wavelength is fun to theorize about, the power density, or irradiance, and the energy density, or fluence, of the laser beam are the most important concepts to master if you are going to be a safe and effective laserist. Here, for completeness, are the only formulas in the book:

$$\text{Irradiance (W/cm}^2) = \frac{\text{Power (Watts)}}{\text{Spot Area (cm}^2)}$$

$$\text{Energy (Joules)} = \text{Power (Watts)} \times \text{Time (Seconds)}$$

$$\text{Fluence (J/cm}^2) = \frac{\text{Power (Watts)} \times \text{Time (Seconds)}}{\text{Spot Area (cm}^2)} = \frac{\text{Energy (Joules)}}{\text{Spot Area (cm}^2)}$$

We will try to stay away from the obligatory discussion of energy, work, radiometric terminology, etc. that often shows up at this point in real textbooks. The key thing is that your laser output has a certain level of mojo and you need to know exactly how to control it.

Look at the last equation for fluence. Note that going up or down on power (Watts) or on exposure duration (Time) creates a linear increase or decrease in the energy delivered. This means that if you are getting a good burn and you decide to, say, double the exposure duration, then you have to decrease the power or you will really cook things. It is hard to imagine why on earth one would want to do this when one is getting a good burn, but this is always mentioned in basic laser texts and it does help ensure that you understand the relationship. The really significant thing is that the clinical effect tends to be very intuitive—a mild increase in the power or duration will give you a mild increase in your burn, and the same is true if you want to turn things down.

However, because we are dealing with a biological system and not a photometer, it turns out that the relationship between the energy delivered and the type of burn that you get is a bit more complex. The exact same energy can result in different burns because the burn depends on how the laser is absorbed and how the heat is transmitted by the tissue. In other words, fiddling with the laser power and duration generally results in a common-sense change in the degree of uptake—a little more time or power results in a little more burn and a lot more time or power results in a lot more burn. But don't depend on this absolutely. Let's take another colorful box break.

> **Colorful Box Break:** *Since you are basically using your laser to warm up the retina, you do need to be careful about using high powers at short duration, because the nice linear relationship breaks down and you can end up microwaving the proverbial poodle of urban legend. (Yes, this is a sophomoric metaphor, but if sleazy skull imagery will help you remember this point it is worth it.) Your "typical" laser burn is determined not only by the energy density but also by the rate of heat transfer out of the burn area. Unfortunately, heat transfer is governed by factors far more complicated than the weenie-pre-med-physics equation above. For instance, heat transfer explains why it is easy to get a burn in the retina but really hard to get a burn on a big blood vessel—the blood "carries" away the heat and you can't get the vessel wall to cook easily. Because you should treat a big vessel exactly never, just remember that if you use a lot of power over a really short duration, there isn't time for the heat to spread out and you can get a much hotter burn than you would expect if the response of the tissue were truly linear.*
>
> *This is not to say that you shouldn't use short durations. Modern lasers, and especially the pattern lasers discussed below, use very short durations, and it is felt that those shorter durations allow careful titration of how far the burn spreads. But you need to internalize the fact that the tissue response to your laser is nowhere near as linear as the fluence equation might suggest. In other words, if you were getting a good burn using 100 milliwatts for 100 milliseconds, and if you decided to decrease the duration by a factor of 10 to 10 milliseconds, the fluence equation suggests that you will need to turn the power up by that same factor of 10 to 1000 milliwatts to get the same burn. But you would never, ever really do that—you would vaporize the retina because the rapid buildup of heat would not have time to dissipate. Instead, you would gradually turn up the power until you had a safe burn. It won't take much experience for this*

to become intuitive—the point is that the basic equations are a guide, but they don't capture the entire essence of lasering a retina.

THE EFFECT OF SPOT SIZE

Going back to the mini-equation above, note that the fluence (or energy density) is an inverse function of the square of the spot size. This is very important to grasp; a small change in spot size can make a big difference in the energy you pour into the retina if you don't compensate by changing the power or duration. With a lot of energy delivered into a small spot, you can create a "YAG effect" because you will raise the temperature so fast and so high that the water in the tissue will actually boil. This is especially likely if you are also using a brief duration (less time for heat transfer, remember). The result is an explosively expanding bubble of water vapor that will cause a hole or hemorrhage or both. Technically, it won't be a true YAG photodisruptive effect—there won't be any plasma formation—but the explosive vaporization of water in the tissue will have the same destructive physical effect, complete with a sickening popping sound that the patient will clearly hear and feel in their head. You can really mess up an eye doing this—and lose lots of style points with your patients and colleagues. We will return to this concept several times in this book to be sure it sinks in—it has to be internalized to your lizard brain parts just like the mental switch that keeps you from engaging phaco when you are next to the posterior capsule.

Anyway, if you make the spot size smaller—even if it is only a little bit smaller—you really have to be religious about decreasing the other parameters so that you don't start punching holes in the retina. For instance, you might be using a strong power to cut through media opacities and you might also be using a short duration to try to make the laser less painful for the patient (no worries—much more on these techniques later). You might then decide to decrease the spot size in order to get an even better burn—a smaller spot will not spread out as much as a large spot if the view is hazy. If you do this, then you must cut back on power and work your way back up to a safe burn; otherwise, you will have increased irradiance and fluence by the square of the difference in spot size, and you will very likely cause a dangerously hot burn. Repeat: You must cut back on power and work your way back up to a safe burn if you decrease the spot size.*

Also, remember that your spot size is not exclusively dependent on the setting you put on the slit lamp adapter. As we will see in the next chapter, each type of contact lens will minify or magnify the size of the actual spot projected on the retina. If you switch to a different contact lens, you might be shrinking the actual spot size without realizing it—thus dramatically changing how much power is focused onto the retina.

There are even more ways the spot size can change unintentionally. When you are working in the retinal periphery, your spot will sometimes shrink down as you treat through the edge of the patient's lens. Or if you are doing a macular laser in an area of swollen retina, the thickened retina will tend to diffuse the beam, and when you move

*Repeat: This concept needs to be so ingrained that if you are captured by aliens and pithed for a science project your decerebrate hands will still reach for the power knob if someone says "smaller spot."

to an area of thin retina, your spot effectively shrinks. Or when you are starting your laser career, it may take way longer than you want to get anything into focus and you may decide to fire away before your focus is crisp because you are frustrated. If the gods of retina then suddenly put your aiming beam into perfect focus, your spot will shrink down and suddenly you will be burning holes in important parts of your patient. This will all be covered in greater detail in upcoming chapters—but the point is that your spot size may change whether you want it to or not, and you have to be ready to anticipate these changes and alter your parameters accordingly.

There is yet another way that the biology of lasering can get you into trouble even without using small spots, and this occurs when you are using powers, for whatever reason, that are causing very hot burns. In this case, the very center of the spot can get hotter than the periphery. Heat building up in the periphery of the burn can at least dissipate into untreated retina, but heat building up in the center of the burn is trapped and cannot spread out much. The result is a sudden hemorrhage at the center of the burn if the uptake increases even a little bit (such as when going into more pigmented areas). As will be discussed in upcoming chapters, it is unlikely that you would be trying to create such a hot burn to treat diabetic retinopathy, but it is important to know all the ways that things can go bad so you don't reinvent complications that your predecessors figured out the hard way.

Time for a Paragraph That Begins With the Phrase "The Bottom Line…"

The bottom line is that you will have three variables that you can control from the front panel of your laser and slit lamp adapter. The power and the duration are mostly linear and tend to be fairly forgiving if you make small adjustments and observe the effect as you treat the patient. Spot size, however, is the one variable that is truly exponential and you have to keep this in mind if you are switching to smaller spots. You must turn down the power and titrate back up. By the way, it may seem daunting when the process of lasering a retina is "unpacked" into all these component parts. One gets a sense that it will take about 30 minutes to line up each shot after tinkering with power, duration and spot size. Actually, there are many tricks to controlling these variables quickly and effortlessly and, well, you are just going to have to read the rest of the book to learn them.

OK. Suppose all of this is just too confusing. Let's get basic and remember what a burn is. The retina is normally a beautifully transparent structure. If the organization of the proteins and cells is disrupted then it begins to lose its transparency, in the same way the cornea begins to become cloudy when it swells. A mild burn means that, literally, the light absorbed by the pigment in the RPE is raising the temperature in the overlying retina enough that the retinal proteins are gently cooked. The retina becomes translucent—it gets a slight grayish color as light begins to be mildly scattered (think of how a poached egg opacifies with increasing heat). You can still see choroidal details through a light gray burn. As the burn gets hotter there is more disruption of the protein matrix and there is more scattering of light and the retina gets whiter and whiter—the choroidal detail is masked by the opaque white retina. If you are treating *a patient and suddenly your burns get very white, please stop immediately and adjust your settings—the easiest thing to do is turn down the power—so that you do not blow things apart or needlessly cook the nerve fiber layer. (See **Figure 2** for an overview—we'll show more examples of what burns should look like in upcoming chapters.)*

Figure 2: An example of how heat spreads up into the retina from the pigmented regions of the RPE and choroid. As the energy is increased, the damage extends higher and higher into the retina. When more of the retina is damaged the clinical appearance of the laser spot becomes whiter as the involved tissue loses its transparency and scatters more light. You can also see how a really hot burn can extend up into the nerve fiber layer, which can cause visual field defects that extend well

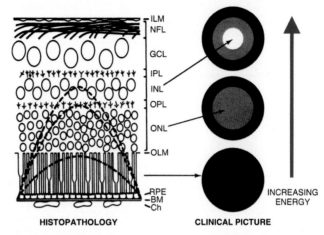

beyond the spot itself. Ch, choroid; BM, Bruch's membrane...Wait...Do you really need those initials spelled out at this point in your career? Hope not. (Modified from Weingeist, T, et al, Laser Surgery in Ophthalmology: Practical Applications, Copyright © 1992;17, with permission of the McGraw-Hill Companies.)

MISCELLANEOUS Odds & Ends

Lasering in the Infrared

Infrared diode lasers tend to be cheaper and relatively bulletproof (their design is simpler than a frequency-doubled green diode laser and they require way less fuss than a gas laser). If cost or logistical considerations are important, you may have no choice but to use infrared. This could be problematic because infrared is much trickier to use. Appendix 3 talks about the special needs of learning this wavelength—best to absorb the basic techniques covered in this book, and then you can read the stuff in the appendix to get ready to use infrared if you are going to use that wavelength.

Micropulse and Other "No Touch" Lasers

There are lots of wondrous things to be found in the halls of diabetic retinopathy treatment. This might be one of them. Not a common technique, micropulse laser involves delivering only a fraction of the requested power over the duration of a burn. It does this by delivering laser energy in pulses rather than continuously, and it brings into the mix a cool new term: duty cycle. This is simply the percentage of time that the pulses are actually delivering laser power relative to the total time of the exposure (Figures 2 and 3). The pulsing keeps the temperature from building up in the same way it would with a continuous wave and allows a gentle subclinical effect without the creation of a visibly identifiable burn.

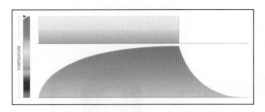

Figure 3: Schematic of the temperature rise associated with a continuous wave laser application. The gray bar represents the duration of the laser pulse and the orange-red represents the rise and fall of the temperature of the treated tissues.

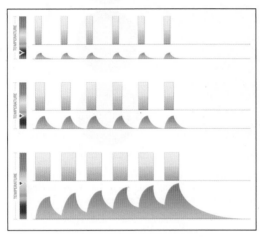

Figure 4: Schematic of micropulse laser. The gray bars represent the effect of "slicing" up the continuous wave laser into small segments, with the wider bars representing larger duty cycles (the laser is on for a greater percentage of the duration of the exposure). You can see that the temperature in the tissue can be finely controlled to create separate elevations or gradually converging and increasing elevations depending on the duty cycle setting. (Figures 3 and 4 courtesy of G. Dorin, Ph.D., Iridex Corporation.)

This approach is felt to create a very localized treatment effect—for instance, warming only the retinal pigment epithelium without affecting the underlying choroid or overlying retina.[1]

How does it work? Well, since no one knows how any retinal laser really works, it is hard to say, but the philosophy would be that if a gnarly scar gets the job done, then perhaps gently heating cells without disrupting them might have some effect without necessarily causing permanent damage. For instance, the heating can stimulate the production of proteins—such as heat shock protein—that can enhance cellular functioning.[2] There are some studies suggesting that this approach can be very effective, but to date there have been no large-scale controlled trials and the technique has not been widely adopted.[3-5] It is worth keeping an eye on this, as well as other non-invasive laser techniques such as nanopulse laser and subthreshold standard laser.[10,11] If future studies demonstrate clear-cut efficacy for non-scarring techniques, you can use a lot of this book for kindling...

Pattern Lasers

These lasers can be programmed to create multiple spots every time they are fired. They use a short duration for each spot in order to rapidly create the desired pattern. The ability to produce multiple spots allows rapid treatment of patients, often with less pain because of the shorter duration of each spot. The shorter duration can also result in a burn that is smaller than the planned size, which means that the number of overall spots may need to be increased relative to a traditional laser.[6] Some have suggested that the burn duration should be increased with pattern lasers in order to be sure effective spots are created.[12] These lasers also tend to be more expensive, and traditional lasers can, to some extent, simulate the effect if they are set at short durations and a rapid repeat mode, but they can't really duplicate what a pattern laser can do. No large study has proven that pattern lasers provide better outcomes in the long run, but doctors that use these feel that the faster, more comfortable treatment makes the extra cost worthwhile.[7]

Navigable Laser

The Navilas laser (OD-OS GmbH, Germany) uses imaging technology to identify pathology such as microaneurysms, and then the physician chooses which lesions to treat. The laser then tracks the fundus to treat the chosen lesions. The laser incorporates a fundus camera and fluorescein angiography, and no contact lens is needed for macular treatment. It is very effective for precise targeting of pathology—something you will greatly appreciate after you have tried to do your first focal laser and surround each microaneurysm with several missed shots! Preliminary studies are promising, and the precise targeting may help decrease the injection burden in patients who need intravitreal treatment. However, the system is expensive and is not in wide use at this time.[8,9]

References and Suggested Reading

1.   Sivaprasad S, Elagouz M, McHugh D, Shona O, Dorin G. Micropulsed diode laser therapy: evolution and clinical applications. *Surv Ophthalmol.* Nov-Dec 2010;55(6):516-530.

2.   Blumenkranz MS. The evolution of laser therapy in ophthalmology: a perspective on the interactions between photons, patients, physicians, and physicists: the LXX Edward Jackson Memorial Lecture. *American journal of ophthalmology.* Jul 2014;158(1):12-25 e11.

3.   Lavinsky D, Cardillo JA, Melo LA, Jr., Dare A, Farah ME, Belfort R, Jr. Randomized clinical trial evaluating mETDRS versus normal or high-density micropulse photocoagulation for diabetic macular edema. *Investigative ophthalmology & visual science.* Jun 2011;52(7):4314-4323.

4.   Luttrull JK, Sinclair SH. Safety of Transfoveal Subthreshold Diode Micropulse Laser for Fovea-Involving Diabetic Macular Edema in Eyes with Good Visual Acuity. *Retina.* May 15 2014.

5.   Othman IS, Eissa SA, Kotb MS, Sadek SH. Subthreshold diode-laser micropulse photocoagulation as a primary and secondary line of treatment in management of diabetic macular edema. *Clin Ophthalmol.* 2014;8:653-659.

6.   Chappelow AV, Tan K, Waheed NK, Kaiser PK. Panretinal photocoagulation for proliferative diabetic retinopathy: pattern scan laser versus argon laser. *American journal of ophthalmology.* Jan 2012;153(1):137-142 e132.

7.   Muqit MM, Marcellino GR, Henson DB, et al. Single-session vs multiple-session pattern scanning laser panretinal photocoagulation in proliferative diabetic retinopathy: The Manchester Pascal Study. *Archives of ophthalmology.* May 2010;128(5):525-533.

8.   Kozak I, Kim JS, Oster SF, Chhablani J, Freeman WR. FOCAL NAVIGATED LASER PHOTOCOAGULATION IN RETINOVASCULAR DISEASE: Clinical Results in Initial Case Series. *Retina.* May 2012;32(5):930-935.

9.   Barteselli G, Kozak I, El-Emam S, Chhablani J, Cortes MA, Freeman WR. 12-month results of the standardised combination therapy for diabetic macular oedema: intravitreal bevacizumab and navigated retinal photocoagulation. *The British journal of ophthalmology.* Aug 2014;98(8):1036-1041.

10.   Casson RJ, Raymond G, Newland HS, Gilhotra JS, Gray TL. Pilot randomized trial of a nanopulse retinal laser versus conventional photocoagulation for the treatment of diabetic macular oedema. Clin Experiment Ophthalmol. 2012;40(6):604-610.

11.   Pei-Pei W, Shi-Zhou H, Zhen T, et al. Randomised clinical trial evaluating best-corrected visual acuity and central macular thickness after 532-nm subthreshold laser grid photocoagulation treatment in diabetic macular oedema. Eye (Lond). 2015;29(3):313-321.

12.   Chhablani J, Sambhana S, Mathai A, Gupta V, Arevalo JF, Kozak I. Clinical efficacy of navigated panretinal photocoagulation in proliferative diabetic retinopathy. American journal of ophthalmology. 2015;159(5):884-889.

Folk JC, Pulido JS. Laser photocoagulation of the retina and choroid. San Francisco: American Academy of Ophthalmology, 1997.

Singerman LJ, Coscas GJ. Current techniques in ophthalmic laser surgery, 3rd ed. Boston: Butterworth-Heineman, 1999.

American Academy of Ophthalmology Laser Surgery Education Center: http://one.aao.org/laser-surgery-education-center

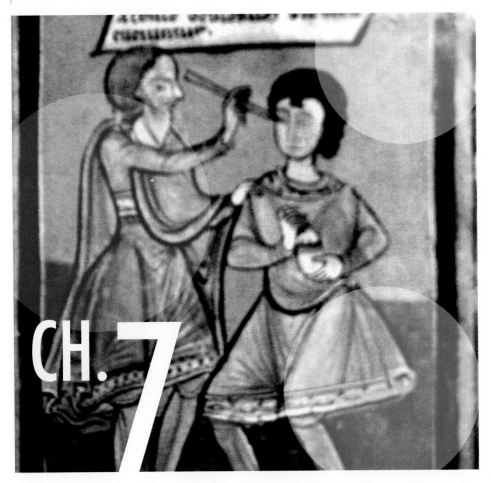

Contact Lenses and the Wrangling Thereof

Give us the tools, and we will finish the job. Winston Churchill

Becoming familiar with the contact lenses that are used to treat diabetic retinopathy is crucial. It is assumed that you have already mastered typical indirect non-contact lenses, such as the 90-diopter lens. But it turns out that contact lenses require a very different skill set, so they get their own chapter. Contact lenses come in two main types: direct view lenses, such as the Goldmann three mirror, and inverted image lenses such as the Rodenstock. But first, a brief editorial...

This chapter will refer to several types of lenses. If you look at the manufacturers' catalogs, you will see that there are zillions of options. How can you try them to see whether they work for you? One option is to go to the manufacturers' exhibits at conventions. You will get a chance to try them all, but they never work as well on patients as they do on the little model eyes they use to demonstrate the lenses.

Another option is to dig around the back of all the drawers where your laser is kept. You will likely find a host of abandoned lenses, especially if you are in a large group practice or academic setting. Sometimes you will quickly realize why a given lens is in the graveyard, but sometimes you will find a real friend that works great for you. This also saves you a trip to the Academy meeting.

Above all, do not be fooled by the advertising that will have you thinking you will be able to treat patients effortlessly if you buy just the right lens. As you begin grappling with contact lenses, it is easy to think that your problems are due to the lens and that, somewhere over the rainbow, there is a perfect lens that will solve all your problems. You need to get over this phase quickly (otherwise, you will be spending a lot of money on lenses). It just takes practice—there is no secret magic lens.

Point-Counterpoint Box *so the Lens Manufacturers Don't Get Too Ticked off by the Previous Box Because We Need and Appreciate Their Constant Innovations*

Although there is no magic lens that flattens the learning curve, there is something to be said for having lenses that differ in subtle ways in order to address different nuances of treatment. Just like some guitarists prefer having a bunch of different instruments and others always use one favorite axe, you may find that you do better with lots of different lenses, or you may be happy with only one or two. Ultimately, this is something you will decide on your own once you have some skills with the basic lenses, so read on.

DIRECT VIEW LENSES

The direct view lenses are the easiest and most intuitive to use. The archetype is the Goldmann three-mirror lens. This is the lens to have if you are stranded on a desert island, because it can do everything reasonably well. The direct (non-inverted) nature of the view means that once you get the lens on the patient, you are simply looking in a straight line through the pupil to the area of interest. The various mirrors then allow you to visualize segments of the periphery. Some Goldmann lenses have a small flange that fits behind the lids and helps to keep the lens in the patient's eye; it is a good idea to take advantage of such a flange when you are learning, because it is harder for the patient to blink the lens out once you get it in the eye. (More specific tips on actually getting the lens where you want it to go are covered in the next chapter.)

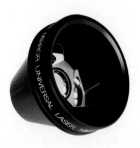

Figure 1: A typical three-mirror Goldmann lens.   (Courtesy of Ocular Instruments.)

The mirrors are set at different angles, with most Goldmann-type lenses having one mirror for the anterior chamber angle and two mirrors for different latitudes of the fundus. There are, however, variations on the Goldmann, which have multiple mirrors at slightly different angles to get better coverage of the retinal periphery (the Karickhoff lens, for instance, has four mirrors).

The direct view makes it relatively easy to line up the lens so you can see the posterior pole, and you do not need to invoke the mental gymnastics that are necessary to use lenses that have an inverted image. Unfortunately, the field of view is rather small compared to the indirect lenses, and you will be more dependent on the patient's cooperation if you need to get to different areas. Also, direct lenses need a widely dilated pupil, and media opacities can be a real pain, because you cannot work around them as you can with an inverting lens.

Because the mirrors are set at a fixed angle and there is a small field of view, you need to make sure that you do not miss areas that lie between the latitudes most easily seen in each mirror. If you cannot quite get the view you need because what you want to see is just outside the limited view provided by the mirrors, you do have some options. You can rock the lens back and forth to get more anterior and posterior exposure as you are treating the retina. The patient can also help you by looking a bit away and toward the mirror to accomplish the same goal. Finally, you can also use the contact lens as a gentle lever to push the eye in different directions. This last option can be done with any type of contact lens, and it is an important skill that will give you a lot of control over the eye. For instance, if the patient has had a retrobulbar block, you have to use the lens to move the eye around to see different areas. You also need to maintain the proper alignment when you do this, though, because if you angle the lens too much as you push the eye in different directions, you will lose your view. You have to fine-tune your finger proprioception so that you automatically know how the lens is oriented as you move it in different directions. (Figure 8 will elaborate on this.)

Important safety tip: If the eye has not been blocked and you are pushing with your lens in order to move it around, you may inadvertently demonstrate the oculo-cardiac reflex—especially if you happen to be treating a patient who is nervous and uncomfortable (and this goes double if they are young males—triple if they have Harley-Davidson tats). Always remind a patient who is about to get their first laser to let you know if they begin to feel light-headed or dizzy, and if they do, stop the laser immediately and have them do the head-between-the-knees thing or even lie down on the floor. For some patients, the time between this light-headed sensation and becoming unconscious is rather short, and you lose many points with the family if your patient's face finds the cross members of the slit lamp table on its way to the ground. This concept is important enough that it is repeated at various points around the book.

Because you cannot get a very big picture with the "keyhole" view through the pupil, you also need to be very careful that your treatment is not extending more posteriorly than you wish. This can occur with the larger mirror and is especially likely if you are working temporally, where there are no large blood vessels to warn you that you are crossing into the macula. It is possible to inadvertently angle the lens and treat into the posterior pole without realizing it, especially if the patient happens to be looking in the direction of the mirror (Figure 2).

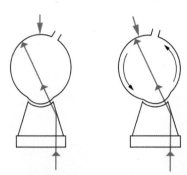

Figure 2: If you are using a Goldmann three mirror, you have to be very careful about where you are treating with the large mirror. It is possible to accidentally get well into the posterior pole, especially if the patient is looking toward the mirror. The red arrow represents the fovea as it moves toward the line of treatment when the eye rotates toward the mirror. As we will discuss repeatedly, it is always worthwhile to confirm your location relative to the fovea multiple times—the adage measure twice and cut once was never truer.

There is another type of direct view lens that is designed exclusively for viewing the posterior pole. In some institutions these lenses are referred to as pancake lenses, presumably because they're smaller than a Goldmann three mirror and because they do not have mirrors (perhaps these qualities make ophthalmologists think of pancakes). An example of this is the Yanuzzi lens, although there are many other types that are available.

These lenses often have a very large flange that really keeps the lens behind the eyelids—you may even be able to let go of the lens so the patient can sit back and rest and it will remain in place. Although the overall field of view is limited by the direct line of sight, and these lenses are more dependent on patient cooperation, they give a breathtaking sense of the thickness of the retina. You should use them as much as possible, especially as you are learning the trade. The axial magnification and clarity of these lenses can really help you comprehend the nature of diabetic macular edema and help you get a feel for the three-dimensional location of the pathology. The patient's retina becomes a wonderland as you gleefully pluck microaneurysms from perches that suddenly seem yards above the underlying RPE. After you have a few exams under your belt with one of

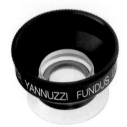

Figure 3: Yanuzzi macular contact lens. Note the very wide flange. This can take a bit of work to get into the eye, but it really locks the lens onto the eye once it is behind the lids. (Courtesy of Ocular Instruments.)

these lenses, you will understand what diabetic macular edema is about in a way that no optical coherence tomography scan can capture. You will also appreciate what a feeble imitation of reality you get when you use a 90-or 78-diopter lens—no matter what the advertisements say. (However, studying a lot of patients with a macular lens like this will enable you to be a much more effective examiner when you decide to cut corners and use a 90 or 78.)

INDIRECT LENSES

The indirect lenses will give you an excellent field of view compared to direct view lenses, but they require more finesse to obtain said field of view. An example of this type of lens would be the various Mainster lenses made by Ocular Instruments or the classic—but no longer manufactured— Rodenstock Panfundoscope (Figure 4). Volk also makes a selection of indirect lenses (Figures 5 and 6). All of these lenses essentially do the same thing that your 90-diopter lens does, but they are stuck to the eye to hold the eyelids open (and they throw in a few more optical elements to kick up the view a notch). You get an inverted image that, once you master the technique, allows you to treat a large area with minimal dependence on the patient's ability to cooperate.

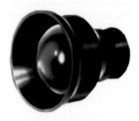 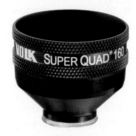 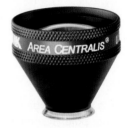

Figure 4: The Rodenstock Panfundoscope. This is a classic lens with an even more classic name. The design is handy because it is long, rather than wide, so it can get under Cro-Magnon brows and the length allows a lot of leverage for torquing the eye. Unfortunately, it is no longer manufactured. Volk makes a substitute, but the newer lens is smaller and works somewhat differently.

Figure 5: This is a more typical contemporary wide-field indirect contact lens. It is much shorter than the Rodenstock and can be a tight fit into a recessed eye, but the field of view does tend to be better. (Courtesy of Volk Optical.)

Figure 6: A typical indirect lens for macular treatment. Note the more subtle flange—not as hard to use, but not as blink-proof. **Figures 5 and 6** are made by Volk, but they are similar to the various Mainster lenses manufactured by Ocular Instruments. (Courtesy of Volk Optical.)

Unfortunately, these lenses can be frustrating. One begins with the preconceived notion that one simply needs to slap on the lens and one will immediately see broad vistas of retina. Just like the first time you tried to ski, snowboard or ice skate, however, the reality is a bit different from the expectations. Strive to overcome your initial disappointment and keep trying—the necessary moves will become automatic with practice, and you will soon become a contact lens Jedi.

Indirect lenses require a much more dynamic approach than the direct view lenses. At all times you need to try to keep a straight line from the patient's retina through the lens and slit lamp and onto your fovea—something that is much easier said than done with this class of lens. (In reality the optics are more complicated, but the straight-line approach is a good mental goal to start with.)

Even if you can get the patient lined up to obtain the best view, you need to continually coordinate movements between the slit lamp, the lens and the eye in subtle ways. This can be very frustrating at first because it feels like you will never succeed. It helps to break this process down into a few separate moves until it becomes automatic...

You have to take full advantage of all the different ways you can shift the lens around the eye. A common problem is not being able to get a good view of what you want to see with both of your eyes—a classic sign that you are not as lined up as you think you are. Try moving the lens in a circle or a cone—this is a handy way of scanning for the best line of sight (Figure 7). Remember, you have to be ready to follow any move you make with the lens by shifting the position of the slit lamp. This last point is really important. An understandable novice move is to concentrate on moving just the lens, because it is difficult enough to manipulate the lens without letting it slide off the eye. However, if you move only the lens without following that inverted image with the slit lamp, you will never get a good view. It helps to affix your lens hand to the patient by spreading your fourth and fifth fingers onto the side of the patient's face or by putting the back of those fingers on the patient's cheek—this gives you more stability and you don't have to exert as much brain power worrying about keeping the lens on the eye. This way you can better concentrate exclusively on moving the lens and the slit lamp as needed in order to get the best view.

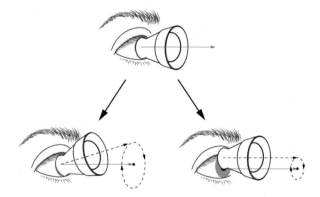

Figure 7: This figure shows slightly different ways of moving the lens around the eye in order to find the best view. These are an exaggeration of the movements required—the real moves are much more subtle. The top image shows a perfectly lined up lens, but this almost never happens spontaneously. The quickest way to find the best view is to rotate the lens around the presumed visual axis. The lower left image shows that you can rotate the axis of the lens so that it creates a cone. In this case, the part of the lens on the eye moves just a little, and the part of the lens facing the slit lamp circles around a lot. The lower right image shows that you can move the lens such that its axis creates a cylinder, with the entire lens moving in the same circular pattern. In reality, you will rapidly learn to combine both moves to scan for the best view—but it helps to realize that each one of these motions will give a slightly different effect, which may come in handy in different circumstances. Remember to follow any moves you make with the lens with corresponding movement of the slit lamp; otherwise you are wasting your time. Note that if you still can't get a great view, you need to recheck where the patient is looking—they may be rotating their eye out of reach.

Don't worry if you aren't getting a perfect view at first—the goal here is to just see what you want to see with both of your eyes at the same time. Once you can do this reliably, it is time for some real finesse: the "Five Point Palm Exploding Heart Technique" of lens wrassling, if you will. It is similar to the technique mentioned in the section on direct lenses, wherein you use the lens to torque the eye in different directions. Sometimes you will do this by translating the entire lens in one direction, and sometimes you will do this in a more subtle way: by slightly rotating the lens around its midpoint (kind of like adjusting the pitch of an airplane). Both moves will slightly change the visual axis of the lens and will slightly rotate the eye at the same time, with the goal being a much more favorable view. (If this is an obtuse paragraph, look at Figure 8, where the proverbial thousand words await.) By the way, if you are having a lot of trouble getting a view, even with all these moves, go back and double check where the patient's fixation is. There is no way, at least at first, that you can get a good view if the patient is rolling their eye up in their head—you will never line things up. (There will be more discussion about enlisting the patient's cooperation in Chapter 8.)

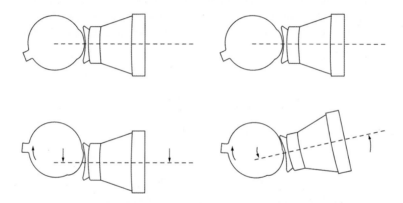

Figure 8: These are exaggerated images of moves you can make to fine-tune your view with an indirect contact lens. On the left, you are moving the entire lens in one direction and keeping the axis of the lens parallel as you move it. At the same time, you are "pulling" the eye with you to try to line up the axis of the lens with whatever you need to see. The image on the right shows a slightly different way of doing the same thing; here, you are torquing the lens through its center as you also rotate the eye, so the axis of the lens is tilting. Both moves accomplish the same goal, but they will give you slightly different views depending on the orientation of the patient's eye. You will rapidly learn to use a combination of both moves to get the best view, but it helps to consciously try them out at first—with practice, your brain will create a macro that automatically moves the lens into the best position using whatever move is necessary. Remember that diabetic corneal epithelium can be fragile, so try not to grind into the eye when doing these maneuvers. You can do these with a light touch, even pulling back a bit on the lens, so you don't rub off epithelium. The patient will not consider eliminating macular edema a success if you manage to give them a non-healing defect.

How do you know which way to tilt the lens to get the best view? At first, you may need to use very gross and even random movements to get a rough view of what you want to see. As things get fine-tuned, you can sometimes let Dr. Sturm and his conoid guide you. Look at your aiming beam. Unless you are a natural, it is likely the aiming beam will be some sort of smeared oval, suggesting that you are out of alignment to a tiny degree. The long axis of the oval tells you which way to rock the lens. Say the long axis is vertical—then tilt the lens up and down around its center and watch the beam—it will shift around and tighten up into a circle as you become more perfectly aligned. Sometimes you have to be more aggressive and move the whole lens up or down to follow the long axis of the aiming beam and then fine-tune with a little gentle tilting. Sometimes you can rotate the eye with the lens as you tilt it and get to your goal even faster. Don't forget to follow your lens moves with the slit lamp, although as you get closer and closer to a good view, you usually do not need to move the microscope as much.

Sadly, there will still be a lot of hit and miss, and you will find that you have to keep iterating and reiterating all of these moves to get in focus and stay in focus. First, get lined up grossly by circling the visual axis. Then try some tilting to offset the long axis of the aiming beam—then do a little more circling and tilting, and ultimately you will be rewarded with a lovely panoramic view that makes treatment very easy. Eventually all these actions will be internalized and, as with indirect ophthalmoscopy, you will begin to automatically make the right moves without thinking. Just don't give up and do keep trying.

You will need different indirect lenses depending on whether you want to treat the macula or the periphery. Macular lenses don't get out very far, but they give you a nice stereoscopic view of the posterior pole. Wide-field lenses, on the other hand, will let you see much more of the periphery (you will have to ignore the impressive marketing names such as Ultra-Quadro-Magnoview, etc., and ask about the field of view as measured in degrees in order to find out exactly how much of the periphery you are supposed to see). The wide-field lenses will allow you to see the posterior pole, but the view is nowhere near as stereoscopic as that obtained with a lens designed to view the macula. Furthermore, there are often a lot of light reflexes when viewing the central retina with a wide-field lens—which make viewing the macula problematic. (Sometimes you can minimize the reflexes by moving your slit beam a bit off axis and/or by decreasing the size of the slit lamp beam.)

Finally, the wider the field of view, the more the lens will magnify the size of your spot, which means that it is hard to safely place small focal burns in the macula with such a lens. (See the next blue box.) All this is why there is not one indirect lens that can be used to treat both the periphery and the macula. Predictably, manufacturers have created a host of different indirect lenses that cover the whole spectrum from very wide-field to very focal macular viewing. As mentioned in the beginning of the chapter, you may want to get comfortable with just one macular and one wide-field lens, and then you can decide whether you want all the more nuanced lenses that are available.

Indirect lenses and spot size

With the direct view lenses, the spot you set on your laser is pretty much the size you will get on the retina, give or take a few microns. The indirect lenses, however, will change the spot size in a manner proportional to the field of view. For instance, a really wide-field lens, like the Mainster 165, can almost double the diameter of your spot setting (a 100-micron spot on the laser turns into a 200-micron spot on the retina). Indirect lenses designed for the macula tend to deliver spot sizes that are closer to the actual laser setting, but they will still vary depending on the width of the field. Some "high-power" macular lenses can actually make the delivered spot smaller relative to the laser setting.

This becomes very important if you are trying to deliver a specific dose of laser energy to a given area (such as with photodynamic therapy for macular degeneration). It is less important in the setting of diabetic lasers, because you will be titrating the energy dose yourself, based on the uptake you see as you do the laser.

Nevertheless, you need to be aware of the effect your chosen lens has on the delivered spot size—lens manufacturers always include this information with each lens and publish it on their websites. If you are trying to, say, follow the Diabetic Retinopathy Study guidelines in terms of spot size and number, you need to realize that if you are using a wide-field lens and you set your laser to 500 microns, you will be placing much bigger burns than you want. Alternatively, if you switch from a wide-field lens to a macular lens, you will make your spot size much smaller. If you do not adjust your power accordingly, you can burn a hole in the retina.

There are two situations in which the wider-field indirect lenses can be useful beyond their ability to allow easy panretinal photocoagulation (PRP). First, if the patient has media opacities, such as a central posterior subcapsular cataract, you may be able to use these lenses to treat the posterior pole. They tend to "reach around" the opacity better than indirect lenses designed for the macula, and certainly better than direct lenses. As mentioned above, you need to do this carefully because you will be creating a large diffused spot, but it may be better than nothing in difficult situations.

The other situation in which the wide-field indirect lenses are extremely useful is when you are looking for retinal breaks in pseudophakic patients. The prismatic effect of the edge of the intraocular lens will often keep you from seeing the far periphery with a direct view lens. A wide-field lens allows better visualization, and such a lens can allow you to find and treat a peripheral tear without the need for a binocular indirect laser or cryotherapy. Of course, sometimes you just can't treat the pathology because of opacities or because it is too peripheral. The binocular indirect laser is handy in such circumstances if you have access to one (the technique is beyond the scope of this book—Chapter 14 has a good reference).

One other weird thing about wide-field indirect contact lenses: The nature of their optics is such that the irradiance can be higher through the patient's lens and cornea than at the retina. This effect is usually insignificant, but it can become a problem with huge (greater than 500-micron) spot sizes—although one would usually not use such large spots. The problem is that if there are a lot of lens opacities the high irradiance through the anterior segment can cause lenticular burns. Corneal burns can also occur with even smaller spots if there is pigment on the surface of the cornea or if you trap an eyelash or mascara under the contact lens. Furthermore, it is likely you won't realize that these burns are occurring because you are not able to easily visualize the anterior segment through an indirect-view contact lens. This is why you need to stop and take the contact lens off and look at the front of the eye if you find that your view of the retina is clouding up. These problems are relatively unusual with modern treatment techniques, but it is good to remember that Murphy's Law can extend far beyond the retina that you are working on. (There will be more on this in Chapter 17, discussing complications.)

What specific lenses should be in your toolbox for retinal lasers? It's a matter of personal taste. There are two main companies that make lenses: Volk and Ocular Instruments (although docs outside the USA may have access to lots of other manufacturers). Both companies make great laser lenses and their product lines tend to be roughly equivalent (although the manufacturers themselves might disagree). They both have return policies, so you can try out different lenses and decide what works for you. Here are some suggestions for a basic lineup:

1. A Goldmann three mirror can do everything reasonably well, but it may take longer to do a treatment and it is not as versatile as separate lenses. Nevertheless, if you can get only one lens, this is the one to have. If you have been good and the Retina Bunny is going to bring you more than one lens, then please read on...

2. A general-purpose indirect macular lens such as the Volk Area Centralis or the Ocular Instruments Standard Mainster will likely become your main lens for focal and grid laser. There are plenty of variations, so you can pretty much choose exactly how much field of view you want—but don't get a field of view that is too big, because the wider the field of view, the harder it is to treat the macula accurately.

3. A pancake lens for an extra-crisp view of the macula (i.e., for diagnosis or very accurate focal treatment of microaneurysms in cooperative patients). Examples would be the Yanuzzi lens by Ocular Instruments or the Fundus 20 by Volk.

4. A wide-field indirect lens for PRPs such as the Mainster 165 by Ocular Instruments or the Super Quad 160 by Volk.

References and Suggested Reading

Mainster MA, Crossman JL, Erickson PJ, Heacock GL. Retinal laser lenses: magnification, spot size, and field of view. Br J Ophthalmol 1990;74:177-9.

Folk JC, Pulido JS. Laser photocoagulation of the retina and choroid. San Francisco:American Academy of Ophthalmology, 1997.

L'Esperance FA. Ophthalmic lasers, 3rd ed. St. Louis: Mosby, 1989.

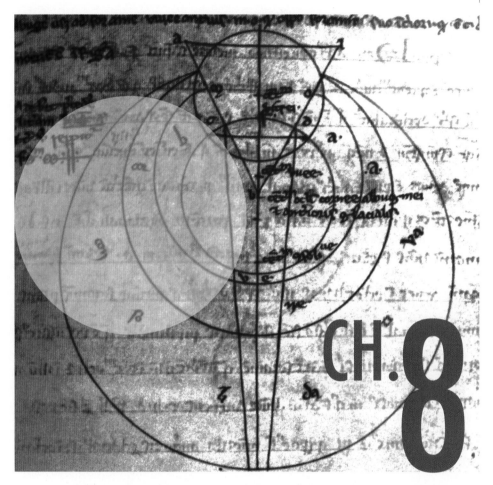

Actually Doing a Laser for Macular Edema

Good judgment comes from experience. Unfortunately, experience comes from bad judgment.
Mulla Nasrudin

GETTING THINGS LINED UP at the Laser

First of all, the patient should be as comfortable as possible under the circumstances. One of the best ways to facilitate this is to allow someone else to stuff a diagnostic contact lens onto your eye at some point during your training. As you experience this, try to study their every move and your response to each move. Based on how it feels you will develop nuances that will allow you to be much gentler with your patients.

The slit lamp table should be at a comfortable height, and check that the patient is not straining to be in position without realizing it because they are nervous and trying to not be a nuisance. Handles on the table are extremely useful—it gives them something to hold on to and steady their torso. Also, make sure their legs are comfortable, even if you have to straddle their feet.

Make sure that you talk the patient through the entire process. Try to proceed slowly and explain each maneuver prior to doing it. There are books written on how to almost hypnotize the patient with a calm, mantra-like repetition of phrases. You can get as new-age as you want, but the important thing is to always tell a patient what you are going to do before you do it.

Remember that for many patients the primary association they have with lasers is the image of the planet Alderaan exploding in the first Star Wars movie. Reassure them that you are using microscopic powers on your laser and that as long as they are reasonably cooperative, they simply cannot make a mistake. This will relieve them of any fear that they may have about having the success of the treatment rest solely on their shoulders—let them know that it does not make any difference if they blink or sneeze and that you are certainly not going to blow their head off no matter what they do.

There is one other thing to discuss, especially if this is their first laser. You need to warn them that when the laser is over, their vision will be essentially black and their eye will feel glued shut. The laser is so bright that most patients see almost nothing for a few minutes, and the methylcellulose makes them feel like their eye is full of paste. These are really important things to mention. You can lay out the most masterful informed consent, but if you have not prepared the patient for this particular moment, you may have a very upset patient. This is particularly true if you have just treated a one-eyed patient. Fortunately, the darkness fades quickly and then they will see the world in shades that are opposite the wavelength of your laser—usually red if you have a green laser. Patients can easily deal with this as long as you let them know about it in advance.

Unless they are laser veterans, they will still be rather anxious at this point. Perhaps the most useless phrase in the world is "try to relax." Nothing can whip a patient into a frenzy faster than an instruction like this. It is much better to offer specific suggestions. For instance, as the patient leans forward to the slit lamp, you may want to put your hand on their neck and shoulder to both guide them and to see how tight their trapezius is. Because it is always as taut as a harp string, you can tell them to try to loosen their neck and shoulders and let the chin rest do the work of holding their head up. By focusing on a specific task, they can have more of a definite goal than just "relax." Another trick that works is to ask them to breathe slow and deep. Lead and let them follow as you breathe a little loudly yourself.

The same is true for the inevitable battle with the contact lens. If you tell them to hold still and try not to blink you might as well inject them with pure methamphetamine and see whether they can shake your slit lamp right off the table. Instead, you may want to consider telling them to blink as much as they want, but to also concentrate on keeping their forehead pressed against the bar. This way, they can focus on this rather simple task, which is far more useful to you than yearning for some fairyland where patients actually open their eyes and stop blinking when you ask them to.

Figure 1 demonstrates a reasonable way to work with recalcitrant eyelids. It is useful if the patient can look down; this allows you to place your thumb over the tarsal plate, which gives you a lot of control over the upper lid. At the same time, you can use the ring finger of the other hand to pull the lower lid down while keeping the contact lens between the thumb and first two fingers. If the patient is truly concentrating on keeping their forehead against the bar, you will be able to generate an effective amount of static friction on the eyelids, and then you can easily separate the lids and get the contact lens inserted. This is where a small flange on the lens is extremely useful, because once you have control of the upper lid and the flange is behind the lower lid, the lens will almost insert itself. Also, with a good flange, the patient will be unable to squeeze the lens out even if they could crush a Volkswagen with their orbicularis. The bigger the flange, the more secure the lens; but there is a balance, because as the flange gets bigger it is harder to get the lens in.

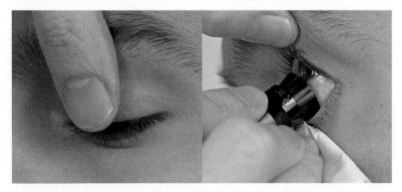

Figure 1: The left photo shows how you can have the patient look down, allowing you to put your thumb in contact with the entire width of their tarsal plate. This gives you maximum traction to pull the lid up and get it out of the way. You can then have them look up in order to make the lower lid more lax and make the patient less likely to see the lens coming. You can then pull the lower lid down with the side of your ring finger, hook the flange over the lower lid, and rotate the lens into the eye. In this case, a tissue is folded up and held between the ring and little fingers to help with traction and to catch any contact lens gel that oozes out of the eye. You want to do this because the gel can run down next to the nose and drive patients nuts during the treatment. (Photos by James Whitcraft, IPFW)

If the eyelids don't get out of the way, you will have an excellent magnified view of the patient's eyelashes at this point. Occasionally you can rescue this situation by having them look in the direction of the eyelid that is under the flange and pushing the lens in the direction of the lid that is properly placed in front of the flange. If the lids are loose enough, you can pull the offending eyelid back over the flange. Most of the time, however, the whole region has been turned into a slippery mess by the contact lens gel, and you have to bail out and start all over again. Make sure you do a Zen breath and wall off any bubbling frustration—patients can detect your irritation with remarkable sensitivity and they will then go into a positive-feedback loop of increasing anxiety and lock their eye shut.

Incidentally, *when you put the methylcellulose on the lens it helps to first squeeze a bit onto a tissue and then continue squeezing what you need on the lens. The first drop often has little bubbles that have a sentient ability to get in your way when you do the laser.*

If you are truly unable to get the lens in you can do a lid block as a last resort, but if you have to do this more than once or twice in your career you may want to reassess how you insert contact lenses—the problem may lie with someone other than the patient. If you are self-aware enough to wonder whether your technique is suboptimal, the best way to find out for sure is to try putting a laser lens on your spouse. Seriously. They will be more than happy to let you know how you are doing it wrong—that is why you married them in the first place.

In any event, once you finally get the lens in place, you should take a moment to congratulate yourself; you have overcome approximately 50 million years of evolution and actually convinced a stranger to let you shove something into their eye. But your job isn't finished.

It is important to continuously check and recheck the patient's positioning. Often while lasering your view can become less and less clear, and double-checking the lens position and the patient's fixation may not solve things. The problem may actually be due to subtle (or not so subtle) changes in the patient's position. Patients can droop—backs that were rigid when the patient was wired during the initial phases of treatment can sag, so the forehead slowly moves away from the band. They can also move side to side and even higher up depending on how they are responding to the laser. Surprisingly, a tech holding the head can be counterproductive—as are those vaguely S&M elastic bands. The patient can be threatened by the feeling of confinement (plus the tech can drift off in the dark!). It's also icky for some techs to touch the back of a sweaty head, and they may fail to keep the patient's head forward. You'll be better off frequently checking head position yourself throughout the procedure, and especially if the view becomes tough. And, again, always be gentle in your reminders. (Just because nothing is simple, there are some patients that actually prefer having their head held in place by a tech—they don't have to think about positioning at all. You can offer the option and see what the patient wants.)

A couple of other points: For a patient who must be lasered in a wheel chair, have a number of firm foam blocks (large enough to fill the entire seat) covered with plastic backed tissue. Getting the patient seated high enough to begin with makes the initial effort of stacking blocks under them worthwhile. And another thing to keep in mind if the view gets hazy is to check the methylcellulose. During a long laser the patient's tears can dilute the slime and the view deteriorates. Removing the lens and reapplying the gel will often clear things up. It may mean another struggle with the lids, but it is worth it.

OK. Now you are ready to begin the real battle.

FIXATION

Getting the patient to look in the right direction can be a daunting task. You will rapidly learn that some patients are utterly precise in their ability to fixate on the target light, and you will thereby learn the art of nailing microaneurysms with barely a whisper of RPE change. Most patients are reasonably accurate, so you can get the job done with minimal fuss. There are occasional patients, however, who make you feel like you are trying to split a diamond during a dune buggy ride, and it is for these that the following section exists.

As with telling them to relax, you have probably figured out that the worst thing you can do is to demand that the patient hold still and stare at the frickin' fixation light. So try a bit of the old word massage: Keep a soothing stream of chatter going—what you say is not as important as how you say it. You can let them know how well they are doing and how well the treatment is going as you chase their perifoveal retina all over the place. (Relax; there was a Papal bull in 1674 saying it is OK to lie to patients while doing a laser.) You can point out that the treatment you are about to apply is so delicate that they wouldn't feel it on their skin, and that everything will be okay if they end up blinking or sneezing or whatever because you can stop anytime. This warm fuzzy stuff does not always work with a fidgety patient, but it provides a good mantra to help you keep your cool.

Other options to encourage fixation include:

1. Sometimes they do not realize that their fixating eye is closed—a gentle reminder will help them realize this, and it may solve the problem.

2. The above is usually too easy; they can't open their eye because they are nervously squeezing both eyes shut. If they can't keep their fixating eye open, then bail out and encourage them keep their fixating eye closed. Sometimes this will get them to relax enough so that even if they aren't quite staring in the right direction, they at least won't be moving all over the place—that is, they won't be futilely struggling with themselves to force their eye open when they simply can't do it. The eye you are working on may Bell up, so you will probably have to shove the lens superiorly to get a better view. Occasionally, patients will have a tendency to look in some weird direction like far right or left when their eyes are closed, so if your view doesn't improve when you push up on the lens, you should lift the eyelid over the "fixating" eye to find out where it is looking. By the way, this is where it is really important to be able to use an indirect contact lens as discussed in Chapter 7—such lenses are much less dependent on patient cooperation and your fixation blues will largely disappear.

3. If your lens has a large flange, you can also try pushing relatively hard on the eye to keep it steady, although sometimes the discomfort makes things worse. As in vasovagal worse. Careful with this one, especially in younger male patients.

4. You can treat all the lesions that are relatively far away from the fovea first. You have to be sure you don't lose your landmarks and accidentally work your way into fovea-land, but sometimes the constant dazzle to these less critical areas will desensitize the patient, so by the time you work your way closer to the center, things are not as jumpy.

5. You can default to a total grid mode and give up on true focal treatment— simply get in spots as safely as you can around the thickened areas. This is less than optimal, especially if there is a lot of focal disease, but it is better than nothing. It is especially important that the laser power in these grid treatments be low – minimal RPE response is the mantra here.

6. Finally, there are some patients who simply need a retrobulbar block to gain control of the situation. You will probably want to consider this sooner, rather than later, in a patient who has clear-cut focal disease but will not hold still. As will be discussed in the next chapter, a carefully applied focal treatment may reverse things tremendously with only minimal changes at the level of the RPE. A shotgun grid performed in desperation on a moving target may chew up a lot of valuable retina that the patient might prefer to have around for the rest of their life. Under these circumstances, it is probably safer to use a block and do a proper focal than to get frustrated and do an overly aggressive grid treatment. Always remember the risk-benefit ratio of an office block, though. The phrase "this is your brain on drugs" takes on a whole new meaning if you squirt lidocaine into someone's brainstem (more on this in Chapter 16).

Some experts recommend using an oral anxiolytic. There are some patients that do prefer some type of sedation, but it is a lot of hassle for a few minutes of laser time. Also, these drugs are often not strong enough to make a difference unless you go for anesthetic doses, which is not a good idea in a laser room. Occasional patients may benefit, though, so don't forget that you were once a real doctor and that you do have this option.

What if they have too much fixation?

The yin to the yang of poor fixation is the tendency for patients to stare directly at your slit lamp light and thereby put the aiming beam right on their fovea at all times. You need to tell them to avoid this, but do so gently, and recognize once again that repetition of this instruction rapidly becomes counterproductive, especially if the pitch of your voice gets higher and higher. Better to tell them once, and then mildly suggest that they imagine they are looking off into the distance while you start treating well away from the fovea to desensitize them, as mentioned above. You have to be really careful as you move closer to the foveal area, because these patients may suddenly swing right into the light—so have a light foot on the trigger. This type of patient can be way more stressful than the patient with poor fixation, because you never know when they might shift their fovea onto your metaphorical hand grenade.

OK, several pages and a few thousand words and we have just reached the point where you can start lasering. Read on...

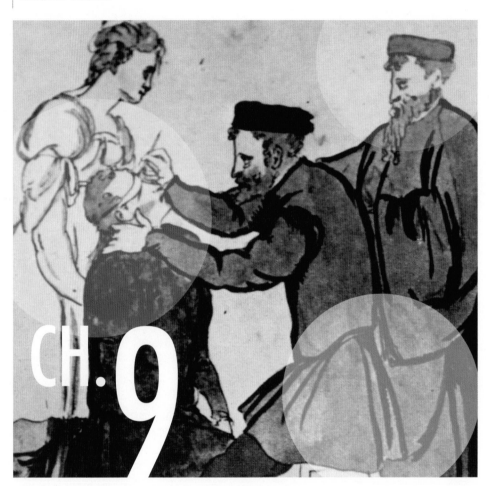

The Chapter That is Really About Actually Doing a Laser for Diabetic Macular Edema

If you're any good at all, you know you can be better. Lindsey Buckingham

If you paid attention to the last chapter you are about ready to start lasering. If you didn't read the last chapter then your surgical pyramid may be on shaky ground—you have to unconsciously be doing everything in Chapter 8 in order to have a fighting chance of actually doing the good stuff in Chapter 9. And here it is...

SPOT POWER and a Little About Spot Size

There are a number of different approaches to the laser treatment for diabetic macular edema. The traditional ETDRS approach was to start with a 50-micron spot and .1-second duration. Then treatment was initiated with a power of 50 milliwatts, and this was gradually increased in 10- to 20-mW increments until a color change occurred in the offending microaneurysm. (This direct treatment of a microaneurysm is referred to as focal treatment.) If there was diffuse leakage without any obvious focal source, then grid treatment was applied, consisting of light burns of 50 to 100 microns spaced >1 burn width apart.

> **For this discussion** it is assumed you are using a duration of .1 second, although as long as you are careful with the other parameters it does not make that much difference—most doctors use something between .05 to .2 seconds. The longer durations use lower powers to get the same effect so the burn builds up slowly and can be titrated easily (recall the energy density equation in Chapter 6). On the other hand, a longer burn gives the patient more time to move and mess up your shot. Shorter durations need more power, but some doctors prefer to obtain a quick hit that is relatively independent of patient movement. However, you have to be very careful to avoid a rapid buildup of the burn given the small spot and the higher power, especially given the variable pigmentation and retinal thickness that can be present in the macula.

Depending on the laser and the eye, you will usually start getting some sort of uptake around 80 to 110 mW, although the actual power requirements may vary a great deal depending on the thickness of the retina, media opacity and fundus pigmentation. For instance, black or Hispanic patients with clear media may need very little power, perhaps as little as 60 to 70 mW. Paler fundi may need frighteningly large powers, especially if there is any sort of cataract or grubby capsule. Clean pseudophakia, on the other hand, can let you get a hot burn very easily, whatever the pigmentation—be very careful and start with a very low power, especially if you have been learning your trade by treating through typical diabetic nuclear and cortical opacities.

Exactly what kind of burn are you looking for? No one knows. Even though the ETDRS called for "light" burns, you can see from Figure 1 that they could still be fairly white and hot (Figure 1 is from a teaching series from the 1980s). Nowadays the philosophy is "less is more" and people use much lighter burns.

Here are just a few reasons why: First of all, Figure 2 reminds you that the spots you put in are like gifts that keep on giving—they can slowly enlarge long after you have moved on. Second, it makes sense to treat with milder burns—simply because you can always go back and apply more treatment, but you cannot undo overly aggressive treatment. Finally, diabetics live a lot longer than they did back when the ETDRS was performed, and they tend to have better control. Better control means that they will respond better to milder treatment, and a longer life means that there is more time for any spots you put in to expand.

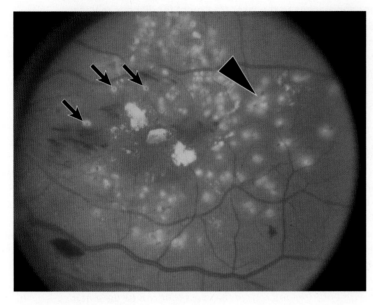

Figure 1: This is from one of the original training slides from over 30 years ago. These burns would be considered quite hot nowadays; upcoming figures will show more typical modern treatment. In spite of the rather aggressive nature of the burns, there are some things to observe. Note the extremely satisfying bombs dropped squarely on some of the microaneurysms (arrows). Ideally, you would want to use a smaller spot to try and treat only the microaneurysm and thereby minimize the dense white collateral damage. Also, notice the classic pattern that occurs when the patient (or doctor) moves just enough to keep from hitting a specific microaneurysm dead on. You can end up peppering the entire area around it in frustration (arrowhead). This is why you want to be careful and not keep firing away at the moving target – you can take out a lot of retina with multiple spots trying to get one little microaneurysm. (Courtesy of the Early Treatment Diabetic Retinopathy Research Group.)

↓ Figure 2: Note enlargement of laser scars – especially the confluence of the scars around the fovea. This is why you need to tread lightly.

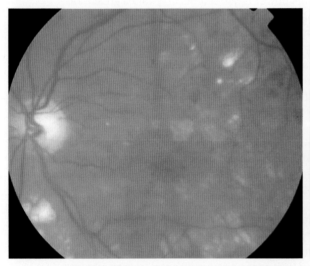
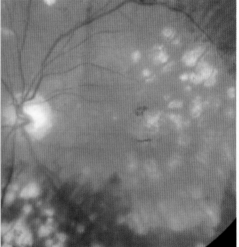

Also, diabetic maculas don't tend to fall apart quickly, and you don't need to feel like your first treatment is the only thing standing between your patient and a white cane—especially if the patient has reasonable diabetic control and the disease is away from the fovea.

Practically speaking, this means that if you are doing a grid the goal is a very subtle, small burn—something that just begins to show some lightening of the RPE. If you are trying to get a specific microaneurysm, the ETDRS wanted you to get some sort of color change within the lesion, either lighter or darker. This is still a nice thing to aim for, but recently there has been more emphasis on just getting the microaneurysm treated and not hammering away until you see a color change.[1] Basically, if you can get a color change, great, but don't go postal trying to get it. Table 1 gives you a nice comparison of the difference between the old-school ETDRS rules and the newer modified ETDRS approach as used by the DRCR.net. If you have been in practice for a while, and were trained on ETDRS techniques, you really need to absorb the new teaching.

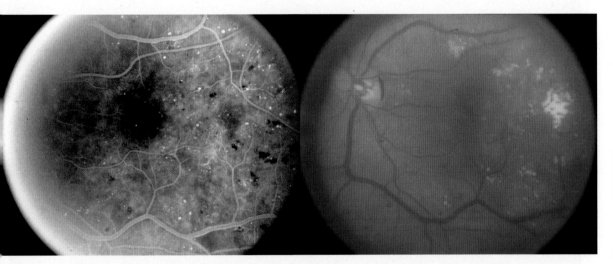

Figure 3: An example of a milder grid. The angiogram shows some microaneurysms but there is a lot of diffuse leakage in the entire temporal half of the posterior pole. Aggressive white laser spots would create a large scar and likely shove edema right into the fovea. A very light grid can be seen in the area of leakage – this is a good degree of uptake to start with, although in retrospect some of the burns are a bit too close together. (Note: this figure, and the other treatment images, are really hard to reproduce in print. You may want to access the online version of the book to get a better view.)

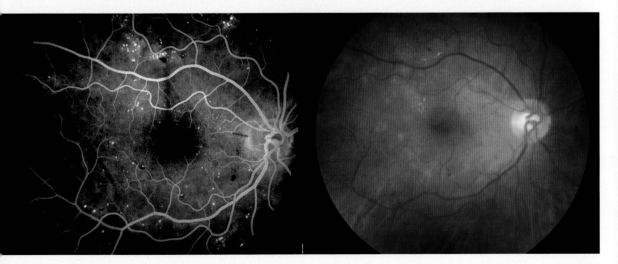

Figure 4a: An example of light treatment to areas of focal leakage. There are light burns and if you are worried they are insufficient you can bring the patient back and repeat as needed. If there is center-involving disease you would likely be solving the problem with intravitreal injections and use the laser as needed for long-term control.

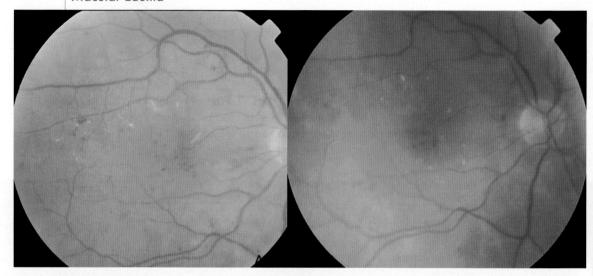

Figure 4b (above) and 4c (below). Here are some more examples of modified ETDRS treatment; pre-treatment photos (not from the same day) are on the left and immediate post-treatment photos are on the right. You can see that the spots are barely visible, especially in **4c**. (Courtesy of the DRCR.net).

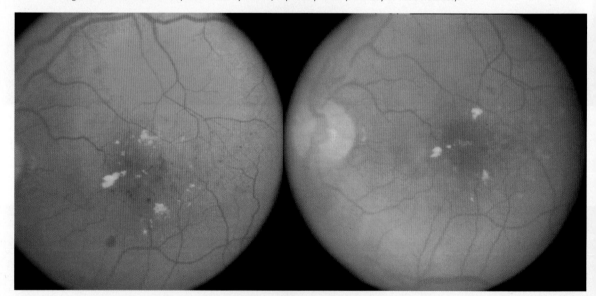

Ultimately, the subtleties of this are learned from clinical experience and not just clinical trials, so understand that these are, at best, guidelines—there is no proven "perfect" burn. Survey the retina people around you and take advantage of any hands-on teaching you can get, and then try to develop a treatment pattern that works best for you. Figures 3 and 4 give examples of milder treatment approaches, and Figure 5 shows the appearance of a mild grid after a number of years.

Whatever burn you are trying for, the first step is to get the tightest focus you can with your aiming beam—if you don't get this first bit right, you will be punching marshmallows and your settings and uptake will be changing all over the place. And don't worry if at first it seems like you are spending hours getting a tight aiming beam and determining an effective power. Review Chapter 8, practice like crazy, and try some of the tricks discussed later in the text. As you develop experience you will be able to rapidly factor in all of the variables and quickly dial in safe and effective settings.

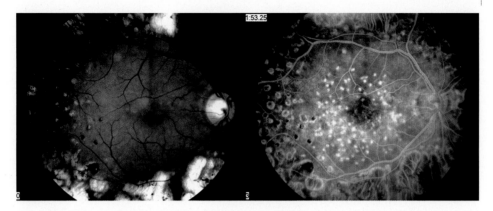

Figure 5: This gives you an idea of how a light grid such as in **figure 4** can look years later. The red-free photograph on the left shows that you can barely see the spots that were placed about nine years prior to these photographs. The angiogram on the right lights up the spots. This patient went from 20/200 to 20/60 with laser combined with better systemic control; he was treated prior to the use of intravitreal medication. Had those medications been available, he might not have needed any macular laser.

Table 1. Comparison of ETDRS and DRCR.net Techniques for the Treatment of Diabetic Macular Edema

Technique	ETDRS	DRCR.NET
Fluorescein angiography	Mandatory	
Optical coherence tomography	Not available at the time. Assessment of retinal thickness depended on clinical exam.	Mandatory to define presence and location of areas of retinal thickening and measure response to treatment.
Laser wavelength	Argon green or blue-green	Green or yellow
Treatment size	50–100 µm for focal treatment 50–200 µm for grid treatment	50 µm for focal and grid
Treatment duration	0.05–0.1 seconds	0.05–0.1 seconds
Determining microaneurysms (MAs) for treatment	All MAs identified by fluorescein angiogram (FA), generally in areas of thickened retina within 3000 µm of center of macula	More emphasis on treating clinically apparent MAs in thickened areas—FA-guided treatment optional
Goal of focal MA treatment	Creating a zone of whitening around the MA with lightening or darkening of the MA itself	Creating a mild grey-white burn at the site of the MA—no change in MA color required
Goal of grid treatment	Light- to moderate-intensity burns 1 burn width apart to areas of diffuse leakage and nonperfusion, generally corresponding to retinal thickening	Barely visible light grey burns no closer than 2 burn widths apart in areas of thickening caused by diffuse leakage. Treatment of thickened areas caused by non-perfusion is optional.
Area treated (After: Walker J, Bressler S. Update on the Management of Diabetic Retinopathy. Focal Point Module 2011, American Academy of Ophthalmology.)	Initial treatment within 500–3000 µm from center of macula. No burns within 500 µm of the disc. If persistent edema and visual acuity ≤20/40, treatment permitted between 300 and 500 µm of the fovea.	500–3000 µm from center of macula for focal treatment. Direct treatment of MA within 300 to 500 µm may be used if center-involved edema persists after initial treatment, but not generally if visual acuity is >20/40. Grid treatment may be extended to 3500 µm from center of macula on the temporal side. No burns within 500 µm of the disc.

SPOT SIZE and a Bit About Spot Power

The main goal is to use the smallest size possible to minimize scar expansion. It is best to start with a 50-micron spot and adjust the power as discussed above (some lasers only go down to 75 microns, which is OK, too). Be warned that 50 (or 75) microns is small, and you need to be very careful that you are not using powers that can accidentally punch through Bruch's membrane.

How do you know if you broke Bruch's? It is usually pretty obvious. First of all, the patient may jump because you will have generated a small popping sound within their head, which is a quick way to lose their trust. Also, did you ever see what happens when an old-fashioned projector breaks and the heat of the bulb melts the film? The frozen frame gets this weird bubbly look, and then it rapidly melts away from the center, leaving nothing but a blank screen and a faint smell of burning celluloid. This is exactly what a burn in Bruch's membrane is like—but way faster and smaller and hopefully without the smell of something burning. Or at least this is what we have been told. This has, of course, never happened to us. Basically, breaking Bruch's is something that you should only imagine; you should never be using settings that are even close to causing this complication.

The problem is that such a burn is really bad. A subretinal hemorrhage may occur and cause permanent loss of vision. (By the way, should there be a hemorrhage, there is something that you should do immediately. Think for a moment about what you would do, because if you end up in this situation, you should be prepared—time is of the essence. If you aren't sure, feel free to do the asterisk thing.*)

A hot burn can also result in the late development of a choroidal neovascular membrane, and you will have given the patient a brand new problem that is way worse than the original disease. By the way, you don't have to break through Bruch's membrane to get a choroidal neovascular membrane to grow—they can occur at any laser spot (although they are more likely with hotter burns closer to the fovea). If a patient starts to get funny-looking pigmentation and edema in a localized area, you need to think about this complication. If you keep treating them with focal laser in a mistaken attempt to treat "diabetic" edema, they will end up with a lot of vision loss that could have been avoided with intravitreal anti-VEGF agents (Figure 6).

---

*Push on the eye like crazy with the contact lens until the bleeding stops! (Warning: This may make some sensitive patients vasovagal—nothing is simple.) There is another technique if the spot keeps bleeding despite tamponade, but this is ONLY if you are well away from the fovea (at least 1-2 disc diameters). You can increase the duration to double of what you have (or at least 0.2 sec) and use a spot size of 200 um and reduce the power to half. This change will lead to a slow and deep burn that can photocoagulate the whole area. Again, this is to be done only if you are well away from the fovea. And when you do this type of photocoagulative burn make sure that you are not seeing a color change in the nerve fiber layer (white on the surface of the retina) – which portends loss of visual field. Mostly, if you find yourself actually using these techniques, you really need to reassess how you are managing your laser settings—you are way too hot.

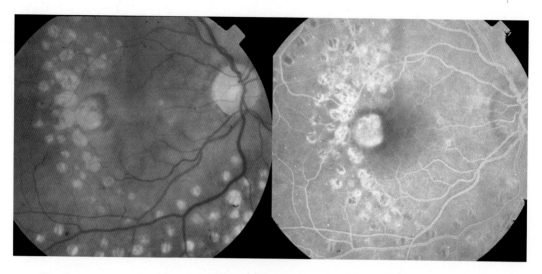

Figure 6: The color shows abnormal pigmentation spreading out from a series of big scars near the fovea. On clinical examination you would see pronounced macular edema in this patient. The FA highlights the presence of a large neovascular membrane growing from the laser scars. This is one of many reasons why you don't want to treat heavily near the fovea, and why we are all very grateful for the ability to use intravitreal injections to control leakage without laser.

Sometimes, using a 100-micron spot will allow you to laser with "training wheels"—the larger size will keep you from punching through Bruch's membrane, and you do not need a high degree of accuracy if you are trying to get a given microaneurysm. A spot this large uses up a lot of ground in the macula, however. If you think you need to use this size, try to use it only for more peripheral treatment to quickly build up experience—you should use the smallest spot you can, as soon as you can.

HAVING PICKED OUT A

Given Spot Size and a Starting Power...

It is probably best to start somewhere beyond the inferior arcade, and well away from the fovea, to test the power; patients are less likely to notice anything in the superior visual field if there is a problem. Once you feel you have a reasonably safe power, you can start to work in toward the meaty areas, but remember that variables like foveal pigmentation and retinal thickness may change your laser uptake significantly from your test spots, so proceed carefully.

It is a good idea to pick an unmistakable set of hard exudates, hemorrhages and/or microaneurysms close to the fovea in order to define The Line That You Must Never Cross. As you begin the great video game of focal treatment, it is all too easy to concentrate on the job of shooting at red things and accidentally move into the edge of the foveal avascular zone, particularly if there is a lot of pathology and if the patient is twitchy. Setting up a mental demarcation line around the fovea will make this much less likely—avoiding the fovea should be the focus of your universe for the duration of the treatment. (By the way, try not to let your aiming beam get near the fovea as you study the lay of the land. The odds are you would never accidentally trigger the laser, but there is no need to tempt the gods of retina to teach you a lesson.)

Be very careful when treating just below the fovea. Before cutting to the blue box to learn why, take a second to try to figure it out for yourself. Hint: This is not something to worry about if the patient has been given a retrobulbar anesthetic.

Remember Bell's reflex and how it can change the position of the fundus. If the patient blinks very hard the front of the eye goes up but the back of the eye goes down. If you are treating just below the fovea, the fovea can flip down into your aiming beam faster than your foot can come off the pedal. And that juicy pigment in the fovea will take up laser really fast. Usually you will have a clue that this might happen based on the patient's behavior at the slit lamp and you can be ready to back off immediately if necessary. Also, just to be confusing, you may notice that in some patients the fovea can actually move up with a blink—perhaps as they squeeze they contract multiple extraocular muscles which makes the ocular movement less predictable. Just be careful around the fovea, period. Besides, with the use of intravitreal injections the need to get close to the fovea is largely eliminated.

OK, now you have set your spot size and power, and your mental GPS has set up a barricade around the fovea. You are now ready to cook pathology. The first step is to treat the obvious microaneurysms in a given quadrant. An even first-er step, though, is to figure out which little red spots are really microaneurysms and which are little dot hemorrhages. This is where it is invaluable to have a projected angiogram available when you do these treatments—especially when you are learning.

You will be surprised at how many little red dots in the fundus are not really microaneurysms at all, and you will also be surprised at how many microaneurysms on the angiogram are almost invisible on fundus exam. Some microaneurysms are even a yellowish color and can simulate a small hard exudate. The point is that indiscriminately treating every red spot can result in a lot of unnecessary damage. Furthermore, it is fairly easy to get a blot hemorrhage to change color, and you can incorrectly think you are doing a great job, when really you are just burning up the nerve fiber layer and not treating the actual leaks. Looking carefully at an angiogram as you treat is a great way to understand the pathology—it will help you fine-tune your ability to perceive microaneurysms and help minimize wasted spots from just "shooting red." If you do angiographically-guided treatment enough, you will find that you will become much better at both your exam and treatments—and ultimately, you even find that you are less dependent on an angiogram because your clinical exam will be so good. (Figure 7 is a good example of how to approach this—and it is not unique. You will find similar differences between the clinical exam and FA in just about any diabetic if you take the time to look.)

Occasionally, microaneurysms may be yellowed from sclerosis, simulating little chunks of hard exudates, which you would not otherwise treat. The only way to learn about this type of stealth lesion is by studying the angiogram and looking at the patient. If you find one, it means you are ready for your black belt (Figure 8).

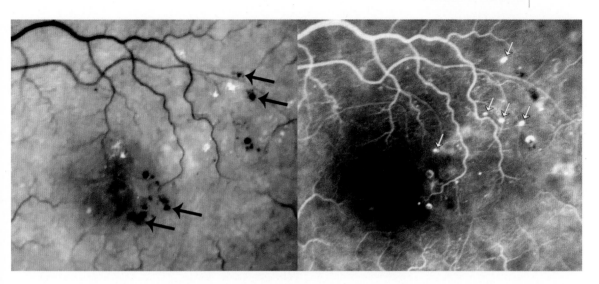

Figure 7: These photos are cool – take some time to study them. First, imagine how you would treat based on the red-free photo on the left. Now look through the arrows, comparing the FA to the clinical appearance. The black arrows show things that you might have treated as microaneurysms but are really just hemorrhages. Note also that there are at least five troublesome microaneurysms that are essentially invisible on the clinical picture (white arrows). If you were studying the patient with a contact lens you would likely see the corresponding microaneurysms as tiny dots; sometimes you can only see them in the back flash of the laser as you treat in the area. Finally, look at the two obvious microaneurysms next to the foveal avascular zone on both the red-free and FA. Although you might be tempted to go after them because they are big and leaky, note that they are part of the few remaining capillaries supplying that side of the fovea. Nailing them could shut down a chunk of the fovea— something to be avoided and a good reason to use injections. (Also note the dark center to some of the microaneurysms, suggesting that their lumen is partially filled with a clot. This is fairly common in large microaneurysms.)

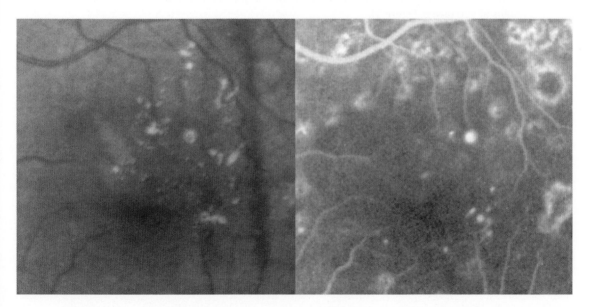

Figure 8: Example of a yellow microaneurysm — in the center of a group of hard exudates. Usually they are not this obvious – they are often much smaller and therefore harder to photograph. They also can be completely yellow; this one has some red showing through the middle. (Extra credit if you can find the other yellowish microaneurysm in the picture.)

Two finesse points: As you study the patient and the FA you will begin to see that there is a clinically detectable difference between a true microaneurysm and a blot heme creating a "pseudo-microaneurysm." You will get a sense that the real microaneurysms can be seen to be little 3-D spheroid globs, while the hemorrhages are more two-dimensional. This is not always the case, and the lesions need to be on the large side to detect the difference, but it is something to look for.

Another finesse point is to look for tiny microaneurysms in the backscatter of your laser shot. If you think you know where a given microaneurysm might be based on the FA but you really don't see anything clinically then treat the area with a spot. If you look carefully you may be able to see the microaneurysm backlit by the bright coherent laser beam. Obviously one does not randomly treat the retina with laser spots just to find hidden microaneurysms. The point of this is to recognize that information is available to you at all times if you look for it and you may be surprised by what you can see if you study the retinal details that are lit up when you fire the laser.

Having found your targets, it is time for the kill. As mentioned above, the traditional goal is to get the microaneurysm to either darken or lighten, which presumably indicates closure or at least sclerosis of the aneurysm wall (refer to Figure 1). Of course, this represents the Platonic essence of laser treatment perfection. In the shadow world where the rest of us dwell, things are a bit more complicated. First of all, unless the patient is very cooperative, it is often difficult to drill a microaneurysm with this degree of precision—even if you are trying just to hit the microaneurysm without getting a definite color change. Most of the time, the first shot misses to one side and then the second shot misses to the other side, and then you are wondering exactly how many shots you are going to take before you convert the region into a charred landscape while the microaneurysm itself cheerfully stays micro-plump and micro-red while it micro-laughs at you (again, Figure 1).

Take heart—you are not alone. If you ask seasoned retina specialists, you will learn that perhaps only 10 to 20% of all shots end up with a truly satisfying direct hit. Sometimes this percentage can go as high as 80 to 90% if the lesions are discreet and the patient is cooperative. If someone tells you that they routinely hit all microaneurysms on all patients then they are either (a) lying; (b) have a navigable laser (see Chapter 6); or (c) they are truly enlightened and you should throw away this book and follow them forever.

In the meantime, we mere mortals are often left in the position of trying to decide what to do once we have used up a few shots and only straddled a given microaneurysm. Discretion is the best part of lasering, and it is probably best to bail out and move on if it looks like you are not making much progress.

This is OK, because no one really knows for sure why focal treatment works. Is it changes in the microaneurysm, or is it changes in the retina and retinal pigment epithelium under the microaneurysm? In other words, does the laser work because you are you sealing the leaks with direct hits, or are you helping the RPE to suck out the fluid faster with misses? The effect of laser is probably a combination of these—and no doubt other effects—and that is why you don't have to be anal with those pesky microaneurysms that dodge your laser spots. Practically speaking, if you do want deliver focal treatment and the first couple of shots miss, it is reasonable to move on to the next location, because it is not in your patient's best interest for you to keep hammering away at each microaneurysm until you have a 300-micron treatment and still no direct hit. Plus—and this is really important—go back to Table 1 and remember that nowadays you don't even need to get a color change in the microaneurysm. The DRCR.net treatment guidelines no longer require it; you just need to get a bit of change in the RPE.

By the way, here is something that is fun to do: Go back and look at microaneurysms that you have treated. Even if you do manage to safely achieve the old ETDRS ideal of a change in color, you may find that a number of the treated aneurysms will have reverted back to a reddish color by the time you have finished treating the last of the line. Should you re-treat them? Some will go back and re-treat obvious big ones, but no one knows if this is worth it—whatever you do, don't go crazy over it.

Sometimes there will appear to be a group of microaneurysms heaped up in one area, almost like a cluster of grapes. These areas are usually deceptive, and you should study the angiogram first before leaping in and treating, because you may think that you have the proverbial fish in the barrel. However, if you look carefully at the angiogram, you will see that there are usually only a few real microaneurysms, and the rest of the red dots are just hemorrhages. If you go in and really cook the whole area, you will cause a big burn that usually goes through some of the nerve fiber cables, and you will have been way more aggressive than necessary.

Some patients will have tons of microaneurysms. If this is the case, do not try to treat every single one—you can end up with far-too-confluent treatment because you are dutifully trying to nail every little leak. Rather, treat obvious large ones and try not to put in more than a spot every three to four spot widths apart. It is better to put in some treatment, then wait and add more, rather than to try to treat everything (Figure 9).

Figure 9: An example of a situation where you do not want to treat every microaneurysm. Aggressive treatment would result in confluent burns – best to go lightly and add more spots over time if necessary. Also note that there are far more microaneurysms on the FA than are apparent clinically. The area in the circle is wall-to-wall microaneurysms. There is almost nothing to see on the color photograph. Of course, if this patient had center-involved disease you would be treating with intravitreal injections first and then going after recalcitrant microaneurysms as needed.

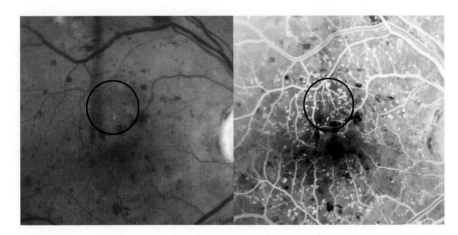

Another occasional finding is a really big microaneurysm (maybe 75 to 100 microns—the large yellow one in Figure 8 is an example). These can be really fun, because you can watch the little bastards shrivel up nicely as you treat them; but there are a few caveats. First, check the angiogram and make sure the lesion is not part of the only remaining vessel supplying the fovea. It would be bad to shut down such a vessel. Second, make sure you are not treating a large microaneurysm with a small laser spot—you can end up puncturing it and making it bleed. Although such a hemorrhage is easy to control, it is still better to carefully increase the spot size and gradually treat the whole lesion, rather than hitting it with a small, hot burn.

As mentioned above, you do not want to waste time treating small hemorrhages that look like microaneurysms. You also need to take special care when treating near large, obvious hemorrhages. Such hemorrhages will take up the laser dramatically, and you can ruin a lot of the patient's nerve fiber layer. This is particularly dangerous when treating in the papillomacular bundle; a burn here can create a scotoma that is far larger than the size of the original laser spot. This same warning applies if you are re-treating a patient who has old laser scars. The extra pigment will increase uptake and you can cause a bad burn very quickly. (You should be staying well away from prior burns in previously treated patients anyway in order to avoid atrophic patches from overlapping treatment.)

Another cool thing, if there is persistent edema, is to repeat an angiogram and look specifically at the microaneurysms that you tried to close with the previous treatment. You may be surprised that these can be frightfully recalcitrant. Note that if you decide to go back and treat the same microaneurysm you need to be careful of the underlying pigment changes caused by the previous laser.

Although it is important not to kill yourself or your patient's RPE in order to nail microaneurysms, you should generally make focal treatment your goal as much as possible. First of all, there are few things more satisfying than toasting succulent microaneurysms with a single laser spot that spares the underlying RPE.* The gratification is even greater because, several months later, these patients usually have a marked decrease in their swelling and hard exudates, with little or no evidence of laser treatment. This represents the Holy Grail of focal diabetic treatment, and it is so rewarding that it brings to mind the old learning psychology axiom, "intermittent reinforcement creates behaviors that are hardest to extinguish." Never extinguish your goal of focal microaneurysm treatment with minimal RPE damage.

Alright, now you have taken out the focal leaks. What if there is a lot of diffuse leakage that doesn't come from obvious microaneurysms? The next step is to perform a light grid to any areas of diffuse leakage, filling in the preexisting focal treatment. Do not get aggressive here—less is definitely way more. *Do not* feel that you have to conquer all the diffuse leakage in one treatment. First of all, many times there are enough microaneurysms that the focal treatment itself creates a sufficient grid. Also, remember that now that the patient is actually being treated for a diabetic complication, he or she

---

*If you don't think this is satisfying you are a real loser. Get outta here and go do clear lens extractions on patients that think glasses are a disease. Jeez.

may get it through their head that their life and vision depend on taking better care of themselves. This will make a much bigger difference than your laser spots, but it will take a while to pay off. To repeat, patience is your most valuable surgical tool.

If there are areas of thickening that have not been treated by focal laser, then put in a grid pattern using a small spot size with a power that gives you a very light burn. Some folks will increase the spot size as the grid is carried out away from the fovea—ranging from 50 microns near the center, up to 200 microns in the periphery. It may be simpler to just use the same small size and place more spots in the periphery, or to defocus the aiming beam to generate a larger spot (more on the latter technique in the next chapter). Regardless of what you may have read, do not put a lot of spots in the thickened area—and try to avoid placing your burns one spot width apart. Maybe go a nice, wide three or four spot widths apart; you can always add more. (Again—all this assumes you are treating disease that is eccentric to the center, or that you do not have access to injectables. You may not need to do any laser in patients who have center-involving disease if you can give them injections.)

BTW, if you need to treat in thickened retina, there are definitely some things to be aware of. First of all, your beam will diffuse out and you will need to increase the power to get a take. Be very careful when you do this—for two reasons:

1. If you go back to thinner retina, you can get a really hot burn, which is not a good thing to do near the fovea. (Vide supra about burning celluloid.)

2. Even if you use a small spot size, the diffusion of the beam through the thick retina can create a large burn that will come back to haunt you as a giant scar.

Another important thing is to be certain you can remember where you have already done parts of the grid. Light, diffuse burns will fade during the course of your treatment, and you can come back to the same area thinking it hasn't been fully treated. If you decide to add just a bit more laser before you call it a day, you can create confluent lesions without realizing it. The result is way too much treatment that will only be apparent to, for instance, every other doctor who sees the patient for the rest of their life. This is definitely a case where "the enemy of good is perfect." Mentally delineate areas that you have gridded so you don't go back over them repeatedly.

Although the ETDRS used a combination of focal and grid treatment, there was another philosophy that espoused the use of pure grid treatment for everything. This approach applied 100 to 200 micron spots throughout all areas of thickening without necessarily treating specific microaneurysms. A DRCR.net study suggested that such an approach—even with much gentler grid treatment—does not seem to be as effective as a focal/grid combination.[1] Although it is easy and tempting to just do a fast grid on everyone, such an approach is neither ideal nor elegant. You should put your shotgun away and concentrate on learning how to treat parsimoniously.

Another thing to keep in mind is that macular edema can actually be exacerbated by overly aggressive treatment. It is natural to want to treat every red spot and swollen area because, well, it is fun to do and you feel you are stamping out blindness. Unfortunately, it is possible to push edema into the fovea with extensive treatment. Patients with fragile vasculature and more diffuse edema are more likely to end up with this problem. It is also more common if there is a "wall" of edema just outside the fovea and you aggressively treat everything in the area of thickening, which can push the wall right into the fovea. You can try to blame this on progression of the patient's underlying disease, rather than a side effect of the laser, and sometimes this will be the case. However, if you really caused the problem there will be no doubt in the patient's mind or in your inner soul that your laser did it—their vision will nosedive and will stay nosedived from the moment you finish the laser.

If you do cause this problem, it will often resolve gradually as your laser reins in the original leakage, but it can take some time. This was a real bummer in the old days, but now you can usually be bailed out with intravitreal therapy. Still, you don't want a reputation for doing things that make patients worse. The key thing to remember is that if you decide a patient needs laser, don't pour in a lot of treatment all at once. For that matter, if you think you have to use a lot of laser to treat disease that has yet to involve the fovea, you may want to rethink your approach and start with injections first. Although there is no data in the literature that clearly defines what to do, injections may help stabilize an eye with lots of perifoveal edema and avoid the need for lots of laser.

But getting back to the treatment...

How far out do you carry your spots? Most people do not treat much beyond the arcades, simply because it is unlikely for there to be any useful effect that far away from the fovea. (This approximates the DRCR.net recommendation to only treat out to 3000 microns from the center—see Table 1). If there are obvious focal areas of leakage that are trying to stream hard exudates and edema toward the fovea from far away, it certainly makes sense to touch them up even if they are outside the arcades. Doing this may help decompress more delicate central structures and buy the patient more time. Also, if there is very diffuse thickening beyond the arcades, it may be reasonable to treat further out, simply to preserve peripheral vision. Don't go nuts and create a mini-PRP all at once, however, because that may undo everything you are trying to accomplish by causing increased macular edema. (Lots more on the effect of a PRP on macular edema in Chapter 14.)

MOVING into the zone

The ETDRS recommended treating up to 500 microns from the center of the fovea, but this is close, and you may want to play it safe and stay 750 microns or more from the center in order to avoid trouble. This is an easy number to define—just mentally split the diameter of the disc in half, and put one end at the center of the fovea. Until you have a lot of experience, or become cavalier (usually they are the same), it is best to avoid getting close to the center. Plus, with ability to use intravitreal injections to treat center-involving disease, there really should be no need to get close unless you don't have access to that modality. Observant patients can really get frustrated with treatment near the fovea, because they can detect your spots more easily. It is also where you can do some serious damage to the perifoveal capillary network if you are not careful. A detailed angiogram is crucial if you work in this close, because you really need to be sure that you are not accidentally treating microaneurysms that happen to supply the few remaining capillaries that supply the fovea.

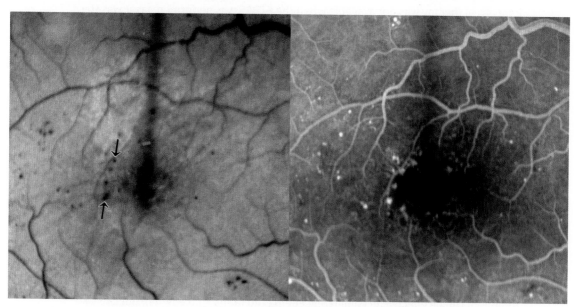

Figure 10: This is why it is good to have an FA before treating near the fovea, if you must do so. The circle represents an estimate of 500 microns from the fovea based on the patient's nerve. The microaneurysms temporal to the fovea (between the arrows) are far enough away to be treatable if you decide to follow old ETDRS guidelines. However, you can see from the FA that aggressive treatment of these little devils could shut down the only vessels supplying the entire temporal side of the fovea – you could cause a lot of vision loss. Patients may have remarkably good vision yet have really large foveal avascular zones—especially if they have poor blood pressure control. So be sure you know what you are doing if you move in close. (Extra credit if you notice that the brightest microaneurysm on the FA is not the same as the most obvious microaneurysm clinically.)

Wait a minute. *Table 1 clearly says that, according to the DRCR.net, a fluorescein angiogram is no longer mandatory for treatment as it was in the ETDRS (although an OCT is).*

But the last few pages have totally emphasized the utility of an FA.

Remember from Chapter 3 that the DRCR.net gang is full of major retina players. If you go on to pursue a career chasing microaneurysms, you too will develop a good sense of what to treat without an FA. Until then, if you are going to put laser into someone's macula, it is useful to have an FA for all the reasons discussed—you learn a lot of stuff to help you do the best treatment. An FA is certainly not mandatory—especially if you don't have access to the test—but it is a valuable tool to make you safe and successful.

Although the ETDRS allowed treatment to within 300 microns of the center of the fovea if necessary, if you really feel that you just have to treat closer than 500-700 microns, you may want to get a second opinion—needles should be replacing photons in your therapeutic hierarchy. Remember that spots this close to the fovea will grow—are you sure that everyone will be happy with the results in five years if they spread into the fovea? You will find an occasional patient that has a few big leakers near the foveal avascular zone, and gentle treatment directed only at the microaneurysms may fix the problem. In general, however, bad leaks in this area don't tend to respond to laser, especially if the fovea is cystic. If you still follow ETDRS guidelines, remember that intravitreal therapy was not available when the ETDRS was performed; laser was the only way to try to dry up foveal edema—hence the more desperate parameters. On the other hand, if you work in a location that doesn't have access to intravitreal drugs, careful treatment up to 300 microns from the foveal center may be your only hope. But if this really is your only option, you are better off trying to figure out a way to get your patients access to injections.

Also, don't forget to look at the individual cuts on your OCT rather than just the pretty colors of the thickness map. Patients may have subtle traction that is keeping the retina thick, and the vascular changes may be secondary to the traction. Finally, never forget that any patient with refractory edema may actually have a bigger problem, such as accelerated hypertension or early renal failure. No perifoveal laser is going to replace nephrons—so think globally before acting locally on juxtafoveal RPE.

CODA...

The goal of life is to seek a balance between extremes. This is very true in the setting of laser treatment for diabetic macular edema. There is no question that very heavy treatment can be effective in eliminating edema (no retina = no edema), but can also create more problems with scotomas, decreased vision, and late complications. Lighter treatment decreases the risks of treatment, but also engenders the risk of damage from progressive edema, especially if the patient is lost to follow-up. Of course, if you are dealing with center-involving disease, you should be primarily treating with intravitreal therapy anyway (Chapter 4).

The best way to judge the needs of an individual patient's retina is experience, and if you end up treating a lot of diabetics you will develop a good sense for this. Until then, take heart—perhaps the most reasonable approach is to be conservative with your lasers. There is probably more damage done by overly aggressive treatment of focal disease than by delayed treatment of focal disease. But now, a colorful box break followed by a mini-chapter on advanced laser techniques.

Sometimes an Angiogram has a Cheatin' Heart

Although the angiogram is usually your friend, there are times it can deceive you. For instance, patients may have "compensated" leakage on the FA. This means that they can have areas of leakage in the later phases, but somehow the retina and RPE are able to pump the leakage out fast enough so that there is no secondary swelling of the retina. In other words, the angiogram may indicate there are areas that need to be treated but if you look closely at the retina with your own eyes there is actually no thickening and therefore no "clinically significant" macular edema. Your OCT will obviously help sort this out, but you should be able to infer with your clinical exam that no treatment is warranted.

Another way an angiogram can mess you up is with the diffuse leakage that can occur at the site of previous laser scars. These areas almost always light up the later phases and you can really chase your tail if you keep hammering laser into these areas thinking that there is still leakage to treat (not to mention the fact that you will create large patches of atrophic retina and RPE). There are also times where the angiogram is not showing leakage, but actually showing a window defect or staining with a central bright spot due to loss of RPE from a previous laser. In some cases, there will be mild nearby leakage that will fool you into thinking that the old microaneurysm that you thought you cooked has sprung a new leak – carefully compare the mid to the late frames of the angiogram in this case. The simplest way to distinguish "staining" from "leakage" is to notice that the borders on the stained retina remain stable and granular through the mid and late phases of the angiogram while the borders on the leaking areas are more diffuse, and progress.

Ultimately, look at the patient. Usually areas of previous laser treatment will be flatter and therefore do not need to be treated—even if they are staining or leaking on the FA. Of course, the OCT will help you here as well—just don't automatically keep shooting at anything that turns white on the FA.

References and Suggested Reading

1. Fong DS, Strauber SF, Aiello LP, et al. Comparison of the modified Early Treatment Diabetic Retinopathy Study and mild macular grid laser photocoagulation strategies for diabetic macular edema. Arch Ophthalmol. Apr 2007;125(4):469-480.

Folk JC, Pulido JS. Laser photocoagulation of the retina and choroid. San Francisco: American Academy of Ophthalmology, 1997.

Photocoagulation for diabetic macular edema: Early Treatment Diabetic Retinopathy Study Report no. 4. The Early Treatment Diabetic Retinopathy Study Research Group. Int Ophthalmol Clin 1987;27:265-72.

Walker J, Bressler S. Update on the Management of Diabetic Retinopathy. Focal Point Module 2011, American Academy of Ophthalmology.)

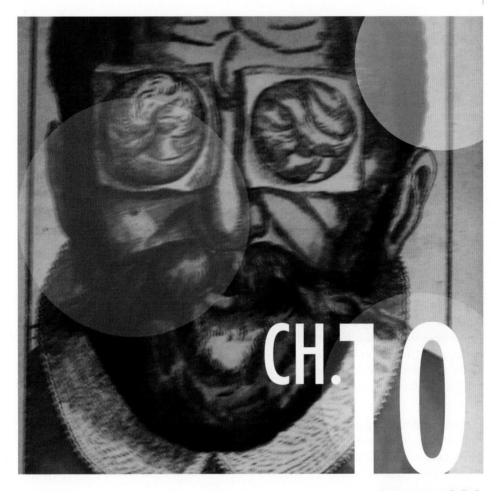

CH.10

Lasers 202

I am still learning. Michelangelo

LASERS 202

It can get quite tedious if you need to constantly adjust your spot size and power in a patient with variably thickened retina and variable pigmentation. Reaching over to change the setting and then relocating yourself on the patient's retina can add a huge amount of time and frustration to the process for both yourself and the patient. There are some tricks you can use to avoid fussing with the laser settings for each spot—but they take a bit of experience. First of all, always strive to get the tightest, most consistent focus on your aiming beam. The energy delivery of your laser is totally dependent on this; if your spot is shifting and blurring, you are wasting your time—and you may even be dangerous if you are turning up the power for a blurry spot, and then suddenly the spot snaps into perfect focus. Everyone in the room will hear the pop of Bruch's membrane exploding.

A consistently good aiming beam can seem impossible at first. Just practice—even if it means putting a contact lens on every patient (as well as family members, friends and each other). You don't even need to do it at the laser—practicing with the lenses in the clinic will readily pay off when you switch to using them in the laser suite. The quicker this skill is internalized, the better it is for everyone. Just. Do. It.

Once you have mastered the art of seeing what you need to see, though, there are some tricks that can come in really handy for enhancing your laser skills. The first technique is to actually undo what you have learned. You have a great deal of control over the energy density when you defocus the spot in a controlled manner. This can be done by either moving the slit lamp back and forth or by throwing a little astigmatism into the lens by tilting it a bit (the former is more predictable and controllable). For instance, if you are doing panretinal photocoagulation (PRP) and moving into the retinal periphery, where the spot is tighter and the retina is thinner, you can just defocus a bit and titrate the uptake without fiddling with the power knob. If you are working in the central macula you obviously do not want to be smearing out and enlarging your spot—it is much better to manually back off on the power—but everywhere else this can be a real time saver. By the way, this technique is easier with an indirect contact lens. A direct lens does not focus and defocus the aiming beam as much, but you can still try it.

Some older lasers are focused in a way that creates a cone of light, and by pushing the slit lamp in, you defocus. When you pull back, the spot size actually gets smaller, with a higher power density. This allows you a great deal of control, but you have to be careful if you tighten up the spot too much—for reasons that should not need mentioning by now.

There is another variable that is even easier to work with, though, and that is the duration of the burn. If you work with a slightly longer time, say .15 or .2 seconds, you will be surprised at how easily you can control, with the pedal, the actual time the laser is on. In fact, if you get good at this, you will find that your foot can be much faster than even shorter durations, such as .1 second. You can then use your foot to titrate the burn—a quick hit for a light burn and more sustained pedal-to-metal for a longer, hotter burn if you run into thicker retina or paler RPE. Remember, however, that if you are using longer durations you may run into trouble if the patient moves during a burn—but if you are light on your foot to begin with, you can usually react in time. Also, this technique is harder to do if you are using really short durations to minimize discomfort.

A variation on the above technique is to use the joystick to rapidly defocus a burn if it seems to be building up too fast. For instance, you can have the aiming beam in focus with the joystick pushed a bit forward. This allows a lot of play in the joystick, so that you can quickly move it backwards to defocus the spot if you are "coming in hot".* You can decide if this works better for you than quickly coming off the foot pedal—but always be ready to do something fast if a burn is starting to look dangerous.

With experience, it is easy to control both of these variables at the same time. You can continuously alter both the spot focus and duration, and you can often do an entire laser without needing to adjust the power setting.

Where can you quickly become experienced in this? Take a look at the PRP chapter. Over there, you can try out these techniques while you are doing several hundred spots and super-accuracy is not crucial. It is also a good way to avoid getting bored while doing a PRP. If you can master these techniques, it will greatly improve your efficiency and safety—because you will have a much more intuitive feel for what the laser is doing and how you can control it. You will also be able to win friends, influence people, have great sex and make your wildest dreams come true. Can doctors who use lasers all day to correct refractive errors make that claim? Not likely...

*Star Wars Episode III, Revenge of the Sith.

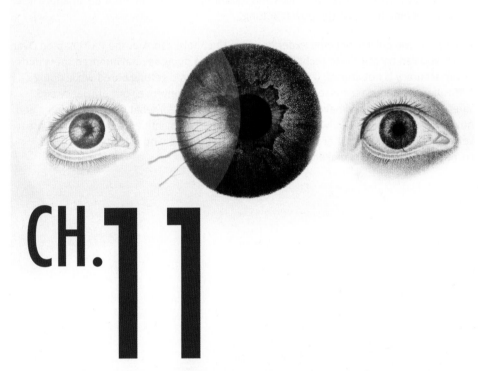

CH.11

Put It Where You Want It. Intravitreal Injections

Confidence is what you have before you understand the problem. Woody Allen

Warning: This chapter is no substitute for hands-on training with people experienced in the performance of intravitreal injections. It is possible to seriously mess up an eye if you don't know what you are doing—and you cannot learn the technique solely from reading a book or watching videos. Nor is this chapter meant to condone the performance of intravitreal injections by non-retinal specialists. If you already have a bunch of retina docs in your community, you will get very little sympathy if you run into trouble, and you will have a hard time showing that your lack of retinal training meets the local standard of care. However, you may be hours away from a retinal specialist, or you may even be the only ophthalmologist for hundreds of thousands of people. So if you are going to take this on because it is the best thing for your patients, then dig in.

Also, this chapter is about performing intravitreal injections for typical adult eyes. If you are going to be treating preemies with ROP, you need to look elsewhere.

Preparing Thine Head

Although putting a needle in the pars plana seems relatively simple in the abstract, there are a lot of things that can go wrong. The journey begins with becoming intuitively aware of all of those bad things.

Think about what happens when you do cataract surgery. There are certain moves that you are planning on doing, but there is also a deeper level of consciousness that is hyperaware of everything that is going on. When you put your phaco tip into someone's anterior chamber, your muscle memory feels how close you are to the endothelium, iris, and posterior capsule, and it goes well beyond mere intellect. You become focused in a way that other mortals don't understand, because you know on a fundamental level the kind of disasters you can create if your moves are off by even a few microns.

Retina specialists develop that same innate sense of where things need to go after doing thousands of vitrectomies. If you are going to take on intravitreal injections as a general ophthalmologist, you need to import that innate awareness.

Figure 1 reminds you that some serious trouble can occur if you enter too anteriorly. The pars plana is the go-to place because it is relatively avascular, but right in front of it is the pars plicata, which has a much more robust blood supply coursing through those plump ciliary processes. You are more likely to create an intraocular hemorrhage if you go through those processes.

Note that if you aim the needle too anteriorly, or if it swings anteriorly once you are in the eye, you can ding or even impale the lens. That will lead to a cataract—and it will happen really fast if you manage to inject drugs directly into the lens. You may feel that you are the god or goddess of cataract surgery, but remember: creating a dense cataract with a hole in the posterior capsule in a diabetic patient is a scenario to be avoided.

You also need to walk in the retina specialist's moccasins for a moment and think about the anatomy of the vitreous base. Recall that the vitreous base is strongly inserted into the retina and pars plana a few millimeters anterior and posterior to the ora serrata (Figure 1). Posterior to the vitreous base the vitreous insertion is not quite as strong, and that is the area that separates when patients have a vitreous detachment. If your needle is swinging around too much in the back of the eye, it is possible to generate tractional forces that can be transmitted to the retina at the vitreous base. Fortunately, the vitreous is springy and is usually forgiving, but a glance at Figure 2 will remind you that if the vitreous insertion at the vitreous base is irregular, it is possible to create traction at a narrow point on the retina and thereby generate a retinal tear—in the same way that patients with predisposing anatomy will get a tear in the retina when they have a vitreous detachment.

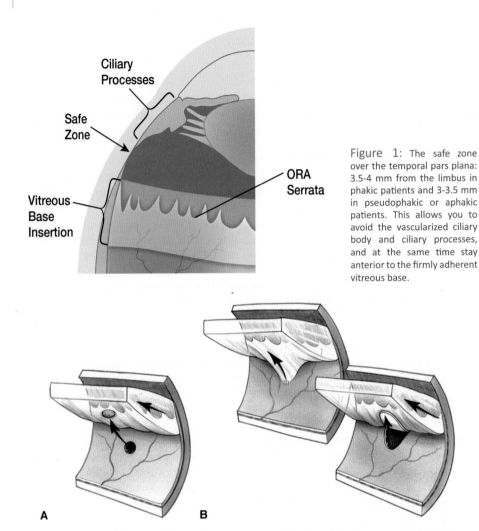

Figure 1: The safe zone over the temporal pars plana: 3.5-4 mm from the limbus in phakic patients and 3-3.5 mm in pseudophakic or aphakic patients. This allows you to avoid the vascularized ciliary body and ciliary processes, and at the same time stay anterior to the firmly adherent vitreous base.

Figure 2: These are well-known images from the retina section of the American Academy of Ophthalmology Basic and Clinical Science Course. They show what happens if there is abnormal adhesion between the vitreous and the retina when the posterior vitreous detaches. Normally, the vitreous separates cleanly from the retina and simply remains attached anteriorly at the vitreous base, floating around like seaweed. But if there is a focal vitreous attachment (A), then the vitreous can pop out an operculated hole. If the vitreous base insertion has a focal area where it extends posteriorly (B), then the forward movement of the vitreous creates localized traction and pulls a horseshoe tear. Keep this heavily in mind when you start sticking needles through the pars plana. (Used with permission; American Academy of Ophthalmology. Artwork by Christine Gralapp after classic drawings done by Tim Hengst.)

This is a major awareness that separates retinal specialists from general ophthalmologists, and this is why retina specialists often feel their gonads retract—wherever they are—when they watch videos of anterior segment surgeons cavalierly swing instruments through the pars plana to assist with anterior segment surgeries. This is not to say that such moves are wrong—there are situations where carefully working through the pars plana can save a case. Still, watching those instruments being swept around, especially in a non-vitrectomized eye, is cringe-worthy for us. Once you get your needle in the eye you want to avoid moving it around back there—do your best to inject and get out as quickly as possible.

Another thing to keep in mind is how far away your activities are from anything that can even remotely generate an immune response. The free-flowing aqueous of the anterior chamber, with the robustly vascularized iris and ciliary body, is like a pristine mountain river thundering over sparkling rocks compared to the middle of the vitreous cavity, which is more like a stagnant swamp. There is some fluid flow through the vitreous, but the avascular matrix of collagen and hyaluronic acid is, for all practical purposes, a free lunch for bacteria. This has been demonstrated in studies showing that the anterior chamber can be contaminated with tens of thousands of organisms and still fight off an infection. On the other hand, in an animal model it took as few as 14 organisms to set up shop and create an endophthalmitis in the relatively unprotected gel-like vitreous.[1,2] Pay really close attention to the advice in this chapter regarding sterile technique. (By the way, this explains why the risk of endophthalmitis goes way up if you bust the posterior capsule during cataract surgery—the anterior chamber can handle some contamination, but if even a few bugs get into the vitreous they will be fruitful and multiply.)

You need to intuitively grasp all of these factors: the vascularized pars plicata, the proximity of crystalline lens, the potential to create traction at the posterior edge of the vitreous base, and the extreme sensitivity of the vitreous to bacterial contamination if you are going to be a safe Impaler of the Pars Plana. And this is also why you should not do intravitreal injections simply because you think you can. A bad injection can turn a problem that interferes with a patient's ability to read the sports page into a problem that interferes with the patient's ability to keep their eye in their head. You need to consider the worst-case scenarios, especially if you are working in a region where patients may be unable to get to a retina specialist in a timely fashion if they develop a retinal detachment or endophthalmitis.

By the way, *this is a good time to remind you to take a peek at the patient's lid margin and ocular surface. If there is a lot of blepharitis you may want to try to address that before jumping into an injection. Since the number of people with some degree of blepharitis is approximately equal to the world's population, you'll have to decide how aggressive you want to be. But given how few bacteria it takes to set up endophthalmitis in the vitreous, you owe it to your patient and your reputation to address this.*

There is one other issue that you need to think about: the injection can significantly raise the pressure in the eye (almost 90% of patients have an IOP rise of 30 mmHg or more 5 seconds after an injection).[3] Most of the time this is not a big deal—studies suggest that a healthy eye can tolerate this easily. However, if a patient has had recent intraocular surgery, or penetrating keratoplasty at any point, you need to warn them about the possibility of a wound rupture. There is also the concern that patients with advanced glaucoma may be much more sensitive to transient pressure elevations. We seem to get away with injections in these patients, but we know that pressure spikes at the time of cataract surgery can snuff out a fragile nerve so it stands to reason that chronic injections could be a problem—especially since glaucomatous eyes tend to take longer for the pressure to lower after an injection.[4]

If you are concerned about this you might consider softening the eye prior to the injection—obviously doing this carefully if the patient had recent surgery. (Warning: some people worry that if you massage the eye using digital pressure over a closed eyelid you might end up expressing potentially infectious secretions from the meibomian glands. Perhaps try avoiding direct pressure over the lid margins and instead have the patient look down and push on the globe above the tarsal plate to avoid this. Another approach is to use a sterile cotton-tipped applicator to push directly on the eye to soften it prior to the injection.[5-7]) You can also give a pressure-lowering drop prior to the injection—this can also help blunt the pressure rise, but you have to give them twice a day before the shot.[8] Finally, many have a low threshold for performing a paracentesis prior to intravitreal injections, but this has its own set of risks and is not done routinely. It may also make sense to monitor patients with fragile nerves and visual fields encroaching on fixation more carefully after the injection to make sure the pressure does come down quickly. (By the way, if you are doing injections on a glaucoma patient that has had filtration surgery, make sure you don't put your needle through anything that is part of the filtration bleb— especially if the patient has a diffuse low-lying bleb that is hard to delineate.)

OK. All that was to get you psyched up for doing an injection. Now let's do it.

The first thing is to get the patient ready—and perhaps the simplest way to ramp up your empathy quotient is to have one of your compatriots put a numbing drop in your eye, insert a speculum and then touch a small blunt object to your conjunctiva. This way you can sense how millions of years of evolution need to be overcome for one human being to let another stick them in the eye with a needle. Pay attention to how their fingers feel on your lids, how the speculum feels, and how tense your neck and shoulders are while someone is invading important parts of your personal space. This will help you anticipate your patients' experiences and make you better able to address their fears.

Also, it is crucial to actually listen to the patient as you give injections. They will provide instant feedback, and if they tell you about something they don't like, you should adjust. In practice situations with multiple doctors, patients may prefer a certain doctor's technique. You definitely want talk to that doc to get pointers. Remember, in medicine (and life) if you think you know the best way to do something, you have immediately lost the ability to learn how to do it better. And if that doesn't motivate you to improve your technique, go read the first paragraph in Chapter 16 for another really good reason.

When doing a laser, a constant stream of soothing chatter helps prepare a patient, and the same applies for injections. Most patients are terrified that they will do something wrong, so it is important to let them know that the weight is off their shoulders; tell them that if they cough or jump you can deal with it. (And your job is to make sure you are ready for whatever they might do.) Finally, it is extremely important to tell the patient what you are going to do before you do it, so that they are not surprised by any moves you make. If you go out of your way to telegraph your actions, you will be rewarded with multiple patients telling you how much they appreciate it, and how their other doctors never tell them what is about to happen. You get lots of warm-fuzzy points...

And don't forget to do all the tedious "time-out" things before you actually get started. Patients that are nervous and scared may become very passive and let you put medicine in the wrong eye before they say something. So mark the eye and make sure you and your staff confirm everything with both the patient and the chart—including the proper medicine. You don't want to make this utterly avoidable mistake.

But back to doing an injection.

There is a big question about whether topical antibiotics are useful during any part of the process. In the early days pretty much everyone would use antibiotics for a few days prior to the injection, then put antibiotics in at the time of the injection, and then have the patient use antibiotics for a few days after the injection. Over the years, data has come out suggesting that such an approach accomplishes exactly nothing and may actually increase the risk of developing resistant organisms on the ocular surface—an unwelcome eventuality if the patient gets endophthalmitis.[7,9-11,47] The weight of opinion is leaning away from the use of antibiotics, but there probably will never be a definitive study given the number of patients that would need to be enrolled.

The one thing you should not do is use antibiotics because you are scared of a lawsuit. It is far better to look at the data available, ask your mentors, and use your noggin to come up with a conclusion you can call your very own. Frankly, if some attorney manages to get a lawsuit started based on the lack of antibiotics at the time of an injection, it is likely that the entire American Society of Retina Specialists would land on his or her head.

Everyone agrees, however, that the use of povidone-iodine (Betadine) is crucial. The standard concentration is 5% povidone-iodine solution, which is the dilution used in cataract surgery. Some people use 10%, which is how it comes straight out of the bottle— but other people feel that concentration is too irritating. Whichever you prefer, there is no well-defined approach as far as exactly how it should be used. Some doctors will put a drop in at the beginning of the process and then add one or two more drops or use a cotton-tip applicator to apply it directly to the site of the injection. Other people will paint the lashes and lids in addition to treating the ocular surface. A recent expert panel suggested that actually scrubbing the lids is probably not necessary given the risk of spreading contaminated debris into the field.[7] Whatever you do, it is important to allow the povidone to sit on the eye to work its magic; give it at least 30 seconds.[12,13] And remember, even povidone-iodine can't completely sterilize the ocular surface, but it does dramatically reduce the bacterial load.[14]

What about patients that tell you they are allergic to iodine? Wykoff, et al. wrote a great review on this. It turns out that most so-called iodine-related reactions, such as seafood allergy and contrast media allergy, are likely unrelated to either povidone or iodine. Although some patients may develop chemical irritation from povidone-iodine, and sometimes even contact dermatitis, a true anaphylactic allergy is extremely unlikely and has never been reported in association with an ophthalmic surgical prep. It seems reasonable to go ahead and use povidone-iodine patients with a vague history of iodine "allergy"—it really is the best choice for surgical antisepsis and there aren't any other great options for the ocular surface. It may also help to irrigate the Betadine out of the eye after the procedure to minimize exposure time. If a careful history indicates that a patient may actually have had a true anaphylactic reaction to iodine or povidone—or if you just aren't sure—then it makes sense to consider an allergy consult. If nothing else, it may put the patient's mind at ease.[7,15]

Should you wear a mask? Intravitreal injection-associated endophthalmitis is different from post-operative endophthalmitis because there is a relatively high incidence of organisms that live in the upper respiratory tract, such as streptococcus species. The presumption is that the needle is contaminated with aerosolized secretions from the doctor and/or patient. This has led some experts to recommend not talking during the injection procedure—but you lose the ability to explain to the patient what you are doing. Plus, the enforced silence gives the whole thing a creepy medieval-dungeon kind of vibe. Try it and see. In any event, you can find support in the literature for both talking[16] and not talking.[17] You decide...

The other option is to wear a facemask and ask the patient to avoid talking once the speculum is in. This allows you to chat amicably about what you are doing, and studies suggest that there are far fewer aerosolized organisms.[17,18] But the use of a mask is by no means a standard of care; and it is not clear how far you should go—it can be argued that if you take this step, then everyone should wear a mask including the assistant, the patient and anyone else present in the room. Still, you might want to consider this as you develop your personal approach; it is unlikely that any study will ever prove the benefit of a mask, but you will feel better if you have done everything you can to avoid an infection when the inevitable occurs. Other variables to consider include the use of a sterile drape around the eye and sterile gloves. There is no proof that any of this makes a difference, but some people feel safer using these things—indeed, some places will only give injections in the operating room.

What about anticoagulation?

Although hemorrhage is always a risk with an injection, it would be unusual to stop a patient's anticoagulation, whether it be antiplatelet agents, warfarin or the newer anticoagulation drugs. No study had identified a significant increased risk of problems when patients on these drugs are treated, and there certainly would be a systemic risk of thromboembolic events if anticoagulants were intermittently discontinued just for an injection. Still, there is always a chance that a hemorrhage could occur—whether a patient is on this type of drug or not—and you don't want to be in the awkward position of telling a patient with an eye full of blood that you decided on your own that they didn't need to worry about their anticoagulation. Patients deserve an informed discussion so they are prepared for any problems, and it is hard to imagine how a patient would prefer the risk of a stroke to the risk of an ocular hemorrhage. See Chapter 26 for a further discussion of anticoagulants in diabetes.

Comfortably Numb

There is absolutely no consensus about numbing the surface of the eye either. Some authors suggest that topical drops, such as standard tetracaine, are sufficient.[19] However, many patients prefer the deeper numbing that occurs with viscous drops. Most clinics will have different types of drops available, and you can try them to see what your patients prefer. There is a concern, at least in the setting of cataract surgery, that more viscous preparations may slightly increase the risk of endophthalmitis. This may not be the case with intravitreal injections.[20] Still, it would be prudent to use povidone-iodine both before and after application of the gel to minimize risk.[21] The gel is typically preservative free, so if you do happen to use it on more than one patient (which would be against the label), make sure to confirm that there was no contamination. Also, definitely throw it away at the end of each day.

Perhaps the best approach is to listen to the patient. You will find that there is a dramatic difference between patients as far as what they can tolerate, and you can begin to get a feel for this if you note how the patient behaves when you do things like applanation tonometry or indirect ophthalmoscopy. The patient that does a lot of squinting and squeezing during these relatively simple maneuvers probably has a whole bunch of wiring between their ocular surface and their cerebral cortex, and they are going to find just about every step of the injection process difficult.

For most patients, and particularly elderly patients, topical anesthesia is usually sufficient, and the viscous preparations seem to be better in our experience. But for patients who are nervous, or younger with a full complement of cranial nerve V nociceptors, subconjunctival anesthesia is the way to go. But you have to do it right. If you just put in some topical drops and then do the subconjunctival injection immediately, the subconjunctival injection can be as painful as the intravitreal injection itself. Instead, it is better to use topical anesthesia and then place a cotton pledget soaked with, say, 2% lidocaine with epinephrine (the epi will blanche the vessels and hopefully minimize the risk of a subconjunctival hemorrhage). Then leave the room and let that sit for a few minutes—when it comes to anesthesia, time is your friend. Remove the cotton and inject a subconjunctival bleb using the same medication. Patients usually do not feel the injection if you give the cotton pledget time to soak in. Then you have to wait a few more minutes to let the subconjunctival anesthetic work; don't just do the intravitreal injection immediately after the subconjunctival injection. All this takes extra time, but hypersensitive patients will really appreciate it because each step is painless. Be aware that you may need to shunt these patients to an unused exam room, because this approach can clog things up on a busy day. By the way, some people feel that the pledget alone allows enough anesthesia that they do the intravitreal injection after removing the pledget without a subconjunctival injection. Finally, no matter how you numb your patient, ask them to keep the numbed eye closed as much as possible until you do the injection. It will make it less likely for them to accidentally scratch the eye or let the ocular surface dry out. Both those things will make both the patient and you miserable (much more on this below).

If you use a subconjunctival injection for anesthesia, make darn sure you get rid of the syringe and needle well before you get ready to inject the intravitreal drug. It is very easy to grab the wrong syringe and you will feel really dumb if you inject local anesthetic into the eye. The small dose probably won't be toxic, but it will likely shut the retina down immediately– you have just numbed the nerve fiber layer (and the double use of the needle increases the risk of infection). It can take up to a day to get vision back and it is a process that makes everyone very uncomfortable. Especially when you now have to convince the patient to let you inject the correct drug!

It is important to tell the patient that the use of a subconjunctival anesthetic increases the risk of a subconjunctival hemorrhage (which some patients will find more traumatic than going blind from their disease, it seems). Patients who receive subconjunctival anesthesia may also be prone to more ocular surface irritation given the longer duration of the numbing. But if you have a patient that has a hard time with topical anesthesia, you should let them try subconjunctival anesthesia at least once—they will probably prefer it. Once you have experience with how different patients respond, you will be able to have a good idea in advance about which patient needs which anesthesia.

What if patients are allergic to the topical anesthetic? A true allergy is rather rare, but you can try an ice pack—see the reference.[22]

Speaking of surface irritation...

When you start doing injections, be prepared to get frantic phone calls later in the evening because the eye hurts and patients are wondering why you personally ruined their life with your stupid awful injection. It is likely that either they accidently rubbed their eye or the surface of the eye dried out because the numbing eliminated the afferent limb of the blink reflex. Fortunately, this problem tends to improve overnight, but it can be very disconcerting to patients.

How do you avoid it? First, look at the patient. If they have a lot of anterior basement membrane changes (and many older diabetics do), then they may be more at risk. Also, do they have baseline dry eyes or blepharitis that will be more likely to contribute to irritation? Finally, how is their blink reflex? Patients with Parkinson disease may let the bottom third of their cornea totally dry out once it is numbed—and they can be really miserable after a shot. A similar problem can occur in patients with exophthalmos, or in those patients who get corneal epithelial breakdown as soon as they are given a topical anesthetic to check the pressure.

As mentioned, one thing is to ask patients to just keep their eye closed as soon as you start putting the stronger numbing medicine in. This way they don't get a chance to let the eye dry out or scratch it. It may help to use a bland ointment after the injection to protect the ocular surface, assuming the patient doesn't mind the extra blurriness and goopiness. Some doctors feel that it helps to wash the eye out after the injection to minimize irritation from residual Betadine; sensitive patients may complain of burning from the Betadine for several hours. At least one study suggested that a nonsteroidal drop right after the treatment can decrease discomfort for quite some time (a trick pioneered by our cornea colleagues for when they heroically destroy corneal epithelium with PRK to spare patients the living hell of glasses).[23]

Another option is to patch the patient for a few hours, especially if they had subconjunctival anesthesia. For patients who have real problems with surface discomfort, it may even be necessary to tape their eye shut as soon as the numbing medicine is placed so the eye doesn't get a chance to dry out, and then patch them once the injection is done. Most patients will balk at the idea of a patch—but if they complain about surface irritation from prior injections you should encourage them to try a patch. They will usually be very grateful.

If you're careful, you should not be bothered by multiple phone calls after a day full of injections. If you are getting lots of calls, then you absolutely need to reassess what you are doing, both to keep your patients comfortable and to keep them in your practice. You may be the most brilliant diagnostician and surgeon in the region, but if you let your patients have too much epithelial keratopathy, there will be tumbleweeds rolling through your waiting room in no time.

By the way, just because nothing is simple, never assume these first night phone calls are always due to surface problems. Although true endophthalmitis usually doesn't show up the first night, you can never let your guard down about it, and even if there is no true infection there are occasional patients who get non-infectious uveitis that can show up really fast. Also, there are rare patients that can have a dramatic pressure spike within a few hours, especially if they received steroids that slosh into the anterior chamber. So you should have a very low threshold for examining patients that call the night of their injection. It may be reasonable to reassure them if their symptoms are mild and clearly surface related—but if there is anything unusual or severe both you and the patient will sleep better if they are checked. More on this at the end of the chapter.

As mentioned above, this chapter should not substitute for hands-on instruction. However, there is a good video at the University of Iowa site if you want to see one approach, courtesy of James Folk and his crew (https://vimeo.com/116066821). If the link does not work, just Google "Iowa intravitreal injection video".

Putting It In

You are now ready to do the actual treatment. If you are going to use a speculum (and most people do—especially at first), you want to make sure you insert it as gently as possible. Patients tend to find a bladed speculum more comfortable than a wire speculum, but this is another situation where you can let the patient try each type and ask them which they prefer. Be careful if you use a wire speculum, though. Sometimes the lashes are not held out of the way with a wire speculum compared to a bladed speculum. It also makes sense to have a pediatric speculum available for people with tiny eyes, or whose eyes have shrunk down in their sockets from aging and/or using prostaglandin analogs to treat their glaucoma. A simple way to put the speculum in, even in an uncooperative patient, is to have them look down and gently elevate the upper lid to place the upper blade of the speculum and then have them look up and pull down the lower lid and do the same thing. At this point you can put in the iodine in the way that you have been trained and get ready to perform the injection.

Note that an occasional patient will consider the speculum the worst part of the process, and at least one study suggests that manually holding the lids is preferable to most patients.[24] If you have enough staff, someone can hold the lids for you for each injection (although some prefer to hold the lids with their own fingers). Be careful the lids aren't pushed in a way that might express debris from the Meibomian glands. Plus, be sure you or your assistant have complete control of the lids—you don't want lids to go back over the injection site once it is prepped, and you especially don't want the lashes to touch the shaft of the needle as you go in the eye. That, as Bill Murray said in Ghostbusters, would be bad.

What about the super-squeezers—the ones that can collapse the speculum in mid-injection? First, they probably need subconj anesthesia to make things easy. Second, if push comes to shove you can always bust out a speculum that locks open (like a Cook speculum), or, in desperate cases, give a lid block. Hard to imaging needing all this, if you go slow, get them numb, and talk them through it.

Getting the Juice

It is easiest when the medication is provided in a prepared syringe with an attached needle (Avastin often arrives this way from compounding pharmacies). Although pulling liquid out of a vial is a skill you have no doubt mastered at this point in your career— be aware that Lucentis and Eylea come in a small volume and it is easy to fail to get everything out of the vial. For up to $2,000 a dose, you would think they would figure out a way to teleport the stuff into your syringe so nary a molecule is lost, but no. The standard move for drawing medicine out of a vial is to invert the vial—but this is tricky when trying to get a small amount. You have to shake the vial down so the fluid is by the cap, and then put the syringe in just enough to visualize the tip of the needle in the pool of fluid and keep it there as you aspirate.

It is a lot simpler to tilt the vial a bit and then stick the needle down into it. That way you can see the needle in the puddle of fluid at the bottom, and it is easier to get out every last bit. Remember, even though the usual dose is .05 milliliters, you need at least .075-.1 milliliter to have enough drug to fill the dead space in the hub of the injection needle. If you don't have enough then the dose will be stuck in the dead space and the patient gets little or nothing. And if you blow it and waste that $2,000 drug, you will be toast. So take some time to mentally plan out the whole process prior to doing your first Lucentis or Eylea injection.

A lot of doctors prefer a Luer-Lok syringe and needle so that the injection needle doesn't have any chance of slipping off the end of the syringe during the process. If you don't have a Luer-Lok syringe then make sure that the injection needle is firmly placed on the end of the syringe and that you don't loosen it when you pull the cap off. It is really annoying to insert a needle into a patient's eye and watch the expensive medication squirt out the needle hub. This is something that the authors have only heard of; none of us would be stupid enough to actually let this happen. Uh-uh. No way.

The most commonly used needle size for an injection is 30-gauge, although some use even smaller gauges such as 31 or 32 to decrease discomfort. (One study looking at this didn't find much difference in terms of pain, but the smaller needles do result in less reflux and a higher post-injection IOP.[51,52]) Although the anti-VEGF drugs and Triesence (the FDA-approved formulation of triamcinolone—more on this below) can easily pass through a 30-gauge needle, the commercially available preparation of triamcinolone acetonide (Kenalog) can get clogged up. And it can do it really fast—you can squirt some out of a 30-gauge needle and think you will be fine and then once you get in the eye the drug can totally lock up and nothing comes out. You will lose many, many style points if this happens. As a result, most people will use at least a 27-gauge needle for Kenalog, even though it may take a little more force to enter the eye.

As for the part of the eye chosen for the injection, some feel that the lower half of the eye is more likely to be contaminated as bacteria and other debris tends to congregate in the lower tear film. (This may explain why inferiorly placed filtering blebs are more likely to get infected.) These doctors prefer to inject in the supratemporal part of the eye. Another reason cited for doing an injection superiorly is that if a retinal tear and detachment occur, it is easier to repair superior pathology with a pneumatic retinopexy. On the other hand, if the patient blinks or squeezes during the process, then Bell's phenomenon is more likely to roll the eye up—making the superior sclera inaccessible. As a result, the infratemporal part of the eye is most commonly used. The one thing that most people agree on, however, is to avoid the horizontal meridians. Therein lie the long ciliary nerves and vessels, and you would want to avoid slicing through those.

Be sure you look at exactly where you are doing the injection. It sounds obvious, but try to avoid any conjunctival vessels to minimize the subconjunctival-hemorrhage-vampire look. In older patients, watch out for those calcified senile plaques (Figure 3). You will find it really hard to get through those—consider going at least 1-2 mm beyond the edge to avoid the calcium barricade.

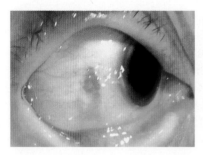

Figure 3: Avoid these dark calcified plaques; they can be impossible to get through.

Performing the actual injection usually involves holding the syringe like a pencil with one hand and stabilizing that hand on the patient's cheek with fourth and fifth fingers so that if they move their head you will automatically follow the movement with your hand (Figure 4). Once the needle is inserted, then the other hand pushes the plunger. (By the way, for medications that are supplied in a preloaded syringe and an attached needle, there is always a chance that the needle is plugged up with desiccated medication. It is a good idea to squirt out a tiny bit of the drug when you uncap the syringe to be sure that the needle is open before you stick it in the eye. Vide supra regarding clogged Kenalog.) Most specialists prefer to inject the drug at a moderate pace—over about a second. A fast squirt may needlessly shake up the vitreous, and a slower rate could leave the needle in too long and give the patient a chance to move and mess things up.

It is important to make sure you are performing the injection at the proper distance from the limbus, and sterile calipers are used for this purpose. Most people use a distance of 3.5-4 mm from the limbus in phakic patients and 3-3.5 mm in pseudophakic or aphakic patients. Both distances will keep you away from the pars plicata and all of its blood vessels, and the larger distance gives you a bit more safety in phakic patients as far as accidentally swinging the needle towards the lens. You don't want to use more than 4 mm because you will

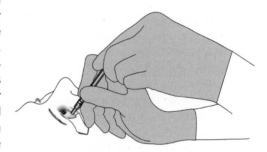

Figure 4: One of many ways to skin this particular cat. The fingers on the patient's cheek help stabilize the hand holding the syringe, and that hand in turn stabilizes the hand pushing the plunger.

be getting deeper into the vitreous base or even put a hole in the retina if you are too far back. Review Figure 1 for the details.

Gee, doc, how many times can you do this before my eye splits open from all the holes?

Fortunately, the sclera tends to be remarkably self-sealing. It can take a lot of sticks; almost like putting a knitting needle through a ball of yarn—it just closes up when you pull the needle out. Still, there are some patients whose sclera can thin, and it makes sense to avoid going through the exact same area every time. Sometimes you can even see where individual injections have been given. This has been referred to as the "pincushion sign", and in such patients it may be a good idea to rotate the site of the injection to avoid obvious thin spots. It would be particularly important to do this in patients that have pre-existing scleral thinning, for instance from old scleritis or surgery.[25]

Some people have proposed a beveled approach—the needle enters at an angle rather than directly perpendicular to the sclera. A variation on this involves entering the eye at an angle and then redirecting the needle to be perpendicular once it is in the eye. When this is done, the wound tends to be more self-sealing and there is less backflow (although a recent study suggested that there is minimal loss of drug when backflow occurs).[26-28] Another theoretical advantage of a beveled entry is that there may be less risk of bacterial access into the eye. If you prefer this technique, remember that if you approach the sclera at too shallow of an angle your needle might not get all the way into the vitreous, especially if the eye rotates away from the needle. Also, try not to torque the needle around inside the eye too much if you want to redirect it after entering obliquely. For better or for worse, most people simply approach the globe in a perpendicular direction—and this is probably the best way to start.

Another method that some doctors use to minimize backflow through the injection site is to roll a sterile cotton-tipped applicator over the site as the needle is removed.[21] This is also something to consider if you hit a conjunctival gusher with the injection, especially if the patient is anticoagulated. Putting some pressure on the vessel will minimize the amount of subconjunctival bleeding, perhaps saving you from a frantic phone call or from ruining any of the patient's family photos for the next 2 weeks. (By the way, it has been suggested that a drop of brimonidine in the eye can decrease the risk of subconjunctival hemorrhages.[29])

Once the injection is in, it is important to remind the patient that the pressure may go high enough that the eye can black out. You have to be careful how you say this because patients can misinterpret your meaning in unbelievable ways. They can think that you mean they will lose consciousness, or they can assume that the blackout can occur at some other point in time, like when they are driving home. So make sure they understand that you are talking about immediate changes in the vision in the eye you just injected. It is customary to check for light perception to be sure that the optic nerve is perfused, or look in the eye to assess perfusion. It is usually not necessary to perform a paracentesis because the pressure does tend to decrease within a few minutes, especially if you are using a volume of 0.05 ml or less. Recall that some people feel that this pressure spike is a potential problem in glaucoma patients, and may even consider softening the eye prior to the injection (see above).

Most doctors don't place any restrictions on patients beyond avoiding touching the eye while the surface is anesthetized. It is a good idea to provide the patients with a note that lists worrisome symptoms and a phone number to call if there are problems. Remind them that it is not unusual to have a subconjunctival hemorrhage, and that the eye may be irritated during the first day and night but it should rapidly improve. They do need to understand that if things gradually worsen over the ensuing days then an infection is much more likely and they should contact you immediately.

The time-honored RSVP handout is a good way to remind patients what to look for. Redness, Sensitivity to light, Vision loss, and Pain—along with your contact info. The "Redness" may get you a few subconj hemorrhage calls, but better to get extra calls than miss early endophthalmitis.

In the past, patients would be brought back after a few days to be checked in the clinic. If you are starting to do injections you may want to do this for a while so you know what to expect, but it is probably not necessary to do this routinely. Many practices will call the patient during the first week after the injection to see how they are doing. As with lasers, you may want to take the time to call the patient yourself after their first injection—they will appreciate the call and it will give you yet another chance to explain why the injection does not automatically allow them to read the phonebook without their glasses. But if you start to do a lot of injections, the logistics of calling every patient for every injection becomes problematic. Plus, as patients get experience with the procedure they get a feel for what to expect; they will know when something bad is happening.

Complications. Or, as they said in Jurassic Park: "What could possibly go wrong?"

Get prepared for first night phone calls—but those are the easy ones. The main concern is, of course, endophthalmitis, and you can't afford to miss that, especially if the cause is some spit-bug that can destroy an eye really fast. So any patient that calls with something other than mild, early onset surface irritation may well need to be seen. Sometimes patients will present with post-injection uveitis that is not truly infectious. If there is only a mild cellular response with no vitritis, pain or hypopyon, you may be dealing with a reaction to the medication and it makes sense to try some aggressive topical steroids to calm the eye down. It is important that you don't use this paragraph to engage in what retina specialists refer to as "EDS" (Endophthalmitis Denial Syndrome): The thought of causing endophthalmitis is so awful that treating physicians will talk themselves into non-infectious uveitis in the face of obvious endophthalmitis, and then things are really bad when the patient is finally referred. If you try the steroid approach, make sure you are being honest with yourself and that it really is not endophthalmitis, and don't hesitate to check the patient within several hours to evaluate for worsening.

A patient with non-infectious uveitis can be problematic, and if it happens with one of the anti-VEGF drugs, you might want to consider switching to a different one. If you can't switch (usually because the patient is taking Avastin and no other drug is affordable), the patient should be warned about a more severe recurrence with repeated use. On occasion you may need to use prophylactic topical steroids, but fortunately most episodes of non-infectious uveitis with these drugs will be self-limited and the problem doesn't tend to recur with repeated use, although that can happen.[30,31]

Intravitreal steroids, however, can be really confusing because they can do four different things when it comes to making the eye look inflamed. First, the steroid particles can enter the anterior chamber and mimic endophthalmitis—the particulate material simulates cells and the drug can even layer out behind the cornea, creating a pseudohypopyon. Usually the lack of pain, rapid occurrence, and the crystalline appearance of the particles at the slit lamp will differentiate this from true uveitis or endophthalmitis. The problem is referred to as pseudo-endophthalmitis, and no treatment is required unless the pressure is elevated from material in the angle.

The next thing that can happen with intravitreal steroids is that patients may paradoxically develop non-infectious uveitis from the steroids. This tends to happen within a day or two of the injection, and patients again tend to not have a lot of pain. Some patients may get a hypopyon that may represent cells or cells and drug crystals. It has been suggested that if the hypopyon readily shifts position when the patient tilts their head, then it may be non-infectious inflammation or even just drug crystals. Infectious hypopyons don't tend to shift easily because of the associated fibrin "glue"[32] (Figure 5).

It is not clear if this inflammatory response is due to the vehicle or the drug, or perhaps even mechanical irritation from the drug particles. The possibility of a reaction to something in the vehicle is why some doctors use preservative-free triamcinolone from a compounding pharmacy, or use the formulation of triamcinolone approved for intravitreal use (Triesence). Whatever the cause, this problem can be dicey because although these patients have true inflammation, all they need is some topical steroids or even just observation since the eye will improve within a few days. But you need to watch them closely and avoid the EDS mentioned above.

Figure 5: A pseudohypopyon consisting of triamcinolone crystals in the anterior chamber. Figure 5B shows the rapid shifting of the crystals with head tilting. Note the relatively quiet eye—a true endophthalmitis with a hypopyon this big would have a steamy cornea and cloudy anterior chamber, as well as marked conjunctival injection. (From Chen, et al. Pseudohypopyon after intravitreal triamcinolone injection for the treatment of pseudophakic cystoid macular oedema. Br J Ophthalmol.[33] Used with permission. Although why one has to ask permission from people that don't even know how to spell edema is beyond us.)

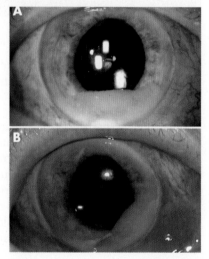

Figure 5

In addition to non-infectious uveitis and pseudo-inflammation from drug crystals, patients can get plain old endophthalmitis from intravitreal triamcinolone—and this requires all the usual treatments such as intravitreal antibiotics and possibly vitrectomy. True endophthalmitis tends to show up a few days later compared to the non-infectious uveitis—usually within the first week rather than the first two days. The vision is often worse than with non-infectious inflammation, and there is more pain with more conjunctival injection and vitreous haze. However, at times the presentation can be atypical because the eye is so full of steroids that the immune response is altered (for instance, the patient may have less pain compared to post-surgical endophthalmitis). And by the way, endophthalmitis is a bit more likely to occur with steroid injections compared to anti-VEGF injections.[48]

Finally, steroids in the eye can shut down the immune system so much that patients can get viral retinitis after an intravitreal steroid injection—and it has even been reported with sub-Tenon's injections. The infection usually occurs a few months after the injection, and is more likely to occur in patients with pre-existing systemic immune-altering conditions such as HIV, immunosuppression, and, well, diabetes. The most common cause is cytomegalovirus, but cases of herpes simplex and zoster infections have been reported. Watch for this in any patient that develops uveitis weeks or months after a steroid injection and be sure to look carefully at the peripheral retina for signs of retinitis (Figure 6).[34,35]

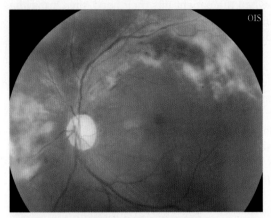

Figure 6: Why is there a picture of CMV retinitis in a textbook on diabetic retinopathy? Go read the text.

Other things that can go wrong with any intravitreal injection include retinal detachment, vitreous hemorrhage and rapid cataract formation if the lens is nicked. All these become self evident when the patient is examined. Don't forget about the risk of wound rupture, too, both for patients that have had recent intraocular surgery and for any patient that ever had penetrating keratoplasty. There have also been cases of ruptured filtering blebs and even ruptured globes after intravitreal injections.[36,37] Patients with thin filtering blebs may also be at risk for endophthalmitis, presumably due to microbreaks in the bleb from either the injection prep or the transient elevated pressure after the injection.[38]

Another finding, particularly in patients who need multiple injections, is the presence of small silicone oil droplets in the vitreous that come from the silicone lubricant in the needle or syringe. These don't tend to cause any trouble, although some patients may see them as floaters.[39] Sometimes you will see other types of particulate debris, perhaps from contaminants in the drug or syringe. Although it has never been formally studied, it also seems that patients who need multiple injections have more vitreous syneresis in the injected eye compared to the fellow eye, and may be more likely to get a posterior vitreous detachment with the attendant risk of a retinal tear.

There are also complications that are specific to the drug chosen, including cataract formation and glaucoma with steroids, or traction retinal detachment with the anti-VEGF drugs. Don't forget that there is a subset of patients who need regular anti-VEGF injections that will develop chronically elevated intraocular pressure. Sometimes this occurs gradually, and sometimes the pressure just jumps up out of the blue after multiple injections. Elevated pressure occurs in perhaps 5-10% of patients, and may be more likely in patients who require more frequent injections or have had a large number of injections. It also seems to occur more often in patients with a preexisting history of glaucoma or ocular hypertension. The effect seems to be shared by all the anti-VEGF drugs—it is not clear if switching drugs will help, but one paper suggests the problem may be less likely with aflibercept.[50] It is not known if the problem is due to contaminants clogging the trabecular meshwork, or some effect that the drugs have on the cells in the meshwork. It could also be due to cumulative damage from all the pressure spikes that occur with each injection. Patients may need topical therapy to control the pressure, and some require laser trabeculoplasty and/or surgery.[40,49]

While we are on the subject of glaucoma and anti-VEGF agents, it is worth noting that some authors have raised the possibility that chronic anti-VEGF use may interfere with healing after glaucoma drainage implant surgery. The concern is that the drugs may inhibit capsule formation around the implant plate, resulting in hypotony. It is not clear if this is a common effect, but if you do glaucoma implant surgery on patients getting a lot of injections, it is something to keep in mind.[41]

Finally, there is the perennial thorn regarding the potential for systemic side effects from the anti-VEGF drugs. This was covered in Chapter 4, where the use of these drugs was discussed in the setting of macular edema.

What about bilateral injections?

Some doctors avoid this, but patients who need frequent treatment in both eyes often find the time and cost commitment of twice as many visits to be burdensome. Studies suggest that this is reasonably safe as long as separate sterile instruments are used for each eye. It is probably not a good idea to give a patient bilateral treatment if it is their first treatment with any drug, though, in case they have some unexpected reaction such as non-infectious uveitis. If a patient is being injected bilaterally, consider using drugs from different lots in each eye, especially with medications from a compounding pharmacy (and ideally lots that have already been used so you know they are OK). This avoids the horrible outcome of injecting a contaminated preparation into both eyes. It has also been suggested that bilateral injections may be relatively contraindicated in patients with bilateral ocular surface or lid problems.

Cash-trash talkin': Most insurance plans, such as Medicare, will only pay half or less for a second injection done on the same day. They argue that you have already done a lot of the set up and discussion for the first injection, so the second one shouldn't be as costly. Some doctors won't give bilateral injections because of this—they make patients return twice as often. If you look into your soul and find that you avoid bilateral injections for this reason alone, then you are a loser. And if you make noise about bilateral infections to rationalize bringing patients back twice as often—but you are simply using that as an excuse to make more money—then you are a real loser.

Dealing in Drugs

Handling the drugs that are designed for intravitreal use—Lucentis and Eylea—is easy because they are supplied in ready to use vials. All you need to do is store them in a refrigerator at the proper temperature, and then figure out how the hell you are going to pay for them.

It gets a lot more complicated when you are using Avastin, which comes in a large vial for use in cancer treatment. Most retina specialists will use Avastin that has been prepared by a compounding pharmacy, and this is probably the safest way to do it as long as the pharmacy is reputable and uses all of the appropriate precautions, such as monitoring for bacterial contamination. The American Society of Retina Specialists maintains a database on pharmacies that have provided this information and have been certified by regulatory agencies.

This may not be an option for doctors that are planning on doing intravitreal injections in regions of the world where compounding pharmacies are not available. When you get your hands on an actual vial of Avastin, you will see that it is very tempting to just draw the medication from the vial as needed, as you might with a local anesthetic. Unfortunately, you are treading on thin ice if you do it this way because there is an increased risk of contamination. And if you are in a situation where you don't have access to an appropriate compounding pharmacy, you may well not have access to an appropriate retina specialist—so endophthalmitis would be a really bad thing. Worse, there have been cases where inexperienced pharmacies have used the wrong drug, and there are even reports of counterfeit Avastin around the world. And remember, it is bad enough if you give a patient a problem with incorrectly prepared Avastin—but if more problems arise around the world from poorly prepared drug, you will make it harder for all of us to continue using the medication as regulatory agencies and plaintiff's attorneys react.

If you have to come up with your own supply of Avastin, you need to review the paper by Gonzalez, et al., wonderfully entitled "Avastin Doesn't Blind People, People Blind People".[42] The paper nicely spells out the standards to follow for compounding the drug, and there are numerous suggestions about how to make sure the process is done safely. You don't have to reinvent the wheel as far as using the drug, and it is a must read for you and the pharmacy if you are the first on your block to bring the drug to your region.*

There is also no consensus about the use of triamcinolone acetonide (Kenalog). In many places, Kenalog is the drug of choice simply because it is so much cheaper than the FDA-approved preservative-free formulation (Triesence). The issue is clouded by the fact that the manufacturer of Kenalog added a specific warning against intravitreal use of the drug in order to be protected from litigation. Boy, were there ever some pissed-off retina and uveitis specialists when Bristol-Meyers did that. So if you are going to use it, remember to review the off-label nature of the drug with the patient.

The problem is that there is concern about toxicity of the vehicle in Kenalog—especially the benzyl alcohol preservative. Some feel that the dose is so small that the drug can be drawn up from the single dose vial directly and injected.[43,44] Others feel that the drug should be separated from the vehicle, and there are several ways to do this in the literature, ranging from letting the drug settle and discarding the supernatant to more sophisticated methods

---

*The title of the paper is poignant as it is, but if you aren't from the USA you may not be aware of the deeper context. There is a constant struggle between the faction in the US that wants open access to guns and the other faction that wants guns to be regulated as a public health measure. Years ago the pro-gun lobby came out with a slogan to defend the right to easily obtain weapons: "Guns Don't Kill People, People Kill People". The idea of a bunch of nerdy eye doctors co-opting that phrase to defend their right to use an off-label drug is, well, amusing. You will know that things are getting really bad, though, if you see a paper using the other expression coined by the gun-lobby: "They can have my Avastin when they pry it out of my cold, dead hands."

using filters, washing and centrifugation.[45] If you need to use Kenalog for whatever reason, perhaps check with your regional specialists to see how they prefer to obtain it so that you are not an outlier—they may have compounding pharmacies that can provide preservative-free formulations, or they may simply draw it out of the commercial vial. If you obtain Kenalog from the vial, note that the drug can harbor pathogens even with the included preservative, so avoid drawing multiple intravitreal doses from the same vial.[46]

References

1.   Records RE, Iwen PC. Experimental bacterial endophthalmitis following extracapsular lens extraction. *Exp Eye Res.* Nov 1989;49(5):729-737.

2.   Shockley RK, Jay WM, Fishman PH, Aziz MZ, Rissing JP. Effect of inoculum size on the induction of endophthalmitis in aphakic rabbit eyes. *Acta Ophthalmol (Copenh).* Feb 1985;63(1):35-38.

3.   Gismondi M, Salati C, Salvetat ML, Zeppieri M, Brusini P. Short-term effect of intravitreal injection of Ranibizumab (Lucentis) on intraocular pressure. *Journal of glaucoma.* Dec 2009;18(9):658-661.

4.   Aref AA. Management of immediate and sustained intraocular pressure rise associated with intravitreal antivascular endothelial growth factor injection therapy. *Current opinion in ophthalmology.* Mar 2012;23(2):105-110.

5.   Gregori NZ, Weiss MJ, Goldhardt R, et al. Ocular Decompression With Cotton Swabs Lowers Intraocular Pressure Elevation After Intravitreal Injection. *Journal of glaucoma.* Apr 29 2013.

6.   Gregori NZ, Weiss MJ, Goldhardt R, et al. Ocular decompression with cotton swabs lowers intraocular pressure elevation after intravitreal injection. *Journal of glaucoma.* Oct-Nov 2014;23(8):508-512.

7.   Avery RL, Bakri SJ, Blumenkranz MS, et al. INTRAVITREAL INJECTION TECHNIQUE AND MONITORING: Updated Guidelines of an Expert Panel. *Retina.* Dec 2014;34 Suppl 12:S1-S18.

8.   Theoulakis PE, Lepidas J, Petropoulos IK, Livieratou A, Brinkmann CK, Katsimpris JM. Effect of brimonidine/timolol fixed combination on preventing the short-term intraocular pressure increase after intravitreal injection of ranibizumab. *Klin Monbl Augenheilkd.* Apr 2010;227(4):280-284.

9.   Milder E, Vander J, Shah C, Garg S. Changes in Antibiotic Resistance Patterns of Conjunctival Flora Due to Repeated Use of Topical Antibiotics after Intravitreal Injection. *Ophthalmology.* Mar 13 2012.

10.   Yin VT, Weisbrod DJ, Eng KT, et al. Antibiotic resistance of ocular surface flora with repeated use of a topical antibiotic after intravitreal injection. *JAMA ophthalmology.* Apr 1 2013;131(4):456-461.

11.   Storey P, Dollin M, Pitcher J, et al. The role of topical antibiotic prophylaxis to prevent endophthalmitis after intravitreal injection. *Ophthalmology.* Jan 2014;121(1):283-289.

12.   Wykoff CC, Flynn HW, Jr., Rosenfeld PJ. Prophylaxis for endophthalmitis following intravitreal injection: antisepsis and antibiotics. *American journal of ophthalmology.* Nov 2011;152(5):717-719 e712.

13.   Friedman DA, Mason JO, 3rd, Emond T, McGwin G, Jr. Povidone-Iodine Contact Time and Lid Speculum Use during Intravitreal Injection. *Retina.* Feb 14 2014.

14.   Gilbard JP, Douyon Y, Huson RB. Time-kill assay results for a linalool-hinokitiol-based eyelid cleanser for lid hygiene. *Cornea.* May 2010;29(5):559-563.

15.   Wykoff CC, Flynn HW, Jr., Han DP. Allergy to povidone-iodine and cephalosporins: the clinical dilemma in ophthalmic use. *American journal of ophthalmology.* Jan 2011;151(1):4-6.

16.   Friedman DA, Lindquist TP, Mason JO, 3rd, McGwin G. Needle contamination in the setting of intravitreal injections. *Retina.* May 2014;34(5):929-934.

17.   Doshi RR, Leng T, Fung AE. Reducing oral flora contamination of intravitreal injections with face mask or silence. *Retina.* Mar 2012;32(3):473-476.

18.   Schimel AM, Scott IU, Flynn HW, Jr. Endophthalmitis after intravitreal injections: should the use of face masks be the standard of care? *Archives of ophthalmology.* Dec 2011;129(12):1607-1609.

19.   Davis MJ, Pollack JS, Shott S. Comparison of topical anesthetics for intravitreal injections : a randomized clinical trial. *Retina.* Apr 2012;32(4):701-705.

20.   Lad EM, Maltenfort MG, Leng T. Effect of lidocaine gel anesthesia on endophthalmitis rates following intravitreal injection. *Ophthalmic Surg Lasers Imaging.* Mar-Apr 2012;43(2):115-120.

21.   Doshi RR, Bakri SJ, Fung AE. Intravitreal injection technique. *Seminars in ophthalmology.* May 2011;26(3):104-113.

22.   Lindsell LB, Miller DM, Brown JL. Use of topical ice for local anesthesia for intravitreal injections. *JAMA ophthalmology.* Aug 1 2014;132(8):1010-1011.

23.   Ulrich JN. Topical nepafenac after intravitreal injection: a prospective double-masked randomized controlled trial. *Retina.* Mar 2014;34(3):509-511.

24.   Rahimy E, Fineman MS, Regillo CD, et al. Speculum versus Bimanual Lid Retraction during Intravitreal Injection. *Ophthalmology.* Feb 26 2015.

25.   Gale RP, Pilly B, Tschuor P. Pincushion sign. *JAMA ophthalmology.* Feb 2014;132(2):161.

26.   Ozkaya A, Alkin Z, Celik U, et al. Comparing the effects of three different intravitreal injection techniques on vitreous reflux and intraocular pressure. *J Ocul Pharmacol Ther.* Apr 2013;29(3):325-329.

27.   Brodie FL, Ruggiero J, Ghodasra DH, Hui JZ, Vanderbeek BL, Brucker AJ. Volume and Composition of Reflux after Intravitreal Injection. *Retina.* Jan 21 2014.

28.   Karth P, Blumenkranz M. Update on Intravitreal Injection Techniques. *Review of Ophthalmology.* 2014(May):81-85.

29.   Kim CS, Nam KY, Kim JY. Effect of prophylactic topical brimonidine (0.15%) administration on the development of subconjunctival hemorrhage after intravitreal injection. *Retina.* Feb 2011;31(2):389-392.

30.   Chong DY, Anand R, Williams PD, Qureshi JA, Callanan DG. Characterization of sterile intraocular inflammatory responses after intravitreal bevacizumab injection. *Retina.* Oct 2010 30(9):1432-1440.

31.   Fine HF, Roth DB, Shah SP, Haque T, Wheatley HM. Frequency and Characteristics of Intraocular Inflammation after Aflibercept Injection. *Retina.* Nov 11 2014.

32.   Mahajan VB, Folk JC, Boldt HC. A head-tilt test for hypopyon after intravitreal triamcinolone. *Retina.* Apr 2009;29(4):560-561.

33.   Chen SD, Lochhead J, McDonald B, Patel CK. Pseudohypopyon after intravitreal triamcinolone injection for the treatment of pseudophakic cystoid macular oedema. *The British journal of ophthalmology.* Jun 2004;88(6):843-844.

34.   Shah AM, Oster SF, Freeman WR. Viral retinitis after intravitreal triamcinolone injection in patients with predisposing medical comorbidities. *American journal of ophthalmology.* Mar 2010;149(3):433-440 e431.

35.   Takakura A, Tessler HH, Goldstein DA, et al. Viral Retinitis following Intraocular or Periocular Corticosteroid Administration: A Case Series and Comprehensive Review of the Literature. *Ocular immunology and inflammation.* Jun 2014;22(3):175-182.

36.   Kahook MY, Noecker RJ, Abdelghani WM, Schuman JS. Filtering bleb rupture after intravitreal triamcinolone acetonide injection. *Ophthalmic Surg Lasers Imaging.* May-Jun 2008;39(3):232-233.

37.   Viestenz A, Kuchle M, Behrens-Baumann W. [Globe explosion due to intravitreal injection]. *Klin Monbl Augenheilkd.* Dec 2008;225(12):1087-1090.

38.   Thoongsuwan S, Dawn Lam HH, Bhisitkul RB. Bleb-Associated Infections After Intravitreal Injection. *Retinal Cases and Brief Reports.* 2011;5(4):315-317 310.1097/ICB.1090b1013e3181f1066bba.

39.   Bakri SJ, Ekdawi NS. Intravitreal silicone oil droplets after intravitreal drug injections. *Retina.* Jul-Aug 2008;28(7):996-1001.

40.   SooHoo JR, Seibold LK, Kahook MY. The link between intravitreal antivascular endothelial growth factor injections and glaucoma. *Current opinion in ophthalmology.* Mar 2014;25(2):127-133.

41.   Hoguet A, Parrish RK, 2nd. Unexpected Hypotony After Glaucoma Drainage Implant Surgery Associated With Anti-Vascular Endothelial Growth Factor Treatment. *JAMA ophthalmology.* Dec 4 2014.

42.   Gonzalez S, Rosenfeld PJ, Stewart MW, Brown J, Murphy SP. Avastin doesn't blind people, people blind people. *American journal of ophthalmology.* Feb 2012;153(2):196-203 e191.

43.   Albini TA, Abd-El-Barr MM, Carvounis PE, et al. Long-term retinal toxicity of intravitreal commercially available preserved triamcinolone acetonide (Kenalog) in rabbit eyes. *Investigative ophthalmology & visual science.* Jan 2007;48(1):390-395.

44.   Li Y, Chen H, Hou J, et al. Further characterization of ocular safety profile of commercially available preserved and preservative-free triamcinolone acetonide. *Retina.* Feb 2012;32(2):364-374.

45.   Garcia-Arumi J, Boixadera A, Giralt J, et al. Comparison of different techniques for purification of triamcinolone acetonide suspension for intravitreal use. *The British journal of ophthalmology.* Sep 2005;89(9):1112-1114.

46.   Bucher RS, Johnson MW. Microbiologic studies of multiple-dose containers of triamcinolone acetonide and lidocaine hydrochloride. *Retina.* Apr-May 2005;25(3):269-271.

47.   Meredith TA, McCannel CA, Barr C, et al. Postinjection endophthalmitis in the comparison of age-related macular degeneration treatments trials (CATT). Ophthalmology. 2015;122(4):817-821.

48.   VanderBeek BL, Bonaffini SG, Ma L. The Association between Intravitreal Steroids and Post-Injection Endophthalmitis Rates. Ophthalmology. Aug 2015. Epub ahead of print.

49.   Bressler SB, Almukhtar T, Bhorade A, et al. Repeated intravitreous ranibizumab injections for diabetic macular edema and the risk of sustained elevation of intraocular pressure or the need for ocular hypotensive treatment. JAMA ophthalmology. 2015;133(5):589-597.

50.   Freund KB, Hoang QV, Saroj N, Thompson D. Intraocular Pressure in Patients with Neovascular Age-Related Macular Degeneration Receiving Intravitreal Aflibercept or Ranibizumab. Ophthalmology. 2015;122(9):1802-1810.

51.   van Asten F, van Middendorp H, Verkerk S, et al. Are Intravitreal Injections with Ultrathin 33-G Needles Less Painful Than the Commonly Used 30-G Needles? Retina. 2015;35(9):1778-1785.

52.   Pang CE, Mrejen S, Hoang QV, Sorenson JA, Freund KB. Association between Needle Size, Postinjection Reflux, and Intraocular Pressure Spikes after Intravitreal Injections. Retina. 2015;35(7):1401-1406.

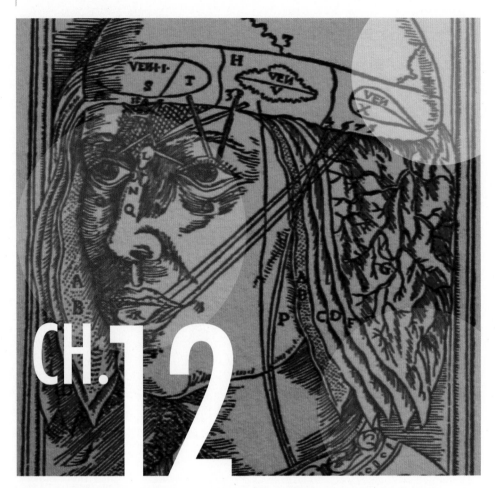

CH.12

Now What? Post-Treatment Management of Macular Edema

After enlightenment, the laundry. Zen proverb

Having finished treating your patient with whatever modality or modalities you have chosen, you then need to decide when to see them again. And this depends on what you did to them.

INJECTIONS

As mentioned in Chapter 11, if they had an injection you should warn them what to expect about having an irritated eye, as well as the signs of an infection and how to reach you. If you are new to injections, you may even want to bring them back in a week or so to check on things and to get a feel for what eyes look like after a shot, although you will rapidly realize that this is usually not necessary.

Speaking about follow up, *here is a really useful tip for injections and lasers (and anything else for that matter): Get on the phone yourself and call the patient a few days after the treatment. Patients may have minor questions that they forgot to ask you, and you can address any issues they have. You will also be surprised by how many patients will say, "Gee, doc, things are not better yet," meaning, "I realize you told me not to expect any improvement and that the goal is to slow things down, but I still thought that I was supposed to be able to throw away my reading glasses." In response, you can once again review the philosophy of treating diabetic retinopathy.*

Patients will be amazed that you took the time to check on them. When you do cataract surgery or Lasik, the patient can see for themselves the benefit of your efforts. Diabetic retinopathy patients do not usually get this type of reinforcement, and it is reassuring for them to know that you are concerned enough to make the extra effort to communicate.

As noted above, the real question is when to plan follow up for the next injection, and that depends on what you gave them. The best way to use anti-VEGF drugs is to follow a plan like the DRCR.net Protocol I discussed in Chapter 4; that usually means monthly visits to repeat the OCT and repeat an injection until the edema is gone or no longer improves. As the eye stabilizes, you can gradually spread out the visits. You will find that, with experience, you will get a good sense for this, and you can anticipate when patients will need to be treated. Patients can get good at this too; they can often recognize when the edema is recurring and get in sooner if need be.

But is it possible to be more specific about the meaning of the phrase "gradually spread out the visits"? To adopt a retina specialist's perspective on this, you have to go back to the beginning of anti-VEGF therapy for age-related macular degeneration. When Philip Rosenfeld at Bascom Palmer blew the world away by trying bevacizumab in macular degeneration, it rapidly became apparent that monthly treatment was the way to go for most patients. But some did OK with fewer injections, so a lot of trials included a "PRN" arm (Protocol I is one such study). In this case, PRN means that patients still came in once a month but doctors could decide whether or not they needed treatment at each visit. Unless they had problems, it would be another month before they were reassessed.

In the real world, it became apparent that PRN dosing was a real hassle for patients, and it doesn't really work that well (as can be seen with the PRN results in macular degeneration trials such as CATT). For instance, say a patient does best with an injection about every 6-7 weeks. On a PRN protocol, that patient would be waiting a couple of weeks before being treated at their scheduled monthly visit, and the monthly cycle and the optimal time for an injection would never quite line up. So many doctors began what is known as "treat and extend"—if a patient was responding to treatment, but still had a smidgen of disease to treat, they would be treated and the next visit would be pushed back a week or two. If things were not worse at the next visit, they would be treated and the interval between visits could be extended yet again. If they were worse, they were treated and brought back at whatever interval had previously kept them stable. This way, unnecessary visits were avoided and the timing of the treatments could be optimized for each patient.[10]

Now, is there any big data that proves this approach is best, either for macular degeneration or DME? Nope. (Or at least not yet—studies are underway.) But treat and extend does seem to work out well, especially in diabetes where the disease can go into remission as patients take better care of themselves. So when we say, "gradually spread out the visits", it means get the patient stable and then see if you can gradually add a week or two to their follow-up interval.

If you also treat age-related macular degeneration, you will have noticed that you can get into trouble really fast if you spread out visits too much and they have a big hemorrhage that can result in irreversible vision loss. DME tends to be a bit more forgiving—the retina seems to tolerate the ebb and flow of swelling much better than it tolerates the disrupted anatomy caused by a neovascular membrane. Some of the recent data from Protocol I (DRCR) shows that some patients can tolerate a certain amount of edema for up to three years without losing vision, so even if the patient is not a good observer you usually can't get into too much trouble as you spread out the visits conservatively. Of course, you will also be hammering them about the need to improve their systemic control at each visit, which is the most important determinant of how often you need to see them.

If the edema stays away for an extended period of time, it is still a good idea to keep checking them at least every three to four months in case they start to get some subtle eccentric edema that is asymptomatic. It is better to catch that sooner than later and it may even be treatable with simple things like a topical non-steroidal. Some patients do very well over time and may be able to go even more months between visits; they are usually the ones that "get it" and take good care of themselves, thereby eliminating their disease.

One other cool thing to be aware of when you use anti-VEGF agents: Because they can get into the systemic circulation, it is possible that as you treat the one eye, you may get a mild treatment effect in the fellow eye.[1] This doesn't always happen, and the effect tends to be mild. But occasionally it will be strong enough to improve borderline DME in the fellow eye. So if you are going to inject one eye, and the other eye is on the fence when it comes to needing treatment, don't automatically treat the second eye. It may improve as the first eye is treated. But be aware that the improvement may only be short-lived, so keep watching the patient. As an aside, some feel that this bilateral response may be more likely with Avastin because of its greater systemic absorption. This is also why some feel that Avastin may pose more risk than Eylea or Lucentis in patients that have had, for instance, a recent stroke or who are undergoing treatment for a foot ulcer (Chapter 4 covered this).

The follow up with triamcinolone is more complicated. You need to see them within a week or two simply to check the pressure, and then follow-up visits may need to be determined by the IOP in addition to retinal morphology. Also, remember that the pressure can rise insidiously, and this may show up well after the drug should have worn off.[2] If there is a concern about the pressure, it is reasonable to check the IOP periodically for six to eight months after the last injection, perhaps even longer if you are worried about them. As a comprehensive ophthalmologist, this is particularly important to remember because your retina specialist may forget about this and let the patient wander off without follow-up.

LASERS, LIKE THE RICH, ARE DIFFERENT.*

If you have done a laser, take a moment to give the patient some post-op "instructions." Even though there really is nothing they need to do or not do after a macular laser, patients may fill this void with all kinds of self-imposed restrictions, depending often on what family and friends tell them. It is important to remind them that there are no activity restrictions subsequent to the laser. Patients are often worried that if they strain or lift they will burst the little blood vessels that you have just sealed. You want to reassure them that this is not the case at all. They have also been told for years that if they use their eyes too much, they will go blind or something. It is amazing how many patients will restrict their lives by trying to "rest their eyes," when it makes no difference whatsoever how they use them. Even if they don't ask you about it, you should always take the time to reassure patients that they cannot hurt their eyes by using them. The concept that one can damage one's eyes by straining them is so ingrained, especially in older patients, that you may find them asking about visual restrictions on a regular basis.

You should remind them that their eyes might be a bit scratchy. (Artificial tear samples come in handy with lasers and injections. Patients may even feel that they actually received something of value if they walk out of the office with a free bottle in their hand.) Their eyes will often be blurry for a few days—and they need to be warned about that as well. You should also remind them, once again, that you aren't doing Lasik and that the goal is to slow things down—they cannot expect to suddenly get better after the laser.

Most of the studies and texts suggest seeing patients three to four months after a laser for macular edema. This is probably reasonable, because usually you will not begin to detect definite changes until this amount of time has passed. On the other hand, if someone just fiddled with your primary sense organ, would you really want to be told to come back in four months and good luck? Especially if you are being treated for something that may not be symptomatic, and that you have been told can get worse without you knowing it?

*Now do you see why they made you read F. Scott Fitzgerald in that one English class you took between p-chem and physics?

Cynically, the three- to four-month time frame is also reasonable from a financial standpoint, because Medicare and most insurance companies won't pay squat for an office visit within three months of a laser treatment. (This is known as a "90-day global"—the surgical fee includes 90 days of follow-up.) As discussed in the next paragraph, it does make sense to see them sooner, but because there are no ironclad guidelines you can decide what you think is best for yourself and the individual patient. The point is that as you develop your own approach to follow-up, you want to be able to periodically look into your soul and feel comfortable that you are always serving the best interests of the patient when you choose a follow-up interval and not just serving mammon. Whatever mammon is...

It is reasonable to bring laser patients back a little bit sooner, perhaps in six to eight weeks, simply to review the nature of the disease and the treatment and to make absolutely sure things are not deteriorating unexpectedly. This is especially important in patients who have one eye that is seeing much better than the eye you have treated— such patients may not know if their bad eye is getting worse, because the brain "covers" any blurriness with the vision from the good eye. The early visit also gives you a chance to head off any unhappiness patients may have with the success of the treatment by reminding them about the goals of treating macular edema. (If you are getting a sense that you have to repeat this every visit, you are right.) Finally, even if you can't detect much difference in the eye, you can at least tell the patient that things are stabilizing, which is always encouraging. As an aside, it usually isn't worth bringing the patient back before four weeks. During this time, even minimal laser can show reactive edema – yes, your careful laser causes inflammation and edema!

Of course, if the patient has worrisome disease that might become center-involving—or if hard exudates are trying to build up in the fovea—you definitely want to bring them back sooner than three months. These are patients who need close follow-up, because if things are going downhill you will need to consider intravitreal injections; you don't want to wait to let chronic damage build up.

One of the tricky things about putting this book together is that it is hard to make specific recommendations—the treatment of retinopathy can be a mixed bag. The next set of paragraphs applies best to situations where laser is the only treatment needed (i.e., peripheral edema) or for places where laser is the only treatment available.

Some of the toughest patients are those who return with some degree of persistent edema after laser. The original ETDRS protocol called for repeat lasers until the edema had resolved—these patients were treated every three months until "the macula was dry." Nowadays, the use of injections makes such an approach unnecessary; even back in the day this philosophy could vaporize the posterior pole pretty fast. (The macular scarring in Figure 10.1 from Chapter 14 is probably due to a doc who had an overly aggressive adherence to this approach.) The decision to re-treat with laser actually is a balancing act between six factors:

1. The patient's perception of how they are doing
   (Yes, this means taking a history. Sucks to be you.)

2. The visual acuity

3. The appearance of the retina relative to the pretreatment appearance

4. Where the swelling is

5. How much treatment has been placed

6. Efforts the patient is taking to improve their control

If you feel the area you have treated is not responding when you see the patient in follow-up, then the traditional approach is to keep treating them with laser. However, recognize that if the patient feels they are doing well (and their vision is stable), it is reasonable to monitor them a bit without treatment. You want to be sensitive to the fact that the patient may be getting frustrated with the whole process—they are going through a lot of effort (and cost) with nothing to show for it as far as they can tell. If you just keep hammering away as a knee-jerk reflex, you may lose your most valuable asset: the patient's trust. You do not want them to get fed up with the process so much that they refuse to come back; they will end up with much worse disease when they finally return in a year or two with symptomatic vision loss.

As a result, careful observation is often the best approach, especially if they are getting their diabetes under better control. You may find that your treatment will work surprisingly well if you just give it more time than the textbooks say, and if your patient's hemoglobin A1c is, uh, sweet.

If you watch such patients closely and re-treat parsimoniously, then the patient is much more likely to understand what you are doing, and is therefore more likely to stick with you for the long term. Your treatment will also be much less destructive than if you had continued to treat at every visit simply because there was some persistent swelling. Obviously, you don't want to wait months if you think the retina is not as good as it should be—you want to bring these patients back soon, so that if they don't improve you can jump in and treat with whatever modality is necessary.

This is where some sort of visual aid, such as a convincing OCT or photos of hard exudates driving towards the macula, can be very helpful. If you have to repeatedly treat a patient who has no symptoms, you can help them to understand the importance of close follow-up by showing them what you are treating. Hopefully they will understand that what they perceive with their vision does not reflect the reality of the situation.

If you think the patient is just not getting it when it comes to additional treatment, it is a good time to consider a second opinion. Even if you don't need one, it is always a good idea to assuage any concerns that the patient might have before they go out and do it on their own.

Please understand that this discussion does not advocate blowing off a retina that is not improving after treatment. There are some patients that simply need recurrent aggressive treatment to keep edema from the fovea. The point is that you need to be flexible with your approach, and keep in mind all of the six factors mentioned above when assessing the patient. Some patients, especially less sophisticated ones, are not as with you as you may think, and you should be prepared to treat the patient's head and not just their retina in order to keep from losing them altogether. As long as you watch the retinal morphology carefully, you can bend the rules and monitor patients without continually treating them just because the ETDRS toldja to.

Another thing to keep in mind is the use of intravitreal injections to control edema that is not center-involving. There really are no studies that address this yet. However, occasional patients have disease that is eccentric to the fovea that is really big and nasty—especially if it is threatening to bring a lot of hard exudates into the center. Under those circumstances you might need to put in a lot of laser to control it, and that can cause a lot of scarring over the long run. A few judicial injections might help control things without the need for extensive laser. Warning: there is no data that supports this, but it is something to keep in mind for problematic patients.

Some screwball things to watch for:

1. Blowing out the macula with too much treatment all at once. This was covered in Chapter 9, but it is worth repeating. Sometimes you can get carried away on a patient with lots of little microaneurysms and put in a ton of treatment because it is, well, fun, and you really feel like you are helping. These patients can come back a lot worse—you can literally push the edema right into the fovea. Usually you do not see these patients at the routine follow up visit. They tend to come in, quite unhappily, a week or two after your treatment. Just remember to go easy if you are starting treatment with laser.

2. A paradoxical increase in hard exudates. There are occasional patients who demonstrate a very annoying tendency to increase their hard exudates subsequent to treatment—even though the retina is actually better (Figure 1). This probably represents transient accumulation of hard exudates as the interstitial fluid is pumped out and protein and fats are left behind. Or perhaps the deposits become more visible as the retina thins and there is less scattering of light. Either way, it is really annoying to put in a beautiful treatment and, two months later, have 50% more hard exudates all over the place. The key here is to look at the retinal thickness and the vision, both of which should be stable to improved. If there is increased retinal thickening, then the hard exudates are worse because the patient is worse, and your treatment is not holding it back. If the retina otherwise looks good and you think you are dealing with this particular situation, it is reasonable to obtain photographs and check the patient in about six weeks. By the way, this paradoxical increase in hard exudates is not limited to laser treatment. It can also happen with anti-VEGF injections.[3] The increase does tend to be transient, though. If your treatment is working, the hard exudates will eventually fade away.[4] And remember that if you do see this phenomenon, it is a good idea to check the patient's lipids—they may be elevated and contributing to the problem.

3. Sometimes patients can have transient worsening of their macular edema subsequent to a severe systemic illness, such as a hospital admission for cardiac problems or for a significant infection. These patients may spontaneously improve over a couple of months as they recover, and it is reasonable to watch such patients a bit before automatically treating them (assuming they do not have a really worrisome morphology).

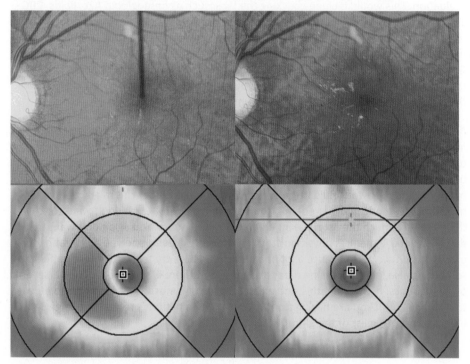

Figure 1: An example of a patient treated with gentle laser that reduced the macular edema as seen on the left and right OCTs, but resulted in a transient increase in hard exudates.

Follow-up testing

What kind of testing do you need to do? With injections, you really need to be doing regular OCTs—that test is crucial to assess treatment efficacy. It may be possible to do it without an OCT, for instance in places where resources are really limited, but that is not ideal.

With disease that is away from the fovea, however, you can often just look at the patient clinically and get a feel for how things are going—it turns out that numbers one through six above come down to simply talking to and examining the patient. Still, most docs will automatically get an OCT to learn the precise morphology, and it can be an invaluable teaching aid for patients.

An angiogram is usually not necessary unless the eye is worsening and one needs to know whether there are a lot of new leaks and where they are (i.e., a bunch of leaks at the edge of the foveal avascular zone mean it is time for intravitreal treatment; a bunch of new leaks to the side may allow precise focal treatment). Of course, if you do not have access to such testing then you have to rely on your clinical skills—which can be almost as good as the most expensive imaging equipment if you are a careful observer.

What if things are going downhill regardless of treatment modality?

This was covered a bit in Chapter 4, but it bears repeating. First, you need to make sure the patient's systemic risk factors are under control. If you are not getting the information you need from the patient or the patient's doctor, you should do your own evaluation. This would include checking the labs, such as hemoglobin A1c, lipids, CBC and renal studies, and checking the blood pressure yourself. Do not ever underestimate the importance of systemic control. It is amazing how a hopeless-looking macula can turn around with a combination of treatment and aggressive systemic management. Conversely, it can be very frustrating to treat patients who are cavalier about their control and listen to them complain that your lasers and shots aren't helping them as their macular capillaries spring leaks like a broken radiator.

Also, don't forget to check whether they are on one of the glitazone family of oral hypoglycemic agents. These can cause fluid retention and heart failure, and are thought to cause worsening of macular edema.[5] Patients whose macular edema is exacerbated by these medications usually have problems with systemic edema, but it can rarely happen without obvious fluid retention so you should consider this in any patient who has refractory cystic macular edema. You have to be careful—you don't want to scare the patient so much they stop taking the med on their own. You also don't want to demand that the medical physician stop these drugs on everyone you are treating for macular edema. You can cause a lot of trouble if doctors try to switch these patients to something else, and there is no data to suggest that there is some sort of universal effect on all diabetics. If anything, this side effect is relatively unusual.[6] The point is to at least think about this if you are having trouble controlling a patient's retinal swelling. Go to blue box land for a list of the glitazones...

The Glitazones (or, more unpronounceably, The Thiazolidinediones):

As monotherapy:	*As combination pills:*
Rosiglitazone (Avandia)	*Rosiglitazone and metformin (Avandamet)*
Pioglitazone (Actos)	*Rosiglitazone and glimepiride (Avandaryl)*
	Pioglitazone and metformin (Actoplus Met)

The handy thing to remember is that these are about the only oral hypoglycemic that start with the letter "A." (OK, for completeness, the other A-pills are: acetohexamide (Dymelor), glimepiride (Amaryl) and acarbose. None of these is associated with macular edema. Plus acetohexamide is no longer available in the USA, glimepiride is not a glitazone and you probably won't see any patients on acarbose because of its minimal efficacy and fun side effects like flatulence and diarrhea.)

And don't forget to rule out some sort of traction that is pulling up on the retina and keeping it swollen. This can be due to an epiretinal membrane that may be very subtle. Or it can be due to vitreomacular traction—the diabetic vitreous tends to be exceptionally sticky, and it can remain attached to the macula as it tries to contract due to normal aging and structural changes caused by the retinopathy. As it tightens it pulls on the macula, creating edema that tends to be very diffuse, cystic, and refractory to laser. Sometimes you can suspect this on clinical examination because there is a golden sheen overlying the retina that is best seen with a contact lens. These patients also tend to have far more leakage on the angiogram than one would suspect from the amount of retinopathy present. There may even be macular distortion if there is an associated epiretinal membrane or incomplete vitreous detachment. OCT testing makes it effortless to spot traction—something mentioned several times in the book but is so important that it is worth a rerun. The presence of traction mandates referral to a retinal specialist, because patients presenting with it may benefit from vitrectomy. (Chapter 19 discusses this and other reasons for referral for vitrectomy.)

Also, it is worth reviewing Chapter 27 on differential diagnosis when faced with refractory macular edema. There are other things—both systemic and intraocular—that can mimic or worsen retinopathy and if you miss them you will feel really stupid.

CHAPTER 12.1 Additional Bits That Don't Quite Fit Anywhere Else

Bit 1

OK. Let's say that you have optimized the patient's retina and they don't need any treatment—just a recheck in a few months. That sounds good to you, but here is something weird that only a patient's brain could come up with:

You say, "Everything looks great, we don't need to do anything, see you in a few months."

But the patient hears: "Well, your eyes are as good as they can get and there is nothing else that can be done. Ever. But we are going to make an appointment to see you in a few months for no reason." So the patient decides to not come back.

Of course, they do eventually come back when things are much worse and their eyes are a mess. And they tell you it's because you said that there was nothing that could be done, so they figured there was no reason to return.

Seriously. This will happen. Perhaps they are just manufacturing an excuse to avoid returning, or maybe they really are obtuse. Or maybe they are afraid of the bill. Or maybe you have the interpersonal skills of an EMR system. Regardless, you need to remind patients that even if they don't need anything at one visit, they will likely need treatment in the future, and if they wait until they have symptoms it may be too late. And don't be surprised if they act like this is brand new information; never underestimate how often you have to repeat the same thing, especially with less educated patients.

Bit 2. Doc, my vision is really blurry in the morning...

If patients develop edema that is in or around the fovea, you will often hear the above complaint. There are a few things you should consider when patients tell you this.

First of all, OCT studies have suggested that macular edema is worse in the morning, presumably because the retina swells during the night, just like someone's ankles swell up if they spend a lot of time standing.[7] Does this mean that they should sleep with a few pillows? No one has looked at this. Maybe you could do an ARVO project...

Another reason may be that their glucose is getting low in the early morning, and by the time they wake up it has rebounded a bit (kind of a mini-Somogyi phenomenon*). You will find that many diabetics, once they have significant retinopathy, will tell you that their vision gets blurry when their glucose gets a bit on the low side—not bad enough to give them the shakes or sweats, but their "weakened" retina seems to become especially sensitive to an otherwise asymptomatic drop in glucose. Indeed, for many patients this becomes a new way to tell that they need to check their sugar. Another factor may be that the dark-adapted retina is more metabolically active and needs more glucose at night.[11] The point is that you may want to suggest that patients set their alarm a few hours earlier than normal to do a fingerstick glucose. If the glucose is on the low side it may be contributing to their morning blur, and they may want to review their management with their medical doctor to see whether they can minimize their symptoms.

Don't forget non-retinal things, too. Sometimes patients will have a bit of dry eye that makes the tear film rusty in the morning—especially if they have superimposed lid problems like a lagophthalmos or floppy eyelid syndrome (the latter is not uncommon in obese elderly diabetics—and don't forget the possible association with obstructive sleep apnea, see Chapter 22). Another possibility could be early Fuchs corneal dystrophy. Your friendly neighborhood retina specialist will usually not think of this kind of stuff, so please protect your patient from our ignorance by being a good generalist and considering these possibilities.

There may be another reason that has no scientific basis whatsoever, but it sounds really good simply because there are sooo many patients—with all types of macular disease—who tell you their vision is blurry in the morning. There seems to be a part of the brain in charge of "Photoshopping" the world, and that part expects to have crisp vision upon awakening—as it has for the bulk of a patient's life. When it is suddenly faced with the kind of crummy vision that damaged maculae provide, it takes it a while to do some image processing to overcome the ragged input it is getting—almost like overcoming morning stiffness by getting up and moving around. (OK, this explanation looks really lame in print, but it plays well with patients—especially if you have ruled out any pathology. Go write your own book if you don't like it.)

---

*Remember, this is the thing where diabetics get low glucose during the night, and then compensatory mechanisms kick in and jack up the sugar by the time they awaken and check their glucose. Because the AM glucose is high, the doctor increases the PM insulin, which only makes the problem worse, and a vicious cycle ensues.

Bit 3

As long as we are talking about weird visual symptoms, here is another one. There are reports of Type 2 diabetics developing a transient hemianopsia in association with non-ketotic hyperglycemia. These resolve with correction of the metabolic abnormality, and are thought to represent focal occipital lobe seizures, perhaps due to localized dehydration. This is not common, but is worth knowing about so you don't just blow off a patient who gives a history suggestive of this.[8]

Bit 4

"But doc, I just need new glasses."

When you hear this, get ready to explain everything about retinopathy again, because it is likely the patient is really saying: "I'll put up with your lasers and injections a bit longer, and then I want to get my new glasses so I can finally see." Don't hesitate to remind them that no pair of glasses can make up for a bad macula, and hopefully that info sinks in before the patient ends up with three pairs of spectacles, none of which help.

But what if they actually do need new glasses because their refraction is old? A recent paper addressed this, indicating that the presence of DME doesn't alter the refraction— the swelling doesn't change the focal plane.[9] So you can try to prescribe new lenses while the patient is being treated for edema. But also remember that if their macula is swollen, they may give you bad answers when you start to do your subjective refraction. Even if we know empirically that the edema doesn't change the refractive status of the eye, you may want to hold off on writing a prescription until the macula is flatter and you are getting consistent results from the patient.

Are there any temporizing measures? Sure. It is amazing how often patients don't think of simple things like reading with a brighter light, using larger print (like on an e-reader), or adding a hand-held magnifier to the mix. Some patients even like to get a cheap pair of readers and put them on over their regular bifocals to make things bigger. Obviously, nothing works as well as a brand new set of eyes, but you can help patients a lot by suggesting simple things like this while you wait for their edema to respond to your ministrations.

CHAPTER 12.2

Refractory Diabetic Macular Edema in Places with No Specialists
(Remember, this book is not just for decadent docs in developed countries.)

What if you only have the option of doing laser—no intravitreal treatment or vitrectomy? One might hope a race of thoughtful aliens will take over our planet and equalize the distribution of healthcare so that no human being is treated worse than another. Until then, however, here are some suggestions.

First of all, if you really are the only one around, then it would be great if you could get some extra training, because your local population would benefit. Can you spend a week at a specialty center and learn some tricks and tips? Can you get a local service club (like the Lions or Rotarians) to help with cost? Some of the resources mentioned in Appendix 2 can help.

Second, it is likely that you are also in a situation where the medical control of your patients is dismal. As mentioned numerous times in this book, anything you do will not work as well if the patients are not well controlled. If there is anything that can be done to help with this, it will make your life a lot easier.

Third, if you are in this situation it is likely that patients are showing up late in their disease course, which only makes your job more impossible. Try to do anything to get them in sooner—patient and doctor education, assistance from service and religious organizations, telemedicine screening—whatever.

As for treating the patient with laser alone, there are not a lot of options beyond adding more spots as patients get worse. You need to do this parsimoniously, though. It has been suggested that once you put about 300 to 400 small spots into a posterior pole, you have done about as much as you can hope for with laser. Numbers like this came from the bad old days—before there were other treatments. Try not to go this high if possible, because this many spots will definitely expand and start to cause problems if the patient lives for many years (although you may not need to worry about this as much in developing countries, where diabetics tend to die sooner). If you are using very small light spots, though, it may be possible to perform multiple treatments, especially if you are just doing focal treatment directed at new microaneurysms.

Sadly, if you really are in this boat you are probably just barely staying ahead of your patient load, and you are also likely seeing lots of really bad, puffed-up maculas. In this situation, you are simply trying to keep eyes in the 20/400 range and not let patients go all the way to hand motions from macular disease. You also need to conserve your resources—if you do gentle, staged treatment on everyone, you can get so backlogged with following them that you can't take care of anyone else. This situation may be the one time when your best option is to do a grid of 100 to 150 spots and hope for the best, and then repeat as needed until you have put in about 300 to 400 spots total. Again, this is not ideal at all, but if there are no other solutions, this approach at least gets enough scarring in to help keep the retina from totally swelling up. Patient expectations are also crucial if you are forced to do this; it will affect not only their own follow up but also the follow up of everyone that they complain to about your treatments. They must understand that they will likely get worse no matter what you do, it is just that by treating them, you will hopefully hold on to as much vision as possible. (The last part of Chapter 5 reviewed this in more detail.)

Reminder: If you are in a situation like this, and you decide to try intravitreal injections, you need to give serious thought to the potential complications. What are your options if a patient gets into trouble? If there is no way to treat it, a case of endophthalmitis or retinal detachment or refractory glaucoma is far worse than count-fingers vision from macular edema. On the other hand, bringing such an excellent treatment modality to your patients would likely do far more good than bad. You just need to carefully balance all the risks if you have limited resources.

Unfortunately, there are some doctors in developed countries who do have access to specialists but act like they don't—until a patient's retina is far-gone. The approach for such folks seems to be: "How can I extract the maximum amount of money from a patient before I refer them out and don't get a chance to bill them again?" One hopes that they are not really thinking this, and that they are simply deluding themselves into thinking they know what is best for the patient without paying attention to the literature (not that thinking this is much of an improvement over greed). If you know someone like this, we can send them a free copy of this book if you wish. Here is the point: Do the best you can but if you think you are getting in over your head don't hesitate to ask for help. You—and your patient—will sleep better.

References

1.   Hanhart J, Tiosano L, Averbukh E, Banin E, Hemo I, Chowers I. Fellow eye effect of unilateral intravitreal bevacizumab injection in eyes with diabetic macular edema. *Eye (Lond).* Jun 2014;28(6):646-653.

2.   Williams CP, Konstantopoulos A, Rowley SA, Luff AJ. Late intraocular pressure rise following intravitreal triamcinolone injection. *Clin Experiment Ophthalmol.* May-Jun 2007;35(4):385-386.

3.   Pemp B, Deak G, Prager S, et al. Distribution of Intraretinal Exudates in Diabetic Macular Edema during Anti-Vascular Endothelial Growth Factor Therapy Observed by Spectral Domain Optical Coherence Tomography and Fundus Photography. *Retina.* Jul 24 2014.

4.   Domalpally A, Ip MS, Ehrlich JS. Effects of Intravitreal Ranibizumab on Retinal Hard Exudate in Diabetic Macular Edema: Findings from the RIDE and RISE Phase III Clinical Trials. *Ophthalmology.* Jan 16 2015.

5.   Idris I, Warren G, Donnelly R. Association between thiazolidinedione treatment and risk of macular edema among patients with type 2 diabetes. *Archives of internal medicine.* Jul 9 2012;172(13):1005-1011.

6.   Ambrosius WT, Danis RP, Goff DC, Jr., et al. Lack of association between thiazolidinediones and macular edema in type 2 diabetes: the ACCORD eye substudy. *Archives of ophthalmology.* Mar 2010;128(3):312-318.

7.   Kotsidis ST, Lake SS, Alexandridis AD, Ziakas NG, Ekonomidis PK. 24-Hour variation of optical coherence tomography-measured retinal thickness in diabetic macular edema. *European journal of ophthalmology.* Sep-Oct 2012;22(5):785-791.

8.   Lavin PJ. Hyperglycemic hemianopia: a reversible complication of non-ketotic hyperglycemia. *Neurology.* Aug 23 2005;65(4):616-619.

9.   Deak GG, Lammer J, Prager S, Mylonas G, Bolz M, Schmidt-Erfurth U. Refractive changes after pharmacologic resolution of diabetic macular edema. *Ophthalmology.* May 2014;121(5):1054-1058.

10.   Freund KB, Korobelnik JF, Devenyi R, et al. TREAT-AND-EXTEND REGIMENS WITH ANTI-VEGF AGENTS IN RETINAL DISEASES: A Literature Review and Consensus Recommendations. Retina. 2015;35(8):1489-1506.

11.   Ramsey DJ, Arden GB. Hypoxia and Dark Adaptation in Diabetic Retinopathy: Interactions, Consequences, and Therapy. Curr Diab Rep. 2015;15(12):118.

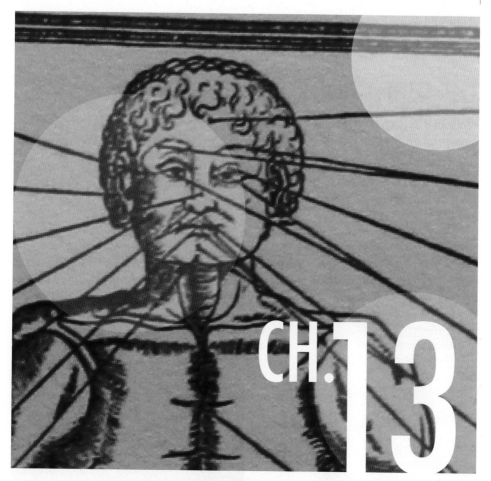

Proliferative Diabetic Retinopathy and Other Things That Go Bump in the Night

Bad news isn't wine. It doesn't improve with age. Colin Powell

THE NUMBERS

Proliferative diabetic retinopathy (PDR) is the real bad boy—it can make an eye stone-black blind. It tends to occur more often and more severely in younger patients with Type 1 diabetes, although no diabetic demographic is free from this problem. In general, the presence of proliferative disease is correlated to the duration of diabetes. For Type 1 patients, the risk is up to 50% if they have had diabetes for 20 years or more. Proliferative disease tends to be less frequent in Type 2 diabetes, perhaps only 10% or so after 20 years. These numbers are older figures; patients with better control have less proliferative disease. Still, depending on the population you care for you will likely have days when you feel swamped with proliferative concerns.

THE DISEASE

In macular edema, the problem stems from blood vessels that are leaky. In PDR, the problem stems from blood vessels that have simply died off. This starts in the periphery and gradually moves toward the center. The dead and dying retina then releases vasoproliferative factors that stimulate new blood vessels to grow (Figure 1).

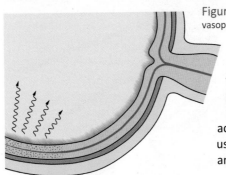

Figure 1: Ischemic peripheral retina emits vasoproliferative factors into the vitreous.

If the blood vessels simply grew in isolation, without any vitreous to latch onto, they would probably form beautiful branching patterns on the retinal surface—which would largely be of academic interest. Unfortunately, the vitreous is usually firmly attached to the retina in diabetics, and the blood vessels love to grow up into it like kudzu on a trellis (Figure 2).

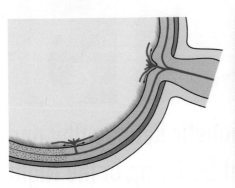

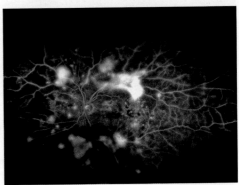

Figure 2: New vessels grow into the vitreous in response to the vasoproliferative substances. The photograph is a wide-field FA showing extensive peripheral capillary dropout and secondary neovascularization at the border of perfused and non-perfused retina. (Courtesy of Raj Maturi, M.D.)

All this would be bad enough, but it gets worse. These new blood vessels are quite leaky, and even if they don't hemorrhage, they allow serum components into the vitreous that the vitreous would normally never see. These compounds cause the vitreous to shrink up sooner than it otherwise would. Although vitreous collapse is a normal aging phenomenon, in proliferative retinopathy the contraction process is accelerated and tends to be more vicious. This is a real problem because the vitreous begins to pull on the new vessels (Figure 3).

Unfortunately, the new vessels are an extension of the retinal vasculature, and as such, they serve to lock the vitreous onto the retina wherever the blood vessels grow. This means that the shrinking vitreous now begins to tug on both the vessels and the retina. Moreover, connective tissue brought in by the new vessels also tends to shrink, which basically turns the vascular frond into the physiologic equivalent of a power winch that contracts in all directions. The result is that vessels at the surface of the retina are placed under constant tension, and the retina itself can be lifted from the pigment epithelium (Figure 4). If left untreated, the final result of this process is for the entire retina to be yanked off of the back of the eye.

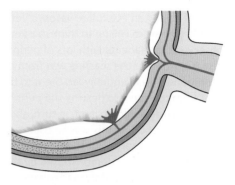

Figure 3: The vitreous contracts and starts to tug on the new vessels.

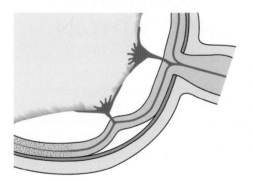

Figure 4: Progressive traction from the vitreous and the vessels begins to pull the retina off the RPE.

As this process is evolving, the stretched blood vessels crack open and bleed, subjecting the patient to periodic hemorrhages. The patient notices these hemorrhages as streaks, cobwebs and/or clouds in their vision. This will usually motivate them to come in for an evaluation if they have been less than diligent in their follow up. Unfortunately, things are usually far advanced by the time the hemorrhages occur. The blood vessels will often be quite extensive and even if they can be controlled with laser and/or injections, it is likely that there will still be a gradual buildup of traction as the vitreous and connective tissue continue to contract.

Such traction may cause anything from mild metamorphopsia (from pulling gently on the posterior pole) to total vision loss (from a tractional retinal detachment). Intermediate problems can include anything from chronic macular edema (due to subtle traction on the macula) to insidious vision loss (from traction on the nerve). If the traction is very severe it may even rip holes in the retina. Once the vacuum-pack seal between the retina and retinal pigment epithelium is broken, the gliotic retina can snap off the back of the eye like a broken garage door spring. These are all Bad Things.

Back in the old days of retinopathy treatment, doctors would shoot at the growing blood vessels on the assumption that the blood vessels themselves were the root of the problem. It quickly became apparent that this approach was worse than useless. Treating the blood vessels alone tends to make them go bananas; they just get revved up by the irritation of the treatment superimposed on the powerful neovascular stimulus created by the dying peripheral retina. Such treatment did not address the more fundamental issue of having an eye full of vasoproliferative substances. Fortunately, there were people who were willing to think in a very open-minded fashion, and these folks observed that patients with lots of peripheral retinal scarring had less active proliferative disease, whether the scarring was from iatrogenic retinal treatment or preexisting ocular conditions. This eventually led them to try using a laser—or a xenon arc, or even focused light from the sun—to destroy the peripheral retina, shutting down the production of vasoproliferative factors and, in turn, shutting down the neovascularization. Apparently the thought of doing this was so counterintuitive that many people thought these pioneers were insane, but they were ultimately vindicated by the success of panretinal photocoagulation as demonstrated by the Diabetic Retinopathy Study. By the way, these last sentences are horribly inadequate to relay the immense effort on the part of the many individuals who have given us this incredible tool to prevent blindness. Every once in awhile, as your foot is stomping away on the laser pedal like a speed-metal drummer, you should think about the broad shoulders upon which we are all standing as we treat diabetics with proliferative disease.

HUNTING DOWN NONPROLIFERATIVE AND PROLIFERATIVE RETINOPATHY IN YOUR PATIENT

Your eternal goal is to try to stop the above chain of events at an early stage before the diabetes can sink too many of its fangs into the retina—before the vessels and fibrovascular tissue have spread all over the place. You should therefore become adept at identifying anything that even remotely suggests the impending arrival of proliferative disease. This means becoming familiar with the various stages of nonproliferative diabetic retinopathy (NPDR). Remember that NPDR can be minimal, mild, moderate or severe (Table 1 shows the standard classification scheme). Severe NPDR is of greatest importance, making it the one you need to be able to recognize unfailingly.

Fortunately, the 4-2-1 rule makes matters relatively easy when it comes to sorting out patients with good-bad retinopathy from those with bad-bad retinopathy. The 4-2-1 part refers to four quadrants of hemorrhages, two quadrants of venous beading or one quadrant of intraretinal microvascular abnormalities (IRMAs). If a patient has any one of these criteria, then they have severe NPDR.

The required amount for each of these findings is defined by the standard photographs used in all of the studies, and you should cram these images into your brain so that you can quickly pick out a patient at risk. (Figures 5-7)

Table 1: Classification of Diabetic Retinopathy

Level	Definition
Minimal nonproliferative retinopathy	Microaneurysms only
Mild nonproliferative retinopathy	Microaneurysms and one or more of the following: • Retinal hemorrhage • Hard exudates • Nerve fiber layer infarct
Moderate nonproliferative retinopathy	Hemorrhages and microaneurysms > standard photograph 2A in at least one quadrant and one or more of the following: • Nerve fiber layer infarct • Venous beading • Intraretinal microvascular abnormality
Severe nonproliferative retinopathy	One of the following: • Hemorrhages/microaneurysms > standard photograph 2A in all 4 quadrants • Venous beading in at least 2 quadrants • IRMA > standard photograph 8A
Proliferative retinopathy	Neovascularization on the disc or elsewhere
High-risk proliferative retinopathy	One or more of the following: • Neovascularization of the disc > ¼ disc area • Any neovascularization of the disc and vitreous/preretinal hemorrhage • Neovascularization > ½ disc area with vitreous/preretinal hemorrhage
Advanced proliferative retinopathy	Proliferative retinopathy with tractional retinal detachment or with extensive vitreous hemorrhage

(Reproduced, with permission, from Fong DS, Ferris FL, Focal Points: Clinical Modules for Ophthalmologists, "Practical Management of Diabetic Retinopathy." American Academy of Ophthalmology, 2003.)

If memorizing the scheme is too painful, you can simplify it this way: if you look in and you can see obvious venous beading and/or definite IRMA, then the patient has severe NPDR or something very close to it. See the next box if you think they have severe NPDR based on hemorrhages alone...

Although the presence of hemorrhages is one of the criteria for severe NPDR, as a practical matter it can be a less reliable predictor in clinical practice. Hemorrhages, like glory, can be fleeting, and they are not quite as dependable as hardcore venous beading and IRMA.[1] Just review the chapter on differential diagnosis to see the many ways hemorrhages may be unrelated to factors that cause proliferative disease. Then look in Chapter 22, where hemorrhages can resolve with institution of good systemic control. Finally, remember how patients on blood thinners may have very dramatic hemorrhages that have nothing to do with NPDR. The real point here is that if you think a patient has NPDR solely because of four quadrants of hemorrhages, and if you are therefore going to treat them with laser, you should be sure they don't have hemorrhages for other reasons. For instance, if they have hemorrhages without the typical venous dilation seen in severe NPDR, you should look for other causes.

When it comes to hunting down evidence of severe NPDR, hemorrhages and venous beading tend to be fairly obvious. IRMAs, on the other hand, can be a bit trickier to identify. IRMAs are tiny, and are usually located in little patches outside the arcades, so it is something that you have to look for with your 90-diopter lens (or 78-diopter or whatever fundus-o-rama lens is being marketed this year by the lens manufacturers). You will need to have the patient look in different directions, similar to the indirect ophthalmoscope exam, but done at the slit lamp. This is something that has to be mastered in order to do a thorough exam for diabetic retinopathy.

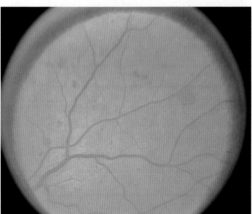

Figure 5: (left) ETDRS Standard Photograph 2a, showing severe hemorrhages and microaneurysms (remember – you need these in four quadrants to get severe NPDR). (Courtesy of the Early Treatment Diabetic Retinopathy Study Group)

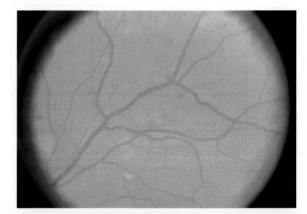

Figure 6: (right) ETDRS Standard Photograph 6a, the criterion for going from mild to moderate venous beading. Notice that you don't need a lot. If you can see obvious venous beading in a patient, then it is bad (but you need two quadrants for severe NPDR). Also, be sure that it is venous beading and not just venous caliber changes or venous narrowing at arteriovenous crossings. With true venous beading, the beaded section must be wider than the normal caliber and because venous beading tends to be a late finding, you should also judge it by the company it keeps – there should be other worrisome findings as well. (Courtesy of the Early Treatment Diabetic Retinopathy Study Group)

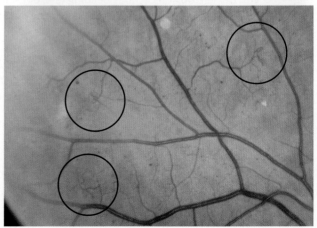

Figure 7: (right) ETDRS Standard Photograph 8a, the circles show the odd, curly Q shape of IRMA. (Courtesy of the Early Treatment Diabetic Retinopathy Study Group)

Late-Seventies programmed-learning moment: What is a skill that has to be mastered in order to do a thorough exam for diabetic retinopathy?

      a. Understanding the conoid of Sturm

      b. Understanding phacodynamics

      c. Understanding Medicare

      d. Using a slit lamp indirect lens to study the midperiphery

      e. Do you see why the Seventies were so much fun?

It is really hard to manage diabetics without being able to do this—a lot of disease starts in the periphery and you not only need to assess for hemorrhages, IRMAs and venous beading, but you also need to look carefully for early proliferative disease. Many patients will get significant proliferative changes in the periphery before you start to see things around the macula and nerve. You don't want to be the last person on the chart to say that they have non-proliferative disease, and have them show up with a vitreous hemorrhage 3 weeks later from peripheral neovascularization that you obviously missed.

When hunting for IRMAs you are looking for fine, irregular vessels that seem to be within or just at the surface of the retina—they do not follow any normal flow pattern and tend to meander around in a tiny area. Sadly, almost every attempt to reproduce photos of IRMAs is foiled by the limitations of the printing process—Figure 7 is a blowup of the standard ETDRS figure, so you get some idea of what you are looking for.

Why bother with this? Eyes with severe NPDR have as much as a 50% chance of developing some degree of PDR within one year, and perhaps a 15% chance of developing high-risk PDR. These averages are from the ETDRS—your mileage may vary with specific patients. If a patient has a long history of good control and very slow progression of their retinopathy, then their risk is much less. If they have poor control and are rapidly going to severe NPDR, then they are far more likely to get into trouble. The point is that knowing the stages of NPDR allows you to determine the patient's risk for progression to PDR and to decide how closely to follow the patient. Staging the patient may also help you decide whether they need panretinal photocoagulation before they get a chance to develop proliferative disease. Vide infra.

WHICH BRINGS US TO PDR Itself...

Although severe NPDR may be the ideal time to identify the potential for trouble, proliferative diabetic retinopathy is your true enemy. Fortunately, PDR does not tend to be subtle, as long as you take the time to look for it. Even very small neovascularization at the disc (NVD) is readily apparent, simply because the vessels weave over the nerve in a path very different from the normal radial capillaries. Remember that NVD does not really need to be exclusively at the disc to be called NVD—vessels within 1 disc diameter of the nerve also qualify.

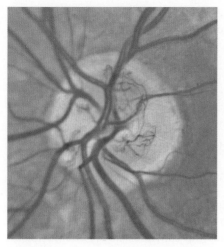

Figure 8: This is the picture that launched a million lasers. It is standard photograph 10a from the Arlie House Classification System – and it shows the size of NVD that qualifies as high risk. (Courtesy of the Early Treatment Diabetic Retinopathy Study Group)

Neovascularization located farther from the disc (known as neovascularization elsewhere—NVE) can sometimes be fainter, and can therefore be difficult to distinguish from IRMA if it is small. IRMA is localized within the retina, and although it may be irregular, it usually does not have a latticework of blood vessels as one sees with neovascularization. NVE is on top of the retina; sometimes it is flat and grows along the surface, while other times it is elevated and grows up into the vitreous. A fluorescein angiogram (FA) is helpful for determining the difference in problematic cases; IRMA may leak a bit, but it doesn't leak anywhere near as much as true neovascularization. On the other hand, an FA will light up small patches of neo like a Broadway marquee. Ideally, you should not need an FA to identify even very early neo—you should have found it with a careful exam of the periphery as discussed above. If the view is hazy, though, or if you are still not sure whether there is any neo present, an FA can be very helpful (Figure 9-11).

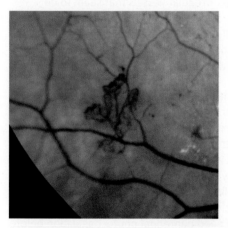

Figure 9: (Left) A typical small patch of NVE. Note how it consists of multiple branching vessels. If you could see it in stereo, you would note that it is growing off the surface of the retina and into the vitreous.

Figure 10: Below the circles highlight patches of IRMA that are obvious on the red-free on the left, but barely leak dye in the late phase in the angiogram on the right. Compare this to the profuse leakage that occurs with true neovascularization (e.g., **Figure 11**).

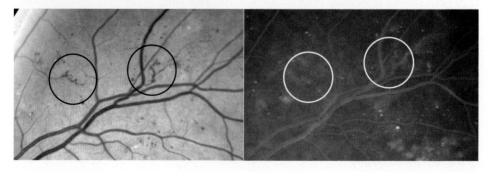

Figure 11 is also notable because it shows a type of retinopathy that can be very deceptive unless you look carefully. Some patients will have what is known as a "featureless retina." This means that the usual signs of disease, such as multiple hemorrhages, are no longer present, presumably because the retina has just plain died off. You will miss the early proliferative disease in these cases if you just quickly screen the fundus with a 20D lens and do not study the retina at the slit lamp.

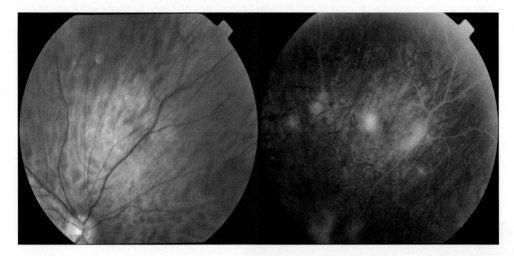

Figure 11: An example of how an angiogram can light up NVE that is not especially visible on clinical exam. Although the color photo does not show the neo, it is likely that a careful 90D exam of the periphery would have identified the small new vessels. Also note that the color shows a very "featureless retina" – the retina is so damaged that the usual signs of worrisome retinopathy are absent; there are no telltale hemorrhages, etc.

Incidentally, if you are doing an FA to look for new vessels, be sure to tell the photographer what you are looking for so they will scan the periphery for anything that lights up. It is easy to focus only on the posterior pole when doing angiograms, but there is a lot of data in the periphery, especially with diabetes. In fact, it makes sense to have your photographer routinely do a survey of the periphery to look for leakage—they get to be a better photographer and you get more info about how ischemic the eye is and where to place panretinal photocoagulation. Newer wide-field angiogram systems automatically provide a view of the periphery that identifies lesions that standard photographs miss. (The photo in Figure 2 is from such a system.) It has also been shown that peripheral abnormalities, such as new vessels and ischemia, are correlated with progression of retinopathy.[5,6] So even if you can't afford a wide-field system, try to get as much info from your standard angiogram as you can.

By the way, it is always a bit embarrassing to order an FA for macular edema, only to find buds of neo at the nerve or along the arcades that you didn't see because you were too busy studying the topology of the macula. Of course, it is even more embarrassing to completely miss the buds of neo on the FA and then spot them when you look at the angiogram three months later because the patient had a vitreous hemorrhage that you could have prevented. Been there, done that.

Missing something obvious is much less likely at the early stages of your career, when everything is new and exciting. It is much more likely to happen when you have some *experience and confidence and you begin to chug along quickly. Develop a systematic way to read an FA in order not to miss anything, and try to stick with it no matter how fast you want to go—it will save you again and again.*

When it comes to sniffing out PDR, another important clue is the presence of some type of vitreous hemorrhage. A big hemorrhage is usually about as subtle as a golf cart in a hotel bathtub—the diagnosis is easy. Sometimes, though, patients will have the symptoms of a hemorrhage (i.e., dots, streaks, cobwebs and/or floaters in their vision) but there is no obvious blood on first inspection. Study such patients carefully. It is possible for patients to have limited hemorrhages, for which they will be very symptomatic, yet you will not see any blood because the amount is small or it has been rapidly washed out. Look at the vitreous with the slit lamp, as you would for a uveitis patient—sometimes the only heme to be found is a few red blood cells in the anterior vitreous. Also, carefully inspect the lower vitreous. Subtle hemorrhages will gravitate down there, and you may need to use a 90-diopter to find faint clouds of blood floating around. Blood can also be identified incidentally as part of the OCT exam, especially with spectral domain machines. You can actually see the red blood cells floating in front of the retina (Figure 12). This is important, because if there is blood, you really have to look carefully for neovascularization—even get an FA, if necessary.

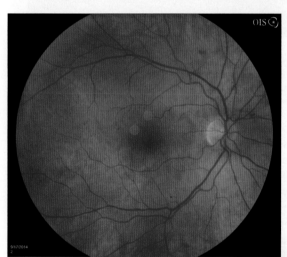

Figure 12: This patient presented complaining of new floaters, but there isn't much to see clinically and there were no blood cells in the anterior vitreous. However, the OCT demonstrates scattered blood cells in front of the retina (the little white dots). The patient had had a partial vitreous detachment, and the separation had torn some superficial retinal capillaries, so he could see the floaters but they were not obvious on exam. There was no proliferative disease. By the way, this technique is also useful for identifying white blood cells in patients with uveitis. (Extra credit if you spot the tiny preretinal hemorrhage just superonasal to the nerve on the photo.)

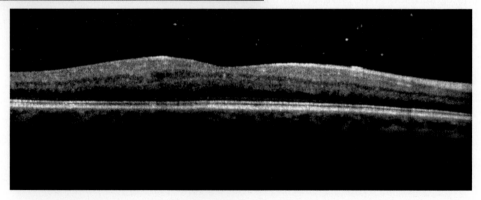

Diabetics can have hemorrhages without neo, though, so don't just look for "clouds of red" and then bust out the laser. First of all, diabetics tend to have a stickier vitreous that doesn't separate as easily. If they do get even a partial age-related vitreous detachment, all of the fragile capillaries on the retinal surface are more likely to bleed as the vitreous peels away. This can create a transient hemorrhage but it does not represent a threat to the patient's vision so no treatment is needed. This partly explains why there was a whole subset of patients in the Diabetic Retinopathy Study who fell into the category of having a vitreous hemorrhage without obvious PDR and why many of these patients did not need any laser (more on this below).

By the way, never forget that diabetics can get non-diabetic problems, such as retinal tears. If a vitreous hemorrhage makes you go into proliferative-disease hunter-killer mode, you can totally miss a tear if you don't also remember to study the far periphery for new breaks. Try to keep an open mind about all the wonderful ways an eye can go bad and do not limit your thinking to diabetic complications just because a patient is diabetic.

Patients who present several months after their symptoms began can also be confusing, because older hemorrhages can decolorize and look like whitish or yellowish globs at the bottom of the vitreous cavity (so-called "chicken fat" hemorrhages). Do not mistake these old hemorrhages for inflammatory vitreous changes such as snowballs or snow banking. Bombing a hemorrhagic diabetic eye with steroids is bad for the patient—and will remove stars from your god-of-ophthalmology score.

PUTTING IT ALL TOGETHER

OK, so now you have scoured the fundus for signs of IRMA or early PDR. Exactly why do you need to memorize the 4-2-1 rule and hunt around for all this stuff, anyway?

There is no question that one of the landmark studies in all of ophthalmology was the Diabetic Retinopathy Study (DRS), which clearly demonstrated the usefulness of laser treatment in avoiding blindness back in the 1970s.[2] (Both the DRS and the ETDRS produced a host of papers; the cited reference is an example.)

As part of this study, proliferative diabetic retinopathy was classified into low-risk and high-risk disease. (Nowadays "low-risk" PDR may be referred to as PDR without high-risk characteristics—see Table 1.) Determining whether a patient has high-risk PDR involves adding up various factors to assign the level of disease. For instance, high-risk vessels at the disc had to be at least one-quarter to one-third disc area (Figure 8 is the standard example chosen for this), and NVE was considered to be significant if it was greater than one-half disc area. Table 2 shows a good summary of how all the different factors were added up to assign the overall risk. For those of us not employed as biostatisticians, however, each one of the following is an admittedly less elegant but simpler approximation for how to call high-risk PDR:

> 1: Any NVD that you can easily see is high-risk PDR.

> 2: Pre-retinal or vitreous blood in the eye with new vessels anywhere is high-risk PDR. 'Nuff said.

Table 2: Definition of High Risk PDR

High-risk PDR was defined as any one of the following:

- Mild neovascularization of the disc (NVD) with vitreous hemorrhage.

- Moderate to severe NVD with or without vitreous hemorrhage (greater than or equal to DRS standard 10A, showing one-quarter to one-third disc area of NVD.

- Moderate (one-half disc area) NVE with vitreous hemorrhage.

High-risk PDR was also defined by any combination of three of the four retinopathy risk factors:

- Presence of vitreous or pre-retinal hemorrhage.

- Presence of new vessels.

- Location of new vessels on or near the optic disc.

- Moderate to severe extent of new vessels.

Adapted from American Academy of Ophthalmology, Basic and Clinical Science Course, Section 12. Retina and Vitreous 2013-2014, page 105-106.

Once you decide a patient has high-risk PDR, you are obligated to treat with panretinal photocoagulation. The reason is that patients tend to do rather horribly on their own once they have reached high-risk disease. In the DRS, treatment cut the risk of severe vision loss by about 50% over the course of the study—and that was at a time when diabetics were not as well controlled medically, and the treatment was often hammered in all at once (and was therefore more likely to decrease the vision). It is likely that these days we obtain even better results with staged treatment, anti-VEGF injections and more emphasis on better medical care. Figure 13 is the classic graph of the overall DRS results.

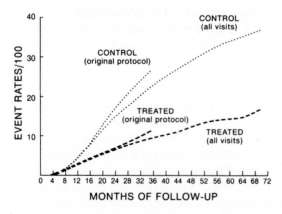

Figure 13: Cumulative rates of severe visual loss for the DRS (the protocol was changed in 1976 to allow more treatment of high-risk eyes). This graph, and the heroic work behind its discovery, is truly awesome (in the traditional, non-surfer sense of the word). (The Diabetic Retinopathy Study Research Group. DRS report #8. Ophthalmology 1981; 88:583-600. Copyright Elsevier 1981)

But deciding to treat definite high-risk proliferative disease is the easy part. The hard part is deciding about treatment in situations that are less black and white...

DRS/ETDRS GAMES When to Do Premature Photocoagulation

Although the DRS clearly demonstrated the need for treatment in patients with high-risk disease, no one was sure how aggressive to be in patients with less than high-risk disease. One aspect of the ETDRS looked at this and found a trend suggesting a beneficial treatment effect if patients were given PRPs at any level of nonproliferative diabetic retinopathy (NPDR).[3] However, the treatment benefits were very small with earlier levels of NPDR. For instance, there was only a dinky subset of patients with mild or moderate NPDR who seemed to benefit from early treatment. Because PRP has definite risks (which will be discussed at length in the upcoming chapters), it is felt that observation is best for these patients.

When the retinopathy progresses to severe NPDR or PDR without high-risk characteristics, it turns out that the treatment benefit was more pronounced—but still fairly small. As a result, the same conservative approach was suggested: Given the hassle and risk of treatment and relatively small benefit, some patients may be better off with careful observation rather than laser. There are, however, other factors that may make you decide to treat. Here are some:

> 1. Severe progressive disease in the fellow eye. Diabetic eyes tend to head down the same path, and the first eye will let you know what the second eye may decide to do.

> 2. The patient's ability to follow up. This may be a very important factor in developing countries, where logistics and economics may prevent careful sequential evaluations, and where early treatment may give a patient much better odds of remaining a functioning member of society.

> 3. Poor control and/or lots of medical problems may warrant earlier intervention, since these patients may go downhill faster and/or may miss appointments.

> 4. A patient who needs to be on Coumadin or other blood thinners may need earlier treatment, given the risk of more pronounced bleeding if more advanced proliferative disease is allowed to develop.

> 5. A very important factor is the rate of change of the patient's disease. A patient who has good control and has smoldered along with mild to moderate NPDR can easily be monitored if they slowly begin to develop severe NPDR or low-risk PDR. On the other hand, a patient who is rapidly going through these stages is at much greater risk for rapid progression to high-risk disease, and should have earlier treatment. (Incidentally, the ability to understand terms like "the rate of change" justifies those calculus classes you took years ago. See? They were worth it.)

6. The type of diabetes also plays a role. A later analysis of the data suggested that patients with Type 2 diabetes, or patients older than 40 years old (which is usually the same thing), are more likely to benefit from scatter photocoagulation when they have severe NPDR or early PDR without high-risk characteristics. This did not seem to be true for patients with Type 1 diabetes who had the same degree of retinopathy. It is not clear why this is the case; perhaps older patients are more likely to get a vitreous hemorrhage once they get neo because their vitreous is more jiggly compared to the more formed vitreous in younger patients. Whatever the reason, this data does support consideration of earlier treatment in older patients.[4]

7. This is a big one, so pay attention. All the above recommendations come from the time before anti-VEGF injections. However, there is growing realization that injections will stop the progression of proliferative disease in its tracks, and actually reverse the overall level of retinopathy. The problem is that injections are transient and laser is permanent. But if a patient is getting regular injections for DME, it may reasonable to delay an early PRP on patients with severe NPDR or early PDR a bit. The injections may change how much laser you need to put in, or perhaps even obviate the need for laser in some cases (although you need to watch such patients closely for progression if the injections stop). This issue starts to get complicated and will be covered in the next chapter—so hold this thought for now.

What if there is a vitreous hemorrhage but no obvious neo?

Although knowing when to intervene earlier is important, it is also good to know when to hold off. Such a situation may occur when you are faced with a patient who has a vitreous hemorrhage but no evidence of neovascularization. The DRS showed that a vitreous hemorrhage alone is generally not an indication for PRP, but this is true only if you are certain there is no neovascularization. If there is a localized preretinal hemorrhage that blocks the view of a section of the retina, or a dense vitreous hemorrhage that allows only a limited view, it is usually best to assume there are new blood vessels somewhere and treat the patient.

Remember *that if the hemorrhage is so dense that there is no view, you have to get an ultrasound to be sure the retina is not being pulled off. You are taking a big risk for both yourself and your patient if you can't see the retina and you don't get an ultrasound; if something is going wrong back there, it is usually bad to do nothing.*

The nature of the retinopathy in the fellow eye can help in such a situation, too. If the fellow eye has already had proliferative disease that required laser, it is worthwhile considering laser in the second eye even if you do not see any obvious neovascularization. On the other hand, if there is only minimal diabetic disease in the fellow eye, observation may be the best course. (Just because nothing is simple, patients may have asymmetric disease as a manifestation of carotid artery obstruction—see Chapter 27 for details.)

If the hemorrhage is mild, though, you need to study the retinal periphery carefully, or even consider fluorescein angiography to help you decide whether there are new vessels. If there are no vessels, then it is definitely better to watch such patients; recall that the diabetic vitreous is sticky and is more likely to break a few capillaries if it separates. You will end up needlessly burning retina if you automatically treat every diabetic with a mild vitreous hemorrhage.

Finally, for the second time in the same chapter, never forget that diabetics can get non-diabetic problems such as retinal tears, so remember to inspect the far periphery closely—don't just look in the midperiphery and quit if you don't see anything.

What if a patient shows up with old, burned-out disease that was never treated?

Although most of your life you will be faced with patients who are in the progressive stages of PDR, remember that if left untreated the neovascular stimulus eventually fades as the retina just plain dies off. Most of the time, if the disease is allowed to run its course the retina ends up like a shriveled orchid in the center of a blind eye (hence the existence of books such as this). You may, however, occasionally see patients in whom this process has occurred with little disruption of the central retina—these patients essentially avoided the typical disastrous outcome and "survived" the proliferative phase of their retinopathy. Such patients often have very broad areas of fibrosis in the periphery, where the old neovascularization involuted and became quiescent. Deciding whether to treat such patients can be difficult—the standard rules do not apply. These patients have somehow achieved a metastable state, and there is always a concern that by going in and aggressively treating with laser you will push them into hemorrhagic or tractional problems that they might not otherwise have developed. In general, however, it is safer to gently work in a PRP, rather than to do nothing. This is because the wide swaths of untreated peripheral retina may become more ischemic with time, and lead to late problems such as recurrent retinal proliferation or anterior segment neovascularization.

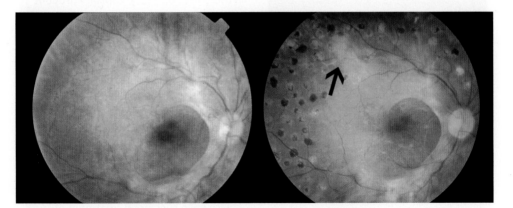

Figure 14: A patient with fibrotic, end-stage PDR. Note how everything seems to be quiescent prior to treatment, but after laser there is an area where subtle neovascularization regressed and became fibrotic (arrow). The omnipresent neovascular stimulus of the ischemic retina makes treatment a safer bet than observation in eyes like this; you are buying the patient insurance that nothing worse happens in the future. Do go slow if you treat such an eye, however. Rapid, carpet-bomb laser will likely scramble things up in such a fragile eye, perhaps even causing a tractional retinal detachment.

If you decide to treat an eye like this, and usually you will, the patient (and you) must understand that there is always a small risk of stirring up trouble. The one thing you don't want to do is to decide that you have to make up for lost time by hammering the entire retina aggressively. This carries a high risk of screwing things up in such a delicate eye. It is much better to treat these patients gradually over a number of sessions, and to avoid heavy burns around the atrophic or tractionally-detached retina, which could lead to hole formation. It is also a good idea to be very careful about doing anti-VEGF injections for macular edema in these patients. As we will see in the next chapter, one of the biggest concerns with using those drugs in a patient with widespread proliferative disease is that all the vascular fronds contract aggressively under the influence of the drug and snap the retina off. This doesn't mean you can't use anti-VEGF agents in these patients—just be sure the patient knows the risks and that you have access to a retina specialist who can do surgery if necessary. (But recognize that he or she is not going to be happy about the problem—these types of detachments are tough to fix.)

Do you have to have an FA before a PRP? No. But...

An FA is not mandatory before treating isolated PDR. The great ophthalmic court in the sky should not frown upon you if you do not get one, especially because in many places it may not be an option. However, if it is available, you should consider doing the test for a few reasons:

1. An FA can give you an idea of exactly where most of the capillary ischemia is in the periphery; this will help you assess how bad the disease is, where to treat, and how aggressive you will need to be with your PRP (Figure 15).

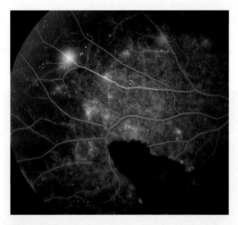

Figure 15: Another example of an FA lighting up neovascularization and defining the border between perfused and non-perfused retina. Note the pre-retinal hemorrhage that does not appear to be near the obvious new vessels. There may be neovascularization underneath the heme, or it may have originated from puffy and swollen vessels inside the perfused retina that are just beginning to sprout new vascular channels.

2. You will get info about the functional status of the macular blood vessels. Sometimes the macula can look fairly decent on clinical exam and OCT, but there may be subtle capillary dropout or leakage on the angiogram, indicating that the macula is more fragile than you would think. These findings suggest that you should go very slowly when you start doing the PRP to avoid stressing out the capillaries and making the patient's central vision worse due to macular edema. Also, if the patient is beginning to develop capillary dropout in the temporal macula you will need to warn the patient about the potential for vision loss that exists with even successful treatment of their proliferative disease. In the manly world of retina specialists, where manly

men and women think up manly names for microscopic problems in order to feel more manly, this particular pattern is sometimes called the flying wedge of death (Figure 16). This pattern does not always progress, and in fact, some patients may be stable for years—especially if they have good control. Still, it is important to let the patient know what you are worried about and what it might mean to their vision. Of note, anti-VEGF agents complementing the laser can be useful with this pattern.

3. A less "medically necessary" but remarkably powerful use of the angiogram is for patient education. If a patient has yet to display symptoms of their retinopathy, you can try to convince them of the impending danger by showing them the fronds of neovascularization surrounding their posterior pole. This is not a reason to subject a patient to an invasive test like an FA, but if a study is done, it is a shame to not use it for this purpose.

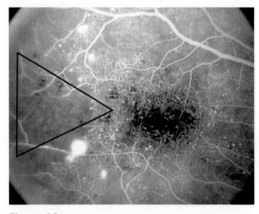

Figure 16: A triangular wedge of ischemia encroaching into the macula.

On the other hand (and the problem with being a conscientious doctor is recognizing that there is always an "other hand"), you may find yourself in a practice where obtaining an angiogram is not a simple thing. If you do not have easy access to an FA, it may be better to go without one if your clinical sense is that the retina does not hold any big surprises. Making the patient jump through hoops to undergo the pleasure of an FA, and to get even more medical bills, may be enough to drive them away from being treated. This is way worse than not having an FA in the first place. Everything is a balance...

References

1.   Wilkinson CP, Ferris FL, 3rd, Klein RE, et al. Proposed international clinical diabetic retinopathy and diabetic macular edema disease severity scales. *Ophthalmology.* Sep 2003;110(9):1677-1682.

2.   Photocoagulation treatment of proliferative diabetic retinopathy. Clinical application of Diabetic Retinopathy Study (DRS) findings, DRS Report Number 8. The Diabetic Retinopathy Study Research Group. *Ophthalmology.* Jul 1981;88(7):583-600.

3.   Early photocoagulation for diabetic retinopathy. ETDRS report number 9. Early Treatment Diabetic Retinopathy Study Research Group. *Ophthalmology.* May 1991;98(5 Suppl):766-785.

4.   Ferris F. Early photocoagulation in patients with either type I or type II diabetes. *Trans Am Ophthalmol Soc.* 1996;94:505-537.

5.   Silva PS, Dela Cruz AJ, Ledesma MG, et al. Diabetic Retinopathy Severity and Peripheral Lesions Are Associated with Nonperfusion on Ultrawide Field Angiography. Ophthalmology. Sept 2015. Epub ahead of print.

6.   Silva PS, Cavallerano JD, Haddad NM, et al. Peripheral Lesions Identified on Ultrawide Field Imaging Predict Increased Risk of Diabetic Retinopathy Progression over 4 Years. Ophthalmology. 2015;122(5):949-956.

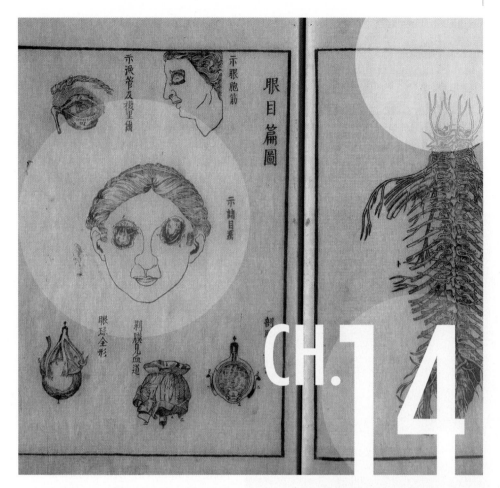

Actually Doing Panretinal Photocoagulation (PRP). Or Not.

As any artist can tell you, it is easier to reach perfection than to stop there. Robert Brault

Performing a PRP is one of those things that seems incredibly simple in the abstract, but actually requires a great deal of finesse to do properly. It is not just a matter of developing the technical skills needed to do the laser. You also have to consider the status of the eye and the systemic medical status of the patient. You even need to take into account far more subjective factors, such as the visual requirements of the patient and even their emotional status.

But first, we need to talk about the role of anti-VEGF drugs in the treatment of PDR. Remember that long, sloppy chapter about the treatment of DME, and how there was no definite paradigm that defined the role of laser versus drugs? Well, things aren't much different in this chapter. The use of these drugs in the setting of PDR is in flux, and different doctors have widely different views on their utility. And, once again, there are variables such as the patient's systemic control and the availability of injectable drugs to consider. So let's try to sort this out...

First, there is no question that bevacizumab and its cousins can totally shut down proliferative diabetic retinopathy.[1] Figure 1 is an example from Avery, et al.'s classic paper—at the time the image was jaw dropping.[2] But the effect is transient, usually wearing off in a few weeks. So the short take would be to use the drug to stop the disease cold and then add laser to get more permanent control. But it is way more complicated than that.

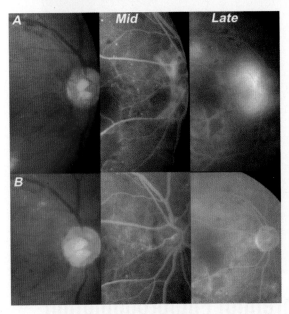

Figure 1: A series of photos showing the effect of intravitreal bevacizumab on PDR—the neovascularization completely disappears in the lower photos. The really exciting thing is that in the midphase photos you can get a feeling that by eliminating the shunting of the new vessels, there is actually some circulation returning to the retinal capillaries. (From: Avery RL, Pearlman J, Pieramici DJ, et al. Intravitreal bevacizumab (Avastin) in the treatment of proliferative diabetic retinopathy. Ophthalmology. Oct 2006;113(10):1695. Used with permission.)

But there is a potential problem with using these drugs in patients with proliferative disease: they result in such rapid involution of the neovascular tissue that one injection can induce a massive traction retinal detachment (TRD), sometimes in days, that can drop the patient's vision and be very difficult to fix. And remember, if you aren't trained in retina, you may think that all one needs to do is snip a few bands of scar tissue and put the retina back on and everything will be fine. Uh-uh. These diabetic detachments can be tough, and the visual recovery may be limited. Plus, if the detachment occurs in the hands of a specialist, they can jump in and fix it quickly. But if the detachment occurs in your hands, and it takes a while to get it taken care of, there is a chance that even with successful surgery the eye will not see as well as it did before you got involved.

This is why retina specialists, when they decide to operate on an eye with bad PDR, will give the injection within a few days of the planned surgery and hope that nothing goes wrong with the patient medically that keeps them out of the OR. Although the injection makes the surgery safer and easier, it is important to get into the eye before everything contracts and the retina is balled up in the center.

Fortunately, this type of massive contraction and detachment is relatively uncommon; a large series found an occurrence rate of 3.5%.[3] It would be great if we knew for sure which patients with PDR were likely to get this complication and which weren't. You could simply refer those with bad problems and start injecting and/or lasering patients below the threshold.

Unfortunately, there is no well-defined amount of PDR that we know will tolerate an injection without pulling the retina off, although it does seem more likely in patients with a lot of proliferative disease rather than patients with early disease. Other risk factors that make a detachment more likely include having diabetes for more than 15 years, poor control, and using a higher dose (2.5 mg) of bevacizumab (recall that the usual dose is 1.25 mg in .05 ml).[3]

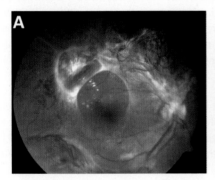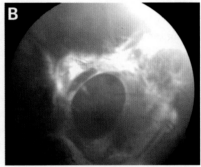

Figure 2: (A) Shows florid neo before bevacizumab. (B) Shows marked resolution of the neo, but there has also been marked contraction of the associated fibrous tissue causing a traction detachment of the macula. The vision went from 20/80 to hand motions, and even with surgery it only recovered to 20/400. AVASTIN IS NOT A TOY. (Arevalo J F et al. Br J Ophthalmol 2008;92:213-216. Used with permission.)

Are there any other guidelines? Nope. Still, there are some things to consider. First, you may be safer in patients with fresh neovascularization—vessels that don't have a lot of associated fibrosis. Once there starts to be noticeable fibrosis (look at Figure 2 again), you start to run into a higher risk. Also, the location of the fibrosis may be important. If it is largely outside the arcades, and mild, then you may be OK. But if it is broad based and within the arcades, and especially if it encircles the macula, then you may want to tell the family to buy a bus ticket and get to a retina specialist rather than giving an anti-VEGF injection yourself. You can certainly put in laser to try and stabilize things as a temporizing measure, but bad disease needs a specialist.

And there is something else to consider:

If you are the only eye doc for an entire region, the risk of stimulating a TRD in a few patients may be worth it compared to the risk of withholding treatment on a bunch of other patients that could have benefited. This is not to give you a license to go crazy—it is just one factor to consider.

On the other hand, if you are a general ophthalmologist in a town full of retina specialists, and you decide to do injections because you think it is a great practice builder, well, you better think real hard about whether you are really helping patients that are at risk for getting a TRD when you could have referred them. Know thyself and thy turf.

Now, if the anti-VEGF drugs get the PDR to disappear so effectively, why bother with a PRP? Why not just treat any macular edema with regular injections, which will automatically control neo, and then if the edema goes away, just give shots if PDR reappears? You can avoid the risks and vision changes associated with a PRP, and you can always add a PRP down the road if you are worried.

These are good points, and some people feel that is a reasonable way to go—there has even been a recent DRCR.net study that showed injections may be better than a PRP, at least over two years (more on this below). In many ways, however, we are all just trying to Feel The Force when it comes to using these drugs for PDR. Right now, most retina docs would be uncomfortable completely withholding a PRP—especially in places where access to care is limited—and here's why:

Retina specialists spend a lot of time trying to put back together eyes that have been needlessly destroyed by progressive and asymptomatic proliferative disease. And sometimes all the king's horses and all the king's men can't save these eyes. It is more reassuring to put in a solid PRP and largely eliminate the risk of bad PDR, rather than depend on patients showing up for regular exams and injecting before things go bad.

Plus, there is always the risk of endophthalmitis with injections, as well as the risk of potential systemic side effects. There is also a feeling that the peripheral ischemia that drives the neovascularization also provides plenty of VEGF to keep the macula swollen, and by doing a PRP you are helping to minimize problems with both PDR and recurrent DME. This is only a "feeling" though. It is by no means proven (see the section on PRP for DME in Chapter 4).

The rest of this chapter will spend a lot of time talking about how to do a safe, careful PRP that minimizes the risk of problems. Although older studies showed plenty of side effects associated with PRPs, modern approaches tend to be much less likely to cause trouble.[4]

Still, the idea of treating with injections alone is really attractive. Remember back in the DME chapter, where we talked about how the use of these drugs actually seemed to reverse some of the peripheral retinal damage that leads to PDR? And how these drugs seemed to alter the course of the retinopathy in a favorable way? For example, go back to Figure 1 in this chapter and note how the capillary non-perfusion was improved with the anti-VEGF injections—perhaps due to elimination of the shunting caused by all the neo.

All these things suggest that chronic anti-VEGF use may undo some of the damage that led to the PDR in the first place, and maybe there are patients that won't need a PRP after treating their DME over time. In fact, the DRCR.net recently released a study that looked at whether chronic injections could obviate the need for a PRP in patients with early proliferative disease, whether they had DME or not (Protocol S).[28] They used ranibizumab and found that over two years patients that had injections did just as well as patients that were treated with PRP. The injected patients also had slightly better vision, had less peripheral field loss, and required fewer vitrectomies. And they needed fewer injections over time—averaging 7-9 injections the first year and 3-5 injections the second year (patients with DME needed the higher numbers).

This is definitely something to consider in appropriate patients, assuming they have the resources and willingness to undergo chronic injections. And for patients and healthcare systems that can't afford years of ranibizumab, it is likely that people will substitute bevacizumab on the assumption that it is likely to work as well. But we don't have long-term data on the use of injections yet, and you have to be darn sure patients will really show up for follow up. We know that when DME resolves and you stop treating them with shots, the proliferative disease can show up rapidly and aggressively.[18,19] And it has been suggested that for a patient to get proliferative disease in the first place they have likely been non-compliant, so you probably can't depend on them to show up for regular injections. (Even in Protocol S, there was only 75% follow up by year 2.) So for now it still makes a lot of sense to get good at PRPs. Hopefully we will soon have long acting delivery systems that will control the disease without the need for laser or repeated injections. But until then, PRPs are a solid way to be certain your patient will stay out of trouble—especially if you are working in a place with non-compliant patients and limited resources.

What about anti-VEGFs and vitreous hemorrhages?

There are several papers that suggest that injecting one of these drugs will speed up the resolution of a vitreous hemorrhage, and it makes sense that getting the neovascularization to shrivel up and stop bleeding would give the eye a chance to clear.[5-7] However, the DRCR.net looked at this with a randomized prospective trial comparing ranibizumab to saline injections, and although there was a mild effect on clearing, it was by no means dramatic.[8] We do know that vitreous hemorrhages will often clear on their own, so maybe we are fooling ourselves thinking that injecting anti-VEGF drugs speeds things up. Still, the anti-VEGF drug will definitely control the proliferative disease while waiting for the blood to clear enough so that laser can be used. This may be useful in patients who can't afford or don't want surgery. Once again, there are no absolute guidelines on this. You have to look at your experience and your patient population and decide for yourself how you want to use these drugs in this situation.

But there is one big caveat if you are not trained in retina, and it goes back to the warning at the beginning of the chapter: you really need to know what is going on in the back of the eye before you inject. You not only need to do the ultrasound to make sure that the retina is where it is supposed to be, you also need to look carefully at what you are seeing on the ultrasound. If there is a lot of fibrosis, with evidence of potential traction and multiple points where the vitreous is stuck to the retina, then it is possible that your injection could stimulate enough traction to pull the retina off. This can make a bad situation unfixable, especially if you don't realize it for a few months while waiting for the hemorrhage to clear. If you don't know what the retina is doing before you inject, you really should refer the patient. You cannot think of your favorite anti-VEGF agent as Vitrectomy-in-a-Syringe.

But back to doing a PRP...

In the Seventies, the original Diabetic Retinopathy Study (DRS) called for a PRP to consist of 1200 to 1600 spots that were 500 to 1000 microns in size at the retina. These were to be placed approximately one-half burn width apart, from the arcades on out. This is a lot of laser. Because such treatment is the traditional standard, one would not be faulted if one ignored the rest of this chapter and just did this to every diabetic that needs a PRP— it is classic treatment from a classic paper. However, it is unlikely you are doing the type of cataract surgery they did back then, so perhaps it is worth looking deeper into why we do what we do...

First, Grasshopper, you must wrap your head around the fundamental contradiction inherent in doing a PRP. It can best be summarized in the following koan:

THE BEST PRP IS THE WORST PRP.

Studies have shown that a powerful, dense PRP gives one the best chance of long-term success. Unfortunately, it also gives one the best chance of having very noticeable side effects: decreased vision, loss of visual field, loss of night vision, glare, etc. The best PRP is the worst PRP. On the other hand, if you go light you are likely to avoid these complications, or the side effects will be so mild that they do not interfere with the patient's life. (For instance, they may be much safer drivers—your actions can have effects that go far beyond your laser room.) Unfortunately, a safer, milder PRP carries a greater risk of problems with recurrent proliferative disease. The best PRP is the worst PRP.

Let's explore this a bit more. If you dig into the ETDRS and the DRS, you will realize that they led to numerous papers looking at all kinds of obscure things. Buried deep in two of these papers are some really useful graphs.[9,10] They are reproduced here in their original pre-Excel glory. They show that the denser the treatment, the more likely it is that patients will avoid severe vision loss. You always need to remember these graphs if you decide to treat less than the standard DRS treatment.

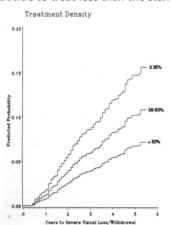

Figure 3: In this case, the authors looked at how dense the PRP was in peripheral photographs versus the probability of severe vision loss. The greater the density, the better the treatment worked (greater than 50% treatment density was best). (Kaufman SC, Ferris FL 3rd, Seigel DG, Davis MD, DeMets DL. Factors associated with visual outcome after photocoagulation for diabetic retinopathy. Diabetic Retinopathy Study Report 13. Invest Ophthalmol Vis Sci 1989; 30: 23-8.)

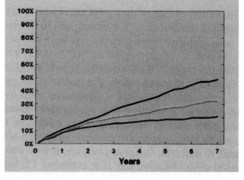

Figure 4: This was an arm of the ETDRS in which patients were assigned to no treatment (black), mild scattered PRP (orange), or standard PRP (dark red). They started with moderate to severe NPDR or low-risk PDR, and the graph shows the probability of developing high-risk PDR. Stronger treatment resulted in much less risk of progression. (Figure 6 is a photo of the standard laser pattern and figure 7 shows the milder pattern.) Yes, this graph was scanned from the original paper; we really like the Old School vibe (Early Treatment Diabetic Retinopathy Study Research Group. Early photocoagulation for diabetic retinopathy (ETDRS report #9). Ophthalmology, 1991; 98: 766-85). Copyright Elsevier.

However, as Chapter 17 will be showing you, you can cause trouble when doing a PRP. Also, remember that the graphs essentially represent dose-response curves, and as with any drug, you do not automatically give the highest dose to everyone just because it seems to work best when you look at the entire population. As a physician, your job is to pick the right dose for each individual patient. You will find that many patients will do quite well with less than a full dose of laser, especially if their control is good. Or, to look at it another way, you are trying to use the lowest dose of laser necessary in order to change the slope of their deterioration, with the goal that their eyes last until they die. (Kind of like treating glaucoma—but things can go bad fast if you make the wrong choice.)

Blue box break for folks treating indigent patients or who are in developing countries, where patients are coming in with awful disease and awful control. These patients just need a ton of laser—often several thousand spots, especially if you have no access to injections or vitrectomy and laser is your only option. You still have to try to break up such heavy treatment into a few sessions to avoid even more side effects, but there is no role for trying the gentler approaches outlined below. Good luck.

In fact, there is a wide assortment of treatments being essayed by retina specialists to try to minimize collateral damage from a PRP, ranging from undetectable micropulse treatment to minimal scatter techniques that only treat areas of angiographic ischemia. The crucial thing is that if you do use a milder treatment, you and the patient have to understand that you are shackled together for eternity. You have to watch these patients and make sure they don't get little nubbins of neo around the areas of lighter treatment, and you have to be prepared to bite the bullet and fill in treatment as needed. You also want to have a good feel for which patients need heavy treatment—sometimes, treatment that is far denser than the DRS guidelines. It is very dangerous to fritter away time doing light treatments in such patients; you have to accept the risk of side effects to get aggressive proliferative disease under control quickly.

So keep the above contradictory koan in mind as you read the following on how to do a PRP...

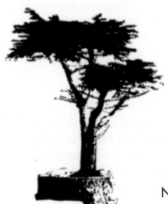

Hey, here is a real Buddhist koan:

A MONK ASKED ZHAOZHOU, "WHAT IS THE MEANING OF THE ANCESTRAL TEACHER'S COMING FROM THE WEST?" ZHAOZHOU SAID, "THE CYPRESS TREE IN FRONT OF THE HALL."

Now how cool is that, and what could it possibly mean?

FIRST, A REVIEW OF SOME BASICS

Take care of any macular edema. You can really mess someone up if you put in an aggressive PRP when they have poorly controlled macular edema; the edema can get much worse. The best way to avoid this is to treat the edema by whatever means you have. If you only have laser, then do that. If the edema is center-involving, then you or someone should be injecting the eye. As discussed in the previous chapter, some people will do injections even if the edema is not center-involving, simply to stabilize the macula and get the PDR under immediate control.[27] Then you can proceed at a gentle pace with the laser in a controlled setting. And keep in mind the previous discussion about how the use of anti-VEGF agents may change how you might apply the PRP, or even if one needs to be done at all. But mostly remember that there are no big studies that clearly define how to work with all the different treatment variables, so keep an open mind and ask your retinal colleagues lots of questions.

In any event, once the macular edema is controlled then you can start doing a PRP (specific techniques to use are discussed below). If the patient has pre-proliferative disease or mild proliferative disease, you definitely have time to do all this slowly and carefully. It gets trickier if the edema is bad and the proliferative disease needs rapid treatment, too—you may have to simply treat the edema and start the PRP at the same time. This is where the anti-VEGF drugs can be a real game changer compared to the bad old days.

Plus, there is one advantage to the use of intravitreal drugs that is not well defined in the literature, and that has to do with the patient's experience. Traditionally, PRPs are miserable for patients, and they usually don't get a lot of reward for the misery—they are blurred up for a while in the best of circumstances and their disease may still drag them downhill in the worst of circumstances. But with an injection they will often notice an improvement in their vision as the macular edema dries up—so you have a patient that gets a laser and actually gets better! That is unusual in the world of retina, and it creates powerful positive reinforcement for the patient to continue with treatment and follow up. This does NOT mean you should use injections like a Pavlovian reward. It does mean, though, that if you are doing injections as part of treating macular edema and proliferative disease, you may be creating a lot more motivation on the part of the patient than you are used to. That is a good thing to be aware of; it is fun to have a patient come back happy and wanting to continue follow up because they can see an improvement.

But back to doing the laser.

The positioning and setup are similar to those discussed in Chapter 8, the chapter that is not really about doing a treatment for macular edema. Because a PRP tends to be much more intense than a macular laser, you really want to make sure the patient is comfortable and you really want to warn the patient about the increased discomfort that accompanies a PRP, especially if their only prior experience is with focal lasers.

Chapter 16 is specifically about controlling pain when doing a PRP, but it is worth discussing a few things right here, because you need to convey some of this to the patient from the start. It turns out that each spot you place—even if it is the exact same type of burn—can vary extremely in terms of discomfort. This is probably due to how close the spots are to the nerves in the suprachoroidal space. The greatest discomfort tends to occur in the mid-periphery, especially in the horizontal and diagonal clock hours where the nerves are more prominent. Although you usually cannot see the nerves themselves, you can often anticipate increased pain when you move toward the vortex veins or more prominent choroidal veins—places where the nerves are more likely to be. This is especially the case if there is extra pigment lying alongside the veins; this makes the burns hotter. Sometimes you can even detect the whiter coloration of a nerve, for instance in the horizontal meridians where the long ciliary nerves run. It makes sense to avoid these areas, or at least go lightly—both for pain control and to minimize effects on pupil function and accommodation. (See Chapter 17 on complications.)

However, even if you follow the above anatomic guidelines, you will find that many times you can be working in an area that is utterly unremarkable and suddenly the patient yelps in pain. You need to warn them in advance that this unexpected change in discomfort can happen. If they are not forewarned about this, and if you do hit a hot spot, they may think that you have cranked up the power and that you are trying to blow their head off—because that is what it can feel like. They can then get very skittish about the rest of the treatment because you hurt them in a way they were not prepared for. It is one thing to tell the patient that a procedure is uncomfortable, and it is another thing to have an unexpected burst of pain when neither you nor the patient expects it.

You should warn them about this and let them know that if it does happen, they should tell you. Then you can avoid the site of discomfort. Even if you warned them, however, it can be difficult to finish because once you hit a spot like this they can get nervous and their threshold of pain can change.

Also, be aware that some patients are exquisitely sensitive to this sudden change in pain, and may rapidly faint due to a vasovagal response. If you warn them about the possibility of both pain and fainting in advance, everyone present will be less frantic if the patient slowly melts down to the ground. If a patient does tell you that they are starting to feel hot or light-headed, you should discontinue the laser immediately and order them to either lower their head between their legs or lie down on the floor. This is really important; once they start to go vasovagal, it may only be a matter of seconds before they convert the potential energy of their head at the slit lamp into kinetic energy—a bad thing given all the sharp edges that are present in your lasering area. Sometimes it helps to put a cool washcloth on their forehead and you can even create a Victorian level of drama if you want to use smelling salts. (On the other hand, don't get cavalier and assume every light-headed patient is simply getting vasovagal. Remember that this group of patients may also be getting hypoglycemic or may even have a true emergency like a heart attack—make sure you monitor such a patient until they improve appropriately.)

GETTING STARTED

Having done all the talk to get the patient ready, it is now time to do the walk. First, you have to choose your weapon, or at least its color. At the beginning of the book it was assumed that you have a green laser, but it is worth noting that the other colors can come in handy when doing a PRP. No study has shown that any wavelength is superior in terms of the ultimate outcome, but just like it is nice to have different wrenches to work on a car, it is nice to know that different colors can be helpful in certain situations. Different wrenches don't cost $40,000, though, so don't feel like you have to run out and get another laser—just be aware of the options.

An example where a different wavelength can be useful is when there are a lot of media opacities, such as a hemorrhage or a nuclear sclerotic cataract. Yellow can get through nuclear sclerosis and a hemorrhage, and a redder wavelength also works because there is less scattering relative to green. An infrared laser can be even more effective at getting through such opacities, but it is trickier to use. (You should check Appendix 3 if you are going to use this wavelength.) Fortunately, you can get most routine jobs done with a green laser. If you really need to use sky-high powers, though, you may want to refer the patient to someone who has other wavelengths in order to avoid some of the complications discussed in upcoming chapters.

Next, remember that the spot size you set on the laser may end up being very different from what you get on the retina, especially if you are using a wide-field indirect lens. Refer back to Chapter 7 for the details—but the important thing is to know the magnification factor for the lens you are using. For instance, a very wide-field lens can double the spot size: If you are set at 500 microns on the slit lamp, you can end up placing 1,000-micron spots on the retina—and these are really huge, painful spots. (It is likely you would be using equally massive powers, and between the power and the pain, you would quickly realize your settings were unnecessarily harsh.) You should also remember that the number of spots you need to use is very dependent on the spot size.

For instance, if you want to do a "standard" Diabetic Retinopathy Study PRP of 1,500 spots that are 500 microns in size—but you are using a smaller spot size—you can't just put in 1,500 spots and quit. You have to increase the number of spots you place so that you cover the same area that would have been covered by 500-micron burns (Figure 5). By the way, knowing how many spots you need can be more complicated when you are using very short durations, such as with a pattern laser that puts in a group of spots with each burst. The tissue response to that technique is different, and even more spots may be needed.[11] An excellent paper by Palanker et al. goes into this deeply and is worth a read if you use such an approach.[12]

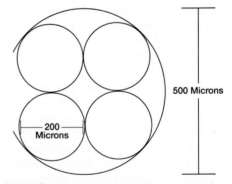

Figure 5: It takes at least four 200-micron spots to fill a 500-micron spot (the π-r-squared thing). If you want to place a certain "dose" of PRP based on the 500-micron burn size, then you have to increase the number of spots you place, depending on how many of your burns it takes to equal the area of a 500 micron spot.

How hot do you make the burns? It is hard to photograph the kind of burn that you actually see when you do a laser, because burns tend to soften rapidly after treatment— they also spread out a bit. The ETDRS asked for medium-white burns as seen in Figure 6, and this is fairly standard. Note the whitening in the center of most burns—if you are getting a much whiter burn, you are probably running too hot, and you should turn down the power.

Figure 7 shows a spread of different intensities. Many specialists feel that you can use lighter intensities (note, in the figure, the milder, grayish burns without any white center). One problem is that over time you will see that milder burns may not form scars as large as the original burn—so you can end up with less area treated than you had planned at the time of treatment. There are no long term studies that prove you can get ETDRS results with burns that are less than the ETDRS standard. However, the DRCR.net uses burns described as mild to medium white burns, which are not as intense as the whiter burns called for by the ETDRS, so there is a tendency to not be quite as aggressive as the old days.[13]

Figure 6 is also the standard density for a full PRP—the spots are about one-half burn width apart (after the burn spreads). Of note, the DRCR.net loosened this up a bit, suggesting that burns could be about a burn width apart prior to spreading.[13] The ETDRS had a "mild scatter" treatment arm, with fewer burns that were spaced further apart, and it is shown in Figure 8 for comparison. This milder pattern resulted in the middle (yellow) line in Figure 4. It is clearly not as effective as a full PRP, and most experts would not go this lightly—or at least not for the full treatment. Still, it gives you an idea of what has been tried and what to expect so you don't have to reinvent the wheel.

Figure 6: This is the ETDRS gold standard for burn intensity and density for a full-scatter PRP. If you do less than this, you could get, burned – but some patients might do quite well with less. Note that laser burns tend to spread out shortly after treatment, so the actual treatment density was a bit less than this (courtesy of the Early Treatment Diabetic Retinopathy Study Group).

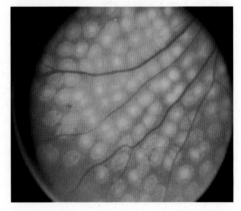

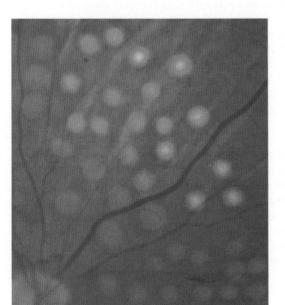

Figure 7: Variable-intensity burns with the upper burns being similar to ETDRS standards and the lower grade of burns representing a milder approach. Note that you can see some of the choroidal detail through the lighter burns, but the whiteness of the heavier burns obscures the underlying choroid. This can help you decide how hot your burns are. Truth in advertising moment: this image was Photoshopped to simulate the burns. It is hard to justify doing this to a patient for didactic reasons.

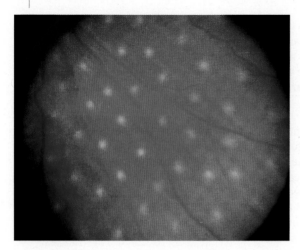

Figure 8: The ETDRS photos showing the pattern used for the "mild scatter" treatment arm. This is a very light pattern, and most people would not go this light even in patients that they think will respond to less laser. It is, however, the pattern that resulted in the middle line in **Figure 4** – not as effective as a full scatter pattern, but still had a treatment effect (Courtesy of the Early Treatment Diabetic Retinopathy Study Group).

Incidentally, when this chapter suggests a given number of spots, it is assumed that these are equivalent to 500-micron spots. You will likely prefer to use smaller spots (for instance, for patient comfort), so you will need to adjust the actual number of spots you place, as outlined above. Also, when this chapter refers to a "standard ETDRS PRP" it means about 1,500 500-micron spots.

AMOUNT, STAGING, & FREQUENCY OF TREATMENT

There is a tendency to feel as though it is some sort of emergency when a patient presents with mild asymptomatic neovascularization. Do not surrender to the temptation to slag the retina simply because you see some vessels that look disturbing. Such vessels are unlikely to change over a few weeks, and most of the acute complications from PRP occur with aggressive treatment delivered all at once. In some ways, the situation is analogous to a patient who presents with long-standing severe hypertension: If you aggressively bring the blood pressure down far and fast you can give them a stroke, but if you gently work it down you can save them safely. It seems as though diabetic eyes function in a similar fashion. Eyes that present with early proliferative disease have been living in an ischemic milieu for quite some time. They can be rather fragile, and if you jump in with 1,500 spots all at once, you might create permanent changes in the macula—as well as an extremely unhappy patient. As will be discussed below, there are times when it may even be best to start slowly with a few hundred spots if you can.

Make no mistake; there are some situations in which time is not your friend. Patients with lots of very angry-looking vessels, very ischemic retinas and active hemorrhaging can go bad fast. The concern is that the extensive neovascularization evolves into dense fibrous tissue, causing severe traction that no vitrectomy can undo. Wasting time doing a slow gentle PRP in such a patient can be disastrous. These patients are often younger Type 1 diabetics with a history of poor compliance, but any demographic can be affected. Such patients do need a lot of laser, even if it means risking side effects, because just about any laser complication is better than where the eye is heading. In this type of situation, you may want to bite the bullet and put in a thousand spots at first, and then repeat weekly until the patient is controlled or hemorrhages and needs surgery. Or at least that is what you do if you don't have anti-VEGF agents. If you do have access to them, you have a lot more control. Often such patients will have macular edema that needs treatment, and even if they don't have definite macular edema, the anti-VEGF drug can help protect the macula from the side effects of the PRP.[14-16] Does this mean that every patient that needs a PRP should have a shot of anti-VEGF juice at the same time, just to be sure the macula stays out of trouble? There is data to suggest that the answer may be yes if you have access to injections, although this is by no means a universal practice.[27] Still, it is good to know that anti-VEGF drugs can help "splint" a precarious macula if you are worried about messing things up with an aggressive PRP.

But it is not as simple as giving a shot and adding PRP. Patients can still have worsening of their macular edema with a PRP even if you are giving them shots, and there is the risk that injections could stimulate a traction retinal detachment if there is a lot of neovascularization (remember the previous discussion). Frankly, if you have a patient who looks bad—where you aren't sure how safe injections are but you need to get lots of laser in fast—you should strongly consider just referring them to a retina specialist. ASAP. This is not to strip you of your prerogatives as a Renaissance Comprehensive Ophthalmologist—but you should recognize that these patients can do abysmally with even specialist care. And more and more data suggests that they need anti-VEGF agents and early surgery to head off a really bad outcome.[17] There will be lots of bread and-butter diabetics for you to treat who don't need subspecialty intervention. If you really, really want to treat such misery, you may need to find yourself a retina fellowship...

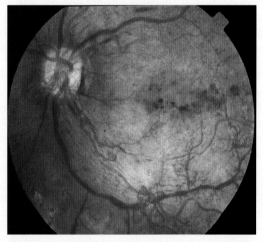

Figure 9: This is a very sick eye – most commonly seen in younger patients with a history of poor control. Note the swollen, beaded veins and all of the smaller intraretinal vessels that seem to start and stop in no clear pattern. Also, note the neovascularization – it is not large, but the vessels are thick and succulent in a way that bodes poorly for the patient. The blotchy hemorrhages in the macula suggest a lot of ischemia, and you are caught between the Scylla and Charybdis doing a fast, aggressive PRP, yet trying not to blow out the fragile macula. This is where anti-VEGF agents can protect the macula and help control the proliferative disease (as long as they do not stimulate traction). Consider referring such a patient if you can – skillfully balancing all the treatment variables in this eye may be very important to the final outcome.

Also, are you waiting for a little chart on spot size, duration and power for a PRP? It would be nice to have a standard setting for all of your PRPs, but hopefully you are realizing that there are so many factors that using one setting for all PRPs is like telling Rembrandt he could only use one paintbrush. With experience you will automatically come up with tailor-made settings for each patient based on a number of variables. These variables will include things such as how aggressively you want to treat the patient, their degree of pigmentation, the presence of media opacities, the location of the treatment and even your estimate of their pain threshold. All of these are discussed at various points in this chapter and throughout the book.

However, you do need to begin somewhere, so here are some basic numbers to try:

Most feel it is best to start with a duration of 0.1 second—this is a nice middling length of time that will not be too likely to let you get in trouble. A good starting spot size is around 350 to 500 microns at the retina (remember the effect of the contact lens on spot size). For the "average" patient, this duration and spot size usually means that you will want to start with a power of about 200 milliwatts and slowly increase it until you get burns similar to those seen in the photos. Don't hesitate to start at an even lower power if the media is crystal clear and/or there is a lot of pigment—you can always turn it up but you can't undo a spot that is too hot.

You can then gradually increase the power—say, by 20- to 50-milliwatt increments—until you start to see a slight graying of the retina. Once you begin to see a change it is likely that you only need to turn it up about 50 milliwatts more in order to get a standard burn. Another clue that you are getting close to the right power is that the patient will often tell you that they are beginning to feel it. You should probably not stray very much from settings like this until you get an intuitive feel for how the retina responds to your treatment, but once you have some experience you will find these settings way too restrictive.

How much do you treat?

This is the question. As the PRP koan implies, less is more—unless they go blind from your doing less. Then less was not enough, and you should have done more—unless they have problems from doing more, in which case you should have done less. You get the point. There are some guidelines, though, to help you decide where to start if you want to do something other than a "one size fits all" PRP.

There are some patients who seem to do well with smaller amounts of laser. These are generally older patients with Type 2 diabetes who do not have a lot of aggressive neovascularization. This is especially true if you are treating an older diabetic at an earlier stage, such as severe NPDR or low-risk PDR. As outlined above, if you decide to go conservative on your treatment, you are obligated to pay close attention to the patient, and the patient must understand that follow up is very important. If there is any sign that things are not responding appropriately, you will simply need to add more laser.

On the other hand, younger patients with more ischemic retinas and aggressive disease may require thousands and thousands of spots to just partially control the process. Accelerated medical problems can add to proliferative disease as well—a patient with renal failure or bad hypertension can kill off retinal vessels in a way that really powers up the neovascular stimulus. Finally, a patient with known poor control (or poor compliance) should get fairly heavy treatment to ensure stopping the disease so they (hopefully) won't go bad even if they never show up again or never check their glucose levels.

For instance, a 70- to 80-year-old patient with Type 2 diabetes who is slowly developing

PDR may only need about a thousand spots to slow things down enough until they exit the Grand Illusion. A 50-ish or 60-ish patient in a similar situation may need something closer to a standard PRP, especially if they have poor control or are progressing quickly. Patients in their 30s to 40s may be fine with this same dose, but often need an extra "half of a PRP dose" for security (say, an extra 500 to 700 spots). Twenty-somethings are likely to be Type 1 patients who were poorly controlled—otherwise they would not get their disease so early. These patients may need two or three times a usual PRP dose, and often quickly.

NOTE: The above are just rough approximations. Each patient is different—gather some experience and use your judgment. And the use of anti-VEGF agents can change the calculus. Injections may allow good neovascular control with a milder PRP. But don't be fooled by the immediate gratification of vessels disappearing with each injection. You may get good control of vessels early on, but as time goes by patients may need fewer injections, for instance if they have less macular edema. If you used a mild PRP, you then need to watch their proliferative disease closely.

This is really important, especially given the promising results of the DRCR.net study suggesting that in selected patients chronic injections can obviate the need for laser. Giving injections can make you think the new vessels are more controlled than they really are. If you are lulled into complacency and end up doing a milder PRP, you have got to watch these patients carefully when you stop doing regular injections—perhaps even consider filling in the PRP regardless of how good they look. If these patients wander off and are not checked, they can get into real trouble.[18] And the same applies for patients who only have DME and are being treated with injections. They will probably not develop PDR while getting regular treatment. But if the DME goes away and they don't need any more treatment, you need to keep bringing them back—don't just send them away for 6 months thinking they will be fine. The injections have been suppressing the VEGF, and once the injections stop the effect of the VEGF will rebound and the proliferative disease can go berserk.[19]

And you aren't just looking for recurrence of their new vessels. Be sure to monitor areas that haven't been treated for worsening of the background retinopathy. In other words, if an area starts to have increasing intraretinal hemorrhages with IRMA and venous beading (as in the 4-2-1 rule) it is likely that area needs additional PRP (or the patient needs to go back on regular injections). An angiogram can be really helpful to identify areas of new non-perfusion that merit treatment. Worsening of background retinopathy is a really important thing to be aware of when patients have untreated retina. This is worth repeating:

Worsening background retinopathy in areas that have not been treated with PRP may indicate that areas of dangerous non-perfusion are developing and additional treatment may be warranted.

Is there a maximum number of spots? A study looking at this considered 6,500 500-micron spots to represent about the upper limit.[20] That is a lot of spots—maybe four to five times the amount of the standard ETDRS PRP—and other studies have gone even higher. The point is that you can put in a lot of laser and still stay away from the important bits of the retina. You can even use the 6,500 number to reassure patients about how much head room you have if they feel that you are destroying their eye *with 1,500 spots. However, if you think you need to keep putting in spots like this in the modern era, you really should refer—with the intravitreal treatments and early vitrectomy it may be possible to spare patients this type of Total War ablation. (By the way, the maximum number of spots reported in the literature is 11,513 from back in the Eighties.[21] It is unlikely you will ever need to go there.)*

Over how many sessions do you put in the treatment?

There is a really short answer to this question, and a much longer answer that is different. Both are correct, depending on your situation and skill. The short one comes from a DRCR.net study looking at the difference in outcome between doing the entire laser in one session or in several, and they clearly found that doing everything in one session was fine.[13] But...

They were treating patients with no macular disease, and those patients were likely better controlled than the average patient you treat. Plus, docs in the DRCR.net posse have done thousands of PRPs and are quite good at it. That means if you have a patient similar to those entered in the study, and you know what you are doing, you will likely be able to do just fine putting everything in during one session. It is good to know that you can do this, because it can save the patient a lot of trips and it can save you a lot of time.

However, many patients have more tenuous macular function, especially if they have poor control and are arriving at your doorstep with more advanced disease. This means that you can make them worse if you treat too much and too aggressively, and you have to default to older approaches that work better in more delicate eyes. Of course, the treatment plan is also affected by the availability of anti-VEGF drugs—as discussed previously, these drugs can stabilize both the macula and the proliferative disease and allow you to treat faster and more aggressively.[22] (Triamcinolone can also stabilize the macula, but it doesn't have the same helpful effect on the overall level of retinopathy that anti-VEGF drugs do.)

If you don't know if an eye can handle a lot of laser at once, it is reassuring that for the "average" patient with early PDR there is not a lot of time pressure. So if you are worried, it makes sense to start with gradual treatment applied over at least two or three sessions. For one thing, one-stop shopping with a PRP may require retrobulbar anesthesia with the attendant risks, and some of the really bad complications of PRP are more likely to occur with single-session treatment in a fragile eye (see Chapter 17 for those complications—things like angle-closure glaucoma and exudative retinal detachments). Even two sessions can be too aggressive in some eyes, and three sessions may be safer for some patients. There is less of a shock to the eye, and patients are more likely to tolerate the discomfort without needing a block.

Another factor that can be very important in deciding how to treat a patient is whether you think they will be compliant. Although a wayward patient is not the ideal patient for risking side effects from aggressive treatment, it may be better to treat such patients quickly over fewer sessions before they wander off and stop seeing anyone. It can be very gratifying to see such patients years later and find that they can still see and function in society thanks to the fact that you put in enough laser before they disappeared (even if they are still bitching about how you messed them up with your laser).

In fact, there are some patients who may be unbelievably sensitive to a PRP. These patients don't turn up very often, but you will certainly know if you stumble across one. Such patients may go from 20/20 to 20/50 for weeks with as few as 200 or 300 gentle laser spots. If you happen to hit one of these patients very hard with the first treatment, you can knock them down to count-fingers and they may never completely recover. Fortunately, this type of severe decreased vision after a PRP is unusual, but it still makes sense to go slowly if you can. At times you may even want to initiate panretinal photocoagulation with as little as 200 to 400 spots, and then plan on adding the full amount over additional sessions, depending upon how the patient tolerates the first treatment. Rare patients may even need to be treated in small doses over six to eight sessions. (Note that these kinds of problems are more likely with sick patients with sick eyes that are in places where there is no access to intravitreal treatment. You will be able to sidestep a lot of this if the patient is also being treated with an anti-VEGF agent or steroid to control macular edema—you will be able to put in more laser more safely.)[23] The important point is to be flexible and never approach the number of sessions with a "one size fits all" mentality.

This blue box likely applies only to docs practicing in America:

Chapter 21 *discusses in detail the socioeconomic issues involved in treating diabetics, but there is one issue that needs to be covered right here. Most insurance companies will pay for a PRP only once every 90 days. The thinking is that they only have to pay once, and that payment will cover as many treatments as are needed for the three-month period. You don't have to have a Nobel Prize in economics to realize that there is, therefore, a strong urge to do every PRP in one session—or as few sessions as possible—in order to maximize revenue per unit of time in the clinic.*

If, for whatever reason, you think a patient is best served with multiple treatment sessions, please ignore this financial urge to stuff all the laser in at once. If you are in the early phases of your training, you are likely untainted and this admonition will seem ridiculous. If you have a practice and a family to pay for, you may notice that a sense of frustration can slowly creep into your soul as you circle the "no charge" line on a bunch of lasers. Recognize that the PRP reimbursement is structured so that these extra visits are taken into account—you are in fact being paid to do several treatments. Consider only what is best for the patient, and pinch yourself strongly if you find that you are even remotely thinking about this as you plan a given patient's treatment.

(As an aside within an aside, you may run across patients treated in the really old days when PRPs were paid for visit by visit. Having a patient tell you that they were brought back 12 times over six months to get a little bit of PRP each time will help you understand that maybe the present payment system isn't so bad.)*

You also have to be flexible about how often you schedule sessions for patients that need to be lasered over several visits. Patients with aggressive PDR may need treatment every week, but treating patients every two weeks is probably best it you are worried about side effects. It has been shown using OCT that even a healthy macula will swell a bit after a PRP. If patients are treated every week, it takes longer for their maculae to

---

* As this book was going to press, there was information that Medicare was going to change the global period for a PRP from 90 days to 10 days, and also decrease the reimbursement accordingly. Perhaps the next edition of this book will be admonishing people to *not* do a ton of PRPs 11 days apart!

recover from this swelling than if the PRP sessions are spread out every two weeks.[24] (And patients in this particular study started with relatively healthy maculae.*) It seems safe to assume that if a patient has a compromised macula, it may be risky to do PRPs spaced a week apart—best to spread things out a bit if the proliferative disease will let you. Again, this may not be as important if you are also giving the patient injections—we are trying to address all the different ways a patient may need to be treated depending on what options are available to you.

Another reason to go with every-two-week treatment is that it is often hard to see where you treated if you bring them back after a week—it often takes about two weeks for the spots to become more visible from scarring. (Finesse point: You can usually identify previous spots—even if you can't see them clinically—in the backscatter of your laser light as described in Chapter 9.)

What if they need bilateral treatment? It is always a bit dicey to do bilateral PRPs right off the bat. If you have one of those patients with really fussy maculae, you can shut down their ability to function for quite a while if you treat both eyes at once. Even if you want to get treatment started quickly in both eyes, it usually makes sense to treat one eye first so you and the patient can see how the eye responds. You can start treating the fellow eye in a few days and adjust your approach depending on how the first eye behaves. If things go well, and the patient doesn't mind having both eyes blurry at the same time, then you can treat bilaterally to save visits. If things don't go well, then you will likely need to alternate eyes at each treatment. This can turn into a lot of visits, but so be it if it makes the treatment safer. And, again, "splinting" one or both eyes with anti-VEGF drugs can buy you time so you can put in the more definitive laser treatment in a way that is more convenient.

What if they have a hemorrhage when they present?

First of all, remember the caveats in Chapter 13—make sure that you are dealing with proliferative disease and not another cause, such as a retinal tear. If the patient does have proliferative disease, then the treatment protocol depends on the amount of blood present. If there is a dense hemorrhage with no view—and they have no history of prior laser—you should refer for early vitrectomy to clear the blood out and get in laser before permanent damage occurs.

One other thing. *You should have a low threshold for doing gonioscopy in these patients. If they are presenting with enough proliferative disease to fill their eye up with blood, there is also a small chance that they could have anterior segment neo, and rarely that only shows up in the angle. More on this in Chapter 20.*

If there is a dense hemorrhage but you can see some retina, you should treat as much as you can (assuming you can be sure the posterior retina is safe with a B scan). The goal of treatment is to get laser in before further hemorrhage obscures your ability to treat the eye. If you can get in enough laser, you may be able to stabilize the eye and give it a chance to clear without the need for vitrectomy. It makes sense to treat all the retina you can see at the first session. This is especially true if there are areas of loculated

---

* One does not get to use a nifty word like maculae very often, yet here it occurs twice in one paragraph. Excellent.

hemorrhage being held in place by the cortical vitreous. These loculations can rupture and if the blood spreads throughout the central vitreous you will lose your ability to treat previously visible portions of the retina. Note, however, that there is one pattern of loculated hemorrhage that can be especially worrisome, and that is if there is a thick, dark and dense layer of blood over the posterior pole. These patients can sometimes do very poorly because of traction you don't see under the blood that damages the retina. Think about sending such patients sooner than later—more on this in Chapter 19.

If you can see most of the retina—i.e., there is only a premacular hemorrhage—you may want to be a bit more conservative in order to avoid complications related to an excessive PRP; perhaps treat in two sessions a week apart using a fairly large number of spots (say 500 to 1,000 to treat the inferior retina, followed by enough to fill in the remaining fundus at the next session). This is more aggressive than usual, but not enough to pulverize the eye. There is often more time than you would expect between hemorrhages in eyes with mild disease, and you are unlikely to "miss an opportunity" by dividing the treatments in patients who are less sanguineous. Although the presence of the blood is often as scary to you as it is to the patient, sometimes the eye does better if you get the laser in gradually. (If you are going to treat over multiple sessions, it does make sense to tell such patients to give you a call if they think the hemorrhage is getting worse—you can bring them in and finish the treatment quickly if necessary.) And don't forget that anti-VEGF agents may help rapidly control the vessels and give you time to get in laser. They may also help stabilize the macula so it is less likely to swell up with the PRP.

Whether you treat all at once or in divided doses, and whether you add anti-VEGF agents, recognize that there really is no incorrect approach as long as you are thinking about what you are doing. (By the way, patients with a vitreous hemorrhage are often best treated first with a wide-field indirect lens to slip around the blood as much as possible, then with a Goldmann three mirror for squeaking treatment out to the far periphery. You will often have a clear view of the far anterior retina because the blood can't get through the vitreous base.)

Also, remember that if you are treating a diabetic with a hemorrhage, you have to remind them that you can only indirectly control their "bad blood vessels" with the laser. They need to know that the blood may get much worse, depending on the capricious nature of their disease. You especially need to remind them that the laser will not make the blood in their vision disappear fast. Don't be surprised if you have to repeat this last point if you call the patient to see how they are doing after the laser. Patients have a strong tendency to assume that the laser will immediately solve a problem that the diabetes has been working for years to create.

As for the anti-VEGF drugs, we know that they can help shut down the neovascularization, but we don't know for sure if those drugs can actually help get rid of the hemorrhage. As mentioned above, there is some data that suggests that they can speed up clearance, but then there is the DRCR.net trial that showed that although ranibizumab had a mild effect on clearing, it was by no means dramatic.[8] Still, it makes sense that getting the neovascularization to shrivel up and stop bleeding would give the eye a chance to clear—especially since we now know from DRCR.net Protocol S that in some patients regular injections can replace the need for laser *and* they protect the macula from swelling up. But don't forget the warning at the beginning of the chapter: you really need to know what is going on in the back of the eye before you inject. If ultrasound shows a lot of fibrosis, with evidence of potential traction and multiple points where the vitreous is stuck to the retina, then it is possible that your injection could pull the retina off and make a bad situation unfixable—especially if a month goes by and the hemorrhage disappears but the retina looks like a crumpled-up carpet. If you don't know what is happening back there, you should consider referring the patient to someone who can figure out what to do.

By the way, it turns out that patients with hemorrhages may end up being some of your most grateful patients if the hemorrhage clears after the laser and/or injection (and it usually does if the disease is relatively mild). They will understand exactly where they were headed, and even if it takes a few months for the blood to wash out, they will greatly appreciate the fact that you saved them with your skills. It makes one wish that every diabetic would just have a little teeny hemorrhage as soon as they start to get some neovascularization. Then they would understand why we do this...

Where should you treat?

The standard DRS protocol called for non-specifically treating from the posterior pole to the equator, but, as with corneas, custom ablation is often the way to go.

For the "standard" treatment, the posterior border usually starts a disc width from the nerve and just outside the major arcades around the macula. The temporal treatment line is usually two to four disc diameters temporal to the fovea (Figure 10). Treatment is then carried out to the point where your contact lens can't easily see through the patient's lens—usually to an area anterior to the equator.

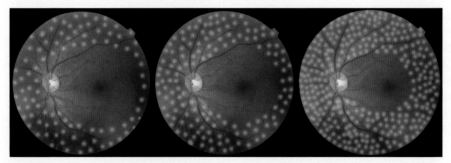

Figure 10: A triptych of approaches to choosing the posterior border of a PRP. These are also Photoshopped – one would be reluctant to put in this much laser all around the posterior pole at one treatment unless absolutely necessary. The middle would be about standard; the one on the left would be light (i.e., an elderly patient with mild disease), and the right would be a very aggressive treatment for refractory disease. Nowadays with the combination of early vitrectomy and intravitreal anti-VEGF agents it is usually unnecessary to apply such a destructive pattern as the one on the right, but in the old days it was not uncommon to have patients with recalcitrant neovascularization that needed harsh laser (and if you don't have access to injectables, you may need to treat like that on the right).

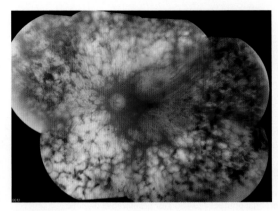

Figure 10.1: Yes, it is possible to do too much of a good thing. Someone, at some point, thought it would be a good idea to do this to an eye. Probably it was done years ago when there were no other treatment options, and the patient has lived a nice long life so there has been plenty of time for the scars to expand more than the treating physician anticipated. Also, to be sure, there isn't enough retina left to get either proliferative disease or macular edema, so by that metric the treatment worked. But nowadays there is no reason whatsoever to do something like this to an eye.

The actual borders that you choose depend on how severe the disease is. There is a common clinical impression that "one spot in the back is equal to two or more on the side," probably because the posterior retina is so much thicker and there are a lot more cells to generate vasoproliferative factors. Bad disease may need treatment that extends further toward the posterior pole, especially if you don't have access to anti-VEGF agents. For instance, some patients need treatment using smaller spots just inside the arcades and two disc diameters temporal to the fovea. Sometimes the treatment needs to be even closer to the fovea (for instance, if the angiogram shows that there is a lot of ischemia temporal to the fovea driving the neovascularization). You can also get a bit closer to the nerve, but most folks stay at least 500 microns away to avoid thermal damage to the disc.

However, moving into areas this close to the center with panretinal photocoagulation is not without risk. If you find that you are considering this, you may want to refer the patient to a retina specialist because the patient may benefit from anti-VEGF treatment and/or vitrectomy to gain control and perhaps avoid the need to ablate retina so close to the center of vision. This is especially true given the Protocol S results discussed above regarding the use of anti-VEGF injections instead of laser. Injected patients had more peripheral vision, and it suggests that your PRP can be more peripheral to minimize field loss if you are using injections.

*It is helpful to use an angiogram with views of the periphery to guide your treatment. The FA will delineate the areas of capillary dropout nicely (especially the newer wide-field angiography techniques, as shown in **Figure 2** in Chapter 13). This allows very targeted treatment. There is, as yet, no study proving that such an approach is better, but it does seem more intuitively satisfying, and photos of the border between dying and normal retina are great visual aids to help patients understand the problem.*

In patients with less aggressive disease, it is possible to stay farther away from the posterior pole. For instance, Blankenship did a study years ago on the effect of bringing treatment just inside the arcades, versus bringing treatment only to within two or three disc diameters of the arcades (Figure 11).[25] Both groups did well, and there were fewer patients with macular problems in the peripheral group. However, the follow up was only six months in this study and patients usually have decades over which they can generate vasoproliferative factors from lightly treated retina. Nevertheless, this is one approach to consider in a patient who needs a lot of PRP but also has a lot of macular edema. The more peripheral treatment can start to get things under control with less risk of worsening the macular edema, particularly if you will also be using anti-VEGF drugs to protect the macula and reverse the overall level of retinopathy. You may need to fill in closer to the center especially if you stop the injections.

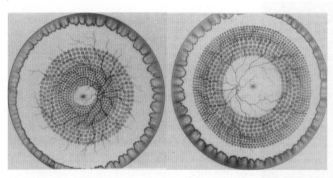

Figure 11: Patterns used in a vintage study comparing central versus peripheral PRP. Over six months the results were similar, and the peripheral group had less macular edema. Nowadays one would not treat as close to the center as is shown in the left image, but it does make sense to try to get more peripheral treatment in all your patients given the lack of useful peripheral vision in the far retina and the fact that that retina serves as a source of vasoproliferative substances. (Blankenship GW. A clinical comparison of central and peripheral argon laser panretinal photocoagulation for proliferative diabetic retinopathy. Ophthalmology 95: 170-7, 1988). Copyright Elsevier.

The temporal area can be problematic, because aggressive treatment in this location seems to be associated with the worsening of any macular edema. However, this area also tends to have a lot of ischemic retina, which can cause trouble if not treated aggressively. In general, there is a tendency for non-retina specialists to be too conservative in treating temporally, and because this area can develop neovascularization years down the road, it should be watched closely if it is not treated (remember if the untreated region "re-acquires" findings associated with severe NPDR, that area may need additional PRP and/or injections).

Getting Way Out There

Most of the time you do not need to go out as far as possible with a PRP; a bit anterior to the equator will do. On occasion you may want to treat everything, for instance in a very ischemic eye with anterior segment neo, or if there is a hemorrhage that prevents treatment of the usual sites. Treating that far out can be tricky, and it is tougher if the patient has had retrobulbar anesthesia and/or is uncooperative. You have some options:

> *1. Use all the lenses at your disposal—generally a Goldmann can go out the farthest in a phakic patient and a wide-field indirect contact lens can go out the farthest in a pseudophakic patient.*
>
> *2. Delivering laser through a binocular indirect ophthalmoscope is a great technique, but is usually not available to a comprehensive ophthalmologist. If this is an option, see the classic paper by Friberg on how to do this.[26] (By the way, this type of laser can be handy in the rare patient that absolutely can't stand the idea of anything touching their eye.)*
>
> *3. Have the patient look in the direction you are treating or, if they are blocked or uncooperative, torque the eye with the lens, as discussed in Chapter 4.*

4. If the eye is blocked, you or someone you trust can push in on the eye to indent the periphery and bring it into view. This often requires three hands, and you can get a very hot burn if you treat right on the hump that is created, so be careful.

5. There is an obscure device known as an Eisner Cone that fits behind the eyelids and provides a way to indent the periphery when using a Goldmann-type lens. This is not easy to use, and it is hard to find, but it is good to be aware of. You would probably be better off getting an indirect ophthalmoscope attachment for your laser if you really want to get this advanced.

6. There is one final move that can be very helpful, and that involves coordinating the position of the patient's head and the angle of your slit lamp. Sometimes, if you have them turn to the side a bit and you swing your slit lamp in the other direction, you can get a few extra degrees of visualization in the periphery. You can also raise and lower the laser table to get a little better view of the superior and inferior retina, respectively, as the patient's head tilts up and down at the slit lamp. Remembering that you have the option of moving the patient's head—even if it is just a few millimeters—can be very helpful with any type of laser treatment.

These techniques don't always work but sometimes they come in handy for diabetics or patients that have retinal tears in the periphery. YMMV.

Another subtlety of panretinal photocoagulation is to use variable spot density in different areas of the fundus. For instance, it seems reasonable to use a lower density of spots superiorly and nasally if the patient does not have severe disease. These areas correlate to the inferior and temporal visual field, which are the most useful portions, particularly in older patients who may have trouble ambulating. You can then treat the inferior retina more confluently (changes in the superior visual field tend to be less noticeable—unless your patient is a fighter pilot or spelunker). You can also treat more confluently in the temporal retina, which is generally compensated for by the nasal retina in the fellow eye.

Targeting neo

Earlier we mentioned that in the old days people would try just lasering the neovascularization, which didn't work at all. At times, however, treatment of vessels has been considered in the setting of a PRP. For instance, the DRS called for the direct, confluent treatment of flat patches of neovascularization in the periphery in order to stamp them out. It is not clear whether this is really necessary, because small patches of flat NVE tend to be benign anyway, and an effective PRP pattern will automatically take care of them. If you feel you have to treat directly, though, do be careful, because very aggressive laser will thin out the retina (it is helpful to increase the duration and decrease power over areas of neovascularization). Be aware that if traction develops, these atrophic areas can tear and allow the retina to detach. Most specialists no longer do this.

Although one may or may not want to treat small patches of flat neovascularization, there is agreement that one should go lightly in areas of pronounced gliosis and extensive neovascularization. These areas will very likely contract with time, and it is important to avoid treating them with heavy confluent burns due to the risk of stimulating aggressive contraction and the risk of eventual hole formation. If traction already exists, or if the retina appears excessively thin, you definitely want to avoid creating a hot spot, because if you poke a hole in one of these taut areas both you and the patient will be sorry very quickly. Repairing combined traction/rhegmatogenous detachments in diabetics is not easy, and the visual results are usually not impressive, even if the surgery is successful. If a hole forms, the vitreoretinal surgeon has to religiously strip off anything that can cause traction—something that is very tricky in areas of retina that are already atrophic. Just be careful when treating around places like this.

Where to stage the treatment

If a patient needs treatment over multiple sessions, most people will treat the inferior fundus at first. Treatment in this area tends to cause fewer symptoms because the inferior fundus corresponds to less useful visual field. This also ensures that the lower fundus is treated in the event that a hemorrhage occurs; the blood tends to settle inferiorly and preclude further treatment. Subsequent treatments will then fill in nasally, superiorly and temporally. Because there is a sense that treating temporal to the fovea is most likely to exacerbate macular edema, it is a good idea to close the temporal loop in at least two steps.

Figure 12 shows how you might treat over two or three sessions. The three-session approach is probably the safest for patients who have early disease and for whom there is no time pressure.

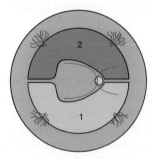 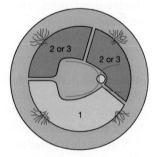

Figure 12: Suggested two- and three-stage PRP patterns. (Reproduced, with permission, from Folk JC, Pulido JS, Ophthalmology Monographs 11: Laser Photocoagulation of the Retina and Choroid, American Academy of Ophthalmology, 1997.)

One of the more difficult things about treating proliferative disease is that, as a conscientious physician, you may find yourself empathizing with your patient in terms of their absolute hatred of panretinal photocoagulation. It can be especially rough if they want to forego retrobulbar anesthesia for whatever reason—you can end up feeling every spot with them. All of this can make you want to try to "help them" by doing the least amount of PRP possible, and it can be easy to grossly undertreat patients by doing this.

Unfortunately, treating proliferative retinopathy usually means you have to be cruel to be kind, and unless you are absolutely convinced that the proliferative disease is mild, you need to harden your heart a bit and put in the appropriate treatment. The next chapter will discuss all sorts of strategies to minimize the patient's discomfort and make the process easier, so you can get the right amount of treatment in with the least amount of pain for both of you.

References

1.   Osaadon P, Fagan XJ, Lifshitz T, Levy J. A review of anti-VEGF agents for proliferative diabetic retinopathy. *Eye (Lond).* May 2014;28(5):510-520.

2.   Avery RL, Pearlman J, Pieramici DJ, et al. Intravitreal bevacizumab (Avastin) in the treatment of proliferative diabetic retinopathy. *Ophthalmology.* Oct 2006;113(10):1695 e1691-1615.

3.   Arevalo JF, Sanchez JG, Saldarriaga L, et al. Retinal detachment after bevacizumab. *Ophthalmology.* Nov 2011;118(11):2304 e2303-2307.

4.   Tsilimbaris MK, Kontadakis GA, Tsika C, Papageorgiou D, Charoniti M. Effect of panretinal photocoagulation treatment on vision-related quality of life of patients with proliferative diabetic retinopathy. *Retina.* Apr 2014;33(4):756-761.

5.   Salam A, Mathew R, Sivaprasad S. Treatment of proliferative diabetic retinopathy with anti-VEGF agents. *Acta Ophthalmol.* Aug 2011;89(5):405-411.

6.   Huang YH, Yeh PT, Chen MS, Yang CH, Yang CM. Intravitreal bevacizumab and panretinal photocoagulation for proliferative diabetic retinopathy associated with vitreous hemorrhage. *Retina.* Sep 2009;29(8):1134-1140.

7.   Sinawat S, Rattanapakorn T, Sanguansak T, Yospaiboon Y, Sinawat S. Intravitreal bevacizumab for proliferative diabetic retinopathy with new dense vitreous hemorrhage after full panretinal photocoagulation. *Eye (Lond).* Dec 2013;27(12):1391-1396.

8.   DRCR.net. Randomized clinical trial evaluating intravitreal ranibizumab or saline for vitreous hemorrhage from proliferative diabetic retinopathy. *JAMA Ophthalmol.* Mar 1 2013;131(3):283-293.

9.   Kaufman SC, Ferris FL, 3rd, Seigel DG, Davis MD, DeMets DL. Factors associated with visual outcome after photocoagulation for diabetic retinopathy. Diabetic Retinopathy Study Report #13. *Investigative ophthalmology & visual science.* Jan 1989;30(1):23-28.

10.   Early photocoagulation for diabetic retinopathy. ETDRS report number 9. Early Treatment Diabetic Retinopathy Study Research Group. *Ophthalmology.* May 1991;98(5 Suppl):766-785.

11.   Chappelow AV, Tan K, Waheed NK, Kaiser PK. Panretinal photocoagulation for proliferative diabetic retinopathy: pattern scan laser versus argon laser. *American journal of ophthalmology.* Jan 2012;153(1):137-142 e132.

12.   Palanker D, Lavinsky D, Blumenkranz MS, Marcellino G. The impact of pulse duration and burn grade on size of retinal photocoagulation lesion: implications for pattern density. *Retina.* Sep 2011;31(8):1664-1669.

13.   Brucker AJ, Qin H, Antoszyk AN, et al. Observational study of the development of diabetic macular edema following panretinal (scatter) photocoagulation given in 1 or 4 sittings. *Archives of ophthalmology.* Feb 2009;127(2):132-140.

14.   Preti RC, Vasquez Ramirez LM, Ribeiro Monteiro ML, Pelayes DE, Takahashi WY. Structural and functional assessment of macula in patients with high-risk proliferative diabetic retinopathy submitted to panretinal photocoagulation and associated intravitreal bevacizumab injections: a

comparative, randomised, controlled trial. *Ophthalmologica. Journal international d'ophtalmologie. International journal of ophthalmology. Zeitschrift fur Augenheilkunde.* 2013;230(1):1-8.

15.   Preti RC, Ramirez LM, Monteiro ML, Carra MK, Pelayes DE, Takahashi WY. Contrast sensitivity evaluation in high risk proliferative diabetic retinopathy treated with panretinal photocoagulation associated or not with intravitreal bevacizumab injections: a randomised clinical trial. *The British journal of ophthalmology.* Jul 2013;97(7):885-889.

16.   Ferraz DA, Vasquez LM, Preti RC, et al. A Randomized Controlled Trial of Panretinal Photocoagulation with and without Intravitreal Ranibizumab in Treatment-Naive Eyes with Non-High-Risk Proliferative Diabetic Retinopathy. *Retina.* Sep 30 2014.

17.   Couturier A, Dupas B, Guyomard JL, Massin P. Surgical outcomes of florid diabetic retinopathy treated with antivascular endothelial growth factor. *Retina.* Oct 2014;34(10):1952-1959.

18.   Michelotti MM, Jain N, Johnson MW. Bilateral Exudative Retinal Detachment in a Diabetic Patient With Severe Peripheral Retinal Ischemia. *JAMA ophthalmology.* Sep 25 2014.

19.   Mookhtiar MA, Carrim ZI. Treating maculopathy at the expense of proliferative disease: an emerging problem in 'macular treatment centres'. *Eye (Lond).* Nov 2014;28(11):1390-1391.

20.   Reddy VM, Zamora RL, Olk RJ. Quantitation of retinal ablation in proliferative diabetic retinopathy. *American journal of ophthalmology.* Jun 1995;119(6):760-766.

21.   Aylward GW, Pearson RV, Jagger JD, Hamilton AM. Extensive argon laser photocoagulation in the treatment of proliferative diabetic retinopathy. *The British journal of ophthalmology.* Mar 1989;73(3):197-201.

22.   Cho WB, Moon JW, Kim HC. Intravitreal triamcinolone and bevacizumab as adjunctive treatments to panretinal photocoagulation in diabetic retinopathy. *The British journal of ophthalmology.* Jul 2010;94(7):858-863.

23.   Margolis R, Singh RP, Bhatnagar P, Kaiser PK. Intravitreal triamcinolone as adjunctive treatment to laser panretinal photocoagulation for concomitant proliferative diabetic retinopathy and clinically significant macular oedema. *Acta Ophthalmol.* Feb 2008;86(1):105-110.

24.   Shimura M, Yasuda K, Nakazawa T, Kano T, Ohta S, Tamai M. Quantifying alterations of macular thickness before and after panretinal photocoagulation in patients with severe diabetic retinopathy and good vision. *Ophthalmology.* Dec 2003;110(12):2386-2394.

25.   Blankenship GW. A clinical comparison of central and peripheral argon laser panretinal photocoagulation for proliferative diabetic retinopathy. *Ophthalmology.* Feb 1988;95(2):170-177.

26.   Friberg TR. Laser photocoagulation using binocular indirect ophthalmoscope laser delivery systems. *Ophthalmic Surg Lasers.* Nov-Dec 1995;26(6):549-559.

27.   Simunovic MP, Maberley DA. ANTI-VASCULAR ENDOTHELIAL GROWTH FACTOR THERAPY FOR PROLIFERATIVE DIABETIC RETINOPATHY: A Systematic Review and Meta-Analysis. Retina. 2015;35(10):1931-1942.

28.   Writing Committee for the Diabetic Retinopathy Clinical Research N, Gross JG, Glassman AR, et al. Panretinal Photocoagulation vs Intravitreous Ranibizumab for Proliferative Diabetic Retinopathy: A Randomized Clinical Trial. JAMA : the journal of the American Medical Association. 2015:1-11.

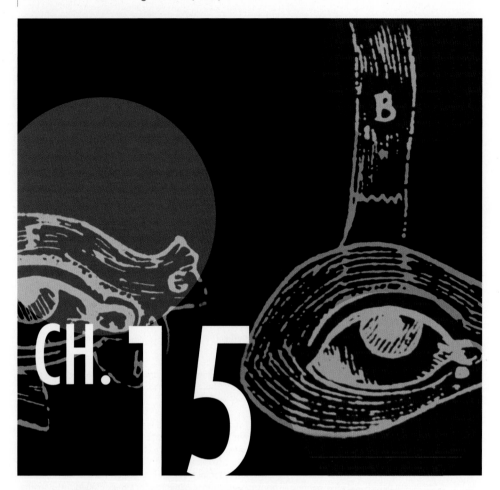

Trust Me, I'm a Doctor / Part Two: The Informed Consent for Panretinal Photocoagulation (PRP)

No man is good enough to govern another man without the other's consent. Abraham Lincoln
No man is good enough to govern any woman without her consent. Susan B. Anthony

Although the mechanics of doing a PRP can be daunting—and will be covered at length in the next chapter—perhaps the most difficult aspect of performing this procedure involves the informed consent. It can be very hard to provide an informed consent that gives the patient a fighting chance of actually understanding what on earth you are about to do to them. The general principles discussed in the section on informed consent for diabetic macular edema also apply here. However, a PRP is much more intense, and the results of treatment are even more likely to confuse the patient, so this chapter will emphasize points specific to doing a PRP.

Of course, there is another variable to consider with your consent, and that is whether you will be using anti-VEGF agents. Right now, the standard treatment for proliferative disease is a PRP, and everything in this chapter applies. But, as discussed previously, when anti-VEGF agents are used for macular edema, they also seem to "reset" the overall level of retinopathy and reverse the progression to proliferative disease. And if you use those agents in a patient with early proliferative disease, there is no question that you will shut it down fast. So in the future, there may be more of a role for injections to prevent and/or stabilize disease and your consent may reflect this—perhaps it will be shown that some injections and a very mild PRP may solve the problem. But the injections do tend to be transient, whereas the laser gives you permanent control—control that is less dependent on the patient's compliance. So it is really good to understand exactly what you are getting into when you try to do this particular treatment to a fellow human being.

THE DISEASE

As with macular edema, you have to start by educating the patient about the nature of the disease. This is easy if you have a sophisticated patient who has already read an entire retina textbook on the internet. If you have such a carriage-trade practice, with nothing but wealthy, educated patients, you don't even need to read this section—just tell them about the pathophysiology of retinopathy and the complications and you are done.

For those who practice in the real world, though, recognize that the nuances of proliferative retinopathy can be quite confusing to patients. So you might as well start with the basics, and this includes pointing out the irreplaceable nature of the retina. (You will find patients that truly believe that they will be able to get a total eye transplant if your laser doesn't work. Really. Educate them about this right at the start, so they are not surprised later—it will also help motivate them to take better care of themselves.)

Next, you need to relay the relentless (and asymptomatic) way that diabetes kills off the distal retinal blood vessels, which in turn causes ischemia and the generation of vasoproliferative factors, which in turn causes bad blood vessels and bleeding, etc., etc. The absolute key is to inform them that the goal of the laser is to get rid of these vasoproliferative factors, and that you are not going to "laser their blood vessels." It is very difficult to convey the "indirect" nature of this treatment, but the importance of making sure they understand this cannot be stressed enough.

First of all, if patients think you are simply going in and cauterizing the bad blood vessels, they will assume—if they hemorrhage subsequent to the laser—that you must have failed in your task. It is hard enough taking care of diabetics as it is; you don't want them thinking you are incompetent for the wrong reasons. Second, if they can understand that the goal is to eliminate the bad chemicals, and that only then will the bad blood vessels start to shrink, they then may be able to understand why they can have hemorrhages even after multiple laser sessions: The blood vessels may not completely disappear in spite of treatment because the laser can only indirectly convince them to go away. It also helps patients to understand why the problem can be controlled for a period of time, but then it can come back. In this case more of their peripheral retina dies off over time and there is a renewed stimulus for vascular growth. As a result, even more laser is required to control the problem.

You have to take the explanation a bit further, though, because some patients will still have hemorrhages with maximal laser. Explain that some of the new vessels can be stuck to the vitreous, and as the vitreous contracts, it can pull at the blood vessels, resulting in recurrent bleeding. This becomes a mechanical problem that no amount of laser can control. The management of this problem is discussed in the chapter on referral for vitrectomy, but this concept has to be conveyed to the PRP patient so they can understand the limits of the laser and why they may still have problems. Sometimes, when they hear this, they will then decide that the laser is a waste of time since they may still need surgery. It helps to point out that without laser their disease will get much worse and that a good laser treatment makes surgery much safer if it becomes necessary.

Conveying all of the above is way harder than doing the stupid treatment. You really need to drive home the point that you will be doing everything you can to control things, but in some ways treating proliferative retinopathy is like making a bed with a 30-foot pole—you can push things in the right direction but it is not clear how well everything will end up.

And this is only the beginning of a complete discussion with the patient...

For instance, depending on the situation there are variations to the consent. The touchiest presentation is if the patient has disease that needs treatment but they have never had any symptoms. You have nowhere to go but down in this case, and education is crucial. Having an angiogram is helpful, because you can at least show them the massive thunderheads of neovascularization that are building up on the horizon of their vision. These patients really need to understand where they are headed without treatment, i.e., severe, permanent vision loss, and they need to understand that the laser does not completely eliminate the risk of transient hemorrhages or gradual blurring over time, though it will very likely allow them to avoid blindness.

Occasional patients will have an annoying problem that is especially bad if you are treating them before they have symptoms: As the new vessels begin to contract from the PRP, they can hemorrhage. In other words, you start with an asymptomatic patient, and a week or two after their first laser they get their first vitreous hemorrhage (which can be truly frightening—these people have been living in dread of both blindness and other complications of their disease; see Chapter 22). If you haven't prepared them for this type of hemorrhage, you may lose the patient to follow up. This would not be so bad if they then just went to someone else; you would deserve to lose patients for being so obtuse. However, the usual pattern is for them to wander off after such a hemorrhage thinking that all doctors and lasers are crazy, and they don't follow up with anyone. They then show up a year or two later with really awful disease that may not be fixable. The point is that treating diabetes is like three-dimensional chess: You have to be able to anticipate not only what the disease might do to the patient, but also what the disease might do after you try to treat it; and then you especially need to anticipate the patient's emotional response to all of this. You may be the best laserist in the world, but if you do not prepare them in advance for hemorrhages and thereby lose the patient's trust, you will end up being the worst laserist in the world.

Another problem occurs when patients show up late in the game with a lot of neovascular tissue. Such patients usually have had at least a few symptoms, but often the symptoms do not give them any idea how bad the situation really is. You have to prepare these patients for a real rollercoaster ride. First of all, any patient with severe disease will usually have intermittent hemorrhaging in spite of laser—big vascular fronds just do not give up without a fight. In addition, any patient who has a great deal of neovascular tissue will inevitably develop tractional forces from the fibroblasts that ride along with the vessels. These forces tend to show up several months after your laser. They may be mild, but with advanced proliferative disease they are usually strong enough to create metamorphopsia, or even a tractional retinal detachment involving the posterior pole. It is important to give the patient advance warning about this. Then if they do need a vitrectomy they are prepared for the possibility and realize that it is a consequence of their proliferative disease and not your laser.

Whatever degree of proliferative retinopathy they have, you have to warn them that things may get darker before the dawn. If you start lasering them without really drilling this possibility into their heads, you can imagine the charitable thoughts they will have about you as you try to explain the above problems after the fact. Then just imagine what they will think if they go on to get tractional problems with permanent changes in their vision—or even if they have a little bit of vitreous haze from a hemorrhage that never completely clears. You will be congratulating yourself on having avoided severe blindness while they are remembering how great they could see before you started lasering them. Welcome to the fundamental disparity in the world of retina—we can be really happy and they think we are monsters. Constant repetition of the nature of the problem and the potential for trouble—even with successful treatment—is your only hope of having the patient at least partially on your side.

Finally, they need to understand something about the time frame of treating proliferative disease. If they have mild disease that you are treating preemptively this is not much of an issue because usually you will treat them and save them and nothing much happens. The time frame is much more of an issue if they have aggressive disease with active hemorrhaging, or if they have big vessels that are likely to hemorrhage and/or scar up. Proliferative disease like this does tend to eventually burn out—but it may take a year or two for things to really settle down.

Of course, this does not mean that they can mark their calendar and assume that in two years they will be done—even burned-out retinopathy needs long-term monitoring and occasional tweaks. This also assumes that their disease is not rampant and that the patient is religious about their follow up and their systemic control. (If they have bad disease the battle can go on forever, but this is usually something that your friendly neighborhood retina specialist will need to deal with, not you.) They need to understand that they are beginning a long-term process and although there is usually light at the end of the tunnel it takes time and effort to get there.

So—all of the above covers what might happen if things go right. What if things go wrong?

COMPLICATIONS

This is an annoying area to bring up, because you can spin an exhaustive tale about the nature of the disease and the importance of PRP, but once you mention that the laser can make things worse, you can pretty much assume that it is the only thing the patient and family will remember. Hopefully by following the teachings of your mentors, and from your own experience, you will be able to treat these patients with only minimal side effects. Still, there is a chance that they could sit back from your laser and be permanently worse—and you cannot avoid discussing this. The actual means by which vision can worsen is discussed at length in Chapter 17—your job is to cover the possibilities in the consent, but never ever have to actually deal with them.

To start with, even if you don't have a true complication there are potential nuisances that patients may notice after a PRP that they need to be informed about. For instance, some patients may notice changes in their side vision, night vision, focusing ability, and increased glare symptoms. If they have already had a hemorrhage, they won't mind these things too much because they have had a taste of what is coming and they tend to view things like needing reading glasses in the proper perspective.

However, if you happen to be treating them prior to their having had any symptoms, and if they develop some of these problems, they will think you are an idiot. They were doing fine before you started lasering them, and now look at the mess you have gotten them into: reading glasses, sunglasses, night driving trouble, etc. You have to prepare them for these side effects, and you have to repeat the rationale for treatment at every laser to remind them what would happen without treatment. If you have done a good informed consent, the patient will understand the need to be treated, and they will stick with you. Fortunately, with careful treatment you can usually avoid inducing these side effects, but you never want anything to come as a surprise to a patient.

It is also worth mentioning that the above problems cannot be blamed entirely on the laser—they are also part of having a sick diabetic eye. In other words, symptoms like changes in side vision, night vision, focusing ability, and resistance to glare are also part of what happens when most of the retina is slowly suffocating due to diabetes. It is one of the great ironies that by discussing these potential side effects of a PRP, you have pretty much guaranteed that if they ever have these symptoms they will blame your laser—even if the laser saved them and even if the laser is only partly responsible for the symptoms. This is why communication and repetition are so important when it comes to treating diabetics. Patients can easily draw unfair conclusions, and you have to anticipate this to keep them from wandering off and getting lost to follow up.

Also, remember that other doctors may look in your patient's eye and demonstrate their examination skills by saying something useless like, "Gee, you would not believe all the laser scars you have in the back of that eye!" (Review Chapter 3 for a full discussion on this.) Even if the patient does not have such an experience, they still tend to imagine that your PRP is gradually steamrolling away all of their retina, so you need to make sure they understand that your treatment is well away from the center of their vision, and that you are treating dead and dying retina that is good for nothing but poisoning the eye.

Finally, when discussing complications, remember to point out that the most feared "complication" is that the laser just plain does not stop their retinopathy, in which case they will definitely get worse—not from the laser, but from the disease.

Wrapping things up so you can get on to toasting retina...

Once again, this is a lot of information. Recognize that patients often want to distill this—or any medical info—into very simple terms. Sometimes, these distillations can be shockingly unrelated to the carefully thought-out reality you have presented. For instance, upon hearing that there may be side effects of the laser, some patients will immediately choose to "take their risks with going blind from the diabetes as opposed to being made blind sooner with the laser." Usually, these thoughts are left unverbalized. If a patient seems unwilling to have treatment, or is poorly compliant, you need to specifically address these concerns by directly asking the patient what they are worried about.

Since understanding the rationale behind doing a PRP can be so counterintuitive, another crucial thing to do is to ask the patient to simply repeat back to you their understanding of what you have said. As discussed in Chapter 5, this a very powerful tool to make sure the patient is really thinking what you think the patient is thinking (which is hopefully somewhat close to what you are thinking).

> **Don't forget** that some patients will incorrectly conclude from your informed consent that they will inevitably go blind, and that the treatment only slows the process down. Watch for this and ask about it—patients can really mess themselves up if they get this into their head. Check back to Chapter 5 for a refresher if needed.

The PRP consent is a bit trickier than a macular edema consent, but the same general pattern applies: Cover the disease, cover the complications, cover the fact that the biggest problem is that the treatment may not stop it, and then talk about the mechanics of the treatment. Recognize that treating macular edema tends to result in smooth curves of response that are easier for the patient to understand—things get slowly better or they get slowly worse, and you do the best you can. Treating proliferative disease is much more of a stuttering, unpredictable process, and you constantly need to anticipate not only everything that can go wrong, but also all the different ways the patient can misinterpret what is happening. Just keep repeating the information and listen carefully for indications that the patient is not getting it. Oh, and last but not least, never miss an opportunity to stress that the patient's systemic control plays a big role in how they respond to your laser. No matter how you do panretinal photocoagulation, it is still a very unpleasant experience and it can be a very powerful motivator if patients clearly understand that better control equals fewer PRPs.

"But Doc, I know somebody who was blinded by the laser..."

Recognize that panretinal photocoagulation is perhaps the most hated and feared treatment amongst diabetics, especially amongst less sophisticated patients. Many diabetics know someone who has been "blinded by the laser," and often it is a PRP that had something to do with it. If you are lucky, the patient will blurt out this concern and you can address it up front. If you are not lucky, you may get a vague sense of reluctance on the part of the patient—a sense that no matter how you try, you can't connect with them. If the patient does seem reluctant, you may need to specifically fish for this issue by asking whether the patient knows other people who have had laser treatment, and what their experiences were.

(Note: Another reason you may get this vague reluctance is because the patient has no money but does not want to admit it—see Chapter 21 on The Big Bucks. A final reason the patient may be reluctant is that you are gradually turning into the jerk doctor you were always afraid you might become and everyone secretly hates and mistrusts you. You are on your own with that.)

If this "blinded by the laser" issue does come up, it can be pointed out that usually any sense that the laser caused a problem is really due to the fact that the patient presented with severe disease and the laser simply could not control the process. In other words, the laser was too little, too late.

Here is a folksy story that might get the point across: Have the patient imagine that a train full of people is headed for a collapsed bridge, and the brakes are broken, so everyone is going to die. Well, suppose that some enterprising soul grabs a big safe, ties it to the train with a big rope, and then throws it out the door to try to slow down the train. The rope breaks and it doesn't work, and the train goes off the cliff. No one would blame the guy who threw the safe out for the fact that the train went off the cliff—it was just a desperate attempt to avoid a catastrophe. Then explain that the doctor who treated the person who "went blind from the laser" was just like the guy with the safe—it is not that the laser caused the blindness, but just that the laser couldn't stop it. Sometimes a parable like this can play big in the laser room.

Unfortunately, as discussed in the next chapter, panretinal photocoagulation is perhaps the one laser that is capable of blinding someone, so you cannot glibly blow off a concern like this with only a parable. Sometimes you can alleviate anxiety by getting more details about this "blinding laser." It may have been a completely different laser—for instance, there was an older treatment for macular degeneration that did indeed blind people by lasering away their fovea (but it was usually better than doing nothing). Still, it is possible that your patient's friend actually had a poorly done PRP. If it sounds like this was the case, all you can really do is point out that you will do everything possible to avoid such a problem. Go slowly with this—you have to be sure you are getting through.

Incidentally, you probably will not be able to tell whether any given "blinded by the laser" story represents a bad PRP or progression of disease in spite of a PRP. Heck, you probably won't even be able to tell whether it was something totally different, like maybe a diopter of astigmatism after Lasik (oh no!). Ultimately, it doesn't make any difference what happened; your goal is to provide a careful informed consent that covers all possibilities, so your patient will recognize that you recognize their concerns and that you are addressing them. You do not want to remotely suggest that their friend, relative, etc. was given a hatchet job of a laser. You were not there, and you do not have any idea about what really happened, so just focus on what you are trying to convey to your patient about their disease and their treatment.

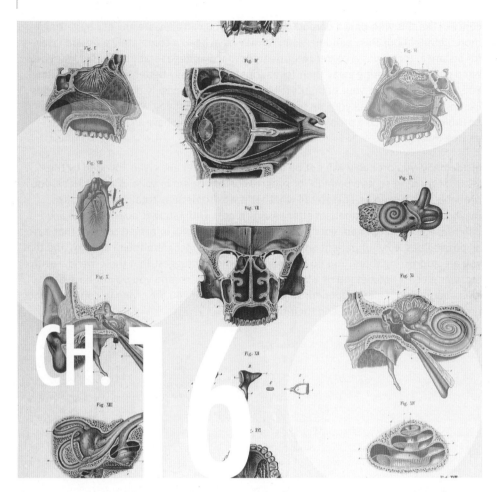

Doc, at Least It's Not as Bad as Having a Baby: Pain Control for PRPs

If you want others to be happy, practice compassion. If you want to be happy, practice compassion.
The Dalai Lama

Pain control can be a real problem, especially on a busy clinic day when all you want to do is cook some retina and move on. It is a good idea to slow down and deal with this thoroughly, though, for three reasons:

    1. It is a nice thing to do.

    2. It is easier to get patients to return for follow up if the experience is not awful.

3. When patients sit around waiting for their endocrinology appointment, they will compare your treatment to the treatment that the other diabetics get. They will dump you if they find out that someone else makes the experience more pleasant than, say, the average Inquisition.

It may well be that as new laser technologies and new laser techniques are brought online, the whole issue of pain control will become much less of a problem. For instance, faster techniques such as the pattern lasers mentioned in Chapter 6 can help minimize discomfort.[1] However, new technology tends to be very expensive, and there will always be patients that are especially sensitive regardless of the technique used. So it is a good idea to know what your options are.

What are your options?

There are a number of variables you can manipulate to make things more comfortable. The first is just to do what was mentioned in Chapter 8: Try to mentally put yourself in the patient's position, and try to anticipate what will scare them or make them uncomfortable. Always inform them about what you are about to do, and try to keep up a calm, soothing chatter while you are doing it—in other words, be a junior hypnotist.

Next, make sure the topical anesthesia has not worn off—especially during a long session. Sometimes the patient can't distinguish the difference between surface discomfort from the lens and pain from the laser. Often the simple act of giving the patient a break as you add more topical anesthesia will help them reset their pain threshold and allow you to get through the procedure.

It can also help to spread the treatment out over multiple sessions. This approach is usually too inconvenient, especially if patients or family members have to take time off of work for each treatment, but this can be effective for some patients as long as the proliferative disease is not progressing.

Some doctors feel that systemic medications will help. You can try anxiolytics or pain medicine by whatever route you feel comfortable. However, when you start tickling the long ciliary nerves it seems as though no amount of systemic medication can help. Nevertheless, remember that you have this option available to you, and you will find an occasional anxious patient who does much better with a hit of Xanax while they are dilating.

There are also some variables on the laser you can play with. The two simplest things are to decrease the spot size and decrease the duration. Some lasers can be set to very brief durations—like .02 seconds—and this seems to help decrease the discomfort.[2] Remember the warnings in the chapter on laser wrangling, though. When you decrease the duration, you will have to compensate by turning up the power. This, in turn, means that there is less time for the heat to spread out in the tissues, and you may be more likely to get a hot burn if you are not paying very close attention to what you are doing—especially if you are also using a small spot and there is a lot of pigment variation in the fundus. You may want to get comfortable with longer durations first, and once you have a more intuitive sense of how the retina responds to your laser you can try going to these much shorter durations.

Also, as mentioned in the previous chapter, you will notice that patients will sometimes complain of a great deal of pain in one location of the fundus and have less pain in another. Most of the time you can correlate this with the location of the various ciliary nerves; for instance, pain is especially common near pigmented areas between the tributaries of vortex veins and when you treat along the horizontal meridians where the long ciliary nerves are. Sometimes the phenomenon is random, and the patient will jump as you are treating a nondescript area of the fundus. You can always treat the less painful areas first and save the more painful ones for fill-in treatment, if necessary.

By the way, there is a situation in which the technique in the previous paragraph can burn you, as well as the patient. If, in follow up, you are seeing a patient who has an odd, patchy PRP pattern, you can bet that the previous treating physician did this very thing as the laser was being placed. If you need to do a PRP fill on such a patient, it is guaranteed that every single one of your spots will be quite painful, no matter how you tweak the settings—and the patient will be convinced that you are a monster and their previous doctor was a saint. It always helps to warn patients that subsequent lasers can be more painful so they understand what is going on.

Another technique is to slow down the rate of fire if you are moving along really fast with your foot on the pedal. Sometimes, rapid laser treatment results in temporal summation and can make the experience more miserable. Slowing down the treatment a lot, however, can make the laser really drag on and on, and it may be better to move on to some sort of anesthetic injection if both you and the patient are getting frustrated by the long process. Note, however, that this suggestion is less likely to apply to a scanning laser. Those devices can put in short duration spots so fast that you can cover a lot of ground very quickly and there is less summation of discomfort.

If you do need to do regional anesthesia, the standard approach tends to be either a retrobulbar or peribulbar injection, depending on your preference. There is a general sense that a retrobulbar injection is more effective and faster, but a peribulbar technique may be safer, with less risk of intracranial spread or damage to the optic nerve. A reasonable approach using the peribulbar route involves a slow and deliberate injection of approximately 6 cc. A few minutes of orbital pressure directly after the injection enhances spread, and you are right there if an orbital hemorrhage develops. A full discussion of regional anesthesia is well beyond the scope of this book—in short, do what works best for you based on your experience.

In addition to full-blown orbital anesthesia, you can occasionally get by with more localized injections. For instance, after numbing the conjunctiva with a pledget, you can place subconjunctival anesthesia, which will do a fairly good job of numbing the anterior portion of a quadrant of the fundus. Another option is to try a sub-Tenon's approach. Although a sub-Tenon's injection is unlikely to give you complete anesthesia of the globe, it can be very effective for treating a larger quadrant of the fundus, and may be safer than a retrobulbar injection. These are not techniques you are likely to use often, but they are good things to keep in your toolbox.

Of course, you need to clearly state the risks of performing local anesthesia, such as globe perforation, retrobulbar hemorrhage and even diplopia from inadvertent muscle injection. All of these things are unlikely, but if you treat a lot of diabetics, you will do a lot of orbital injections, and the odds will tend to catch up with you at some point. You do not want such a complication to come as a surprise to the patient. Usually, however, if the patient is miserable from the laser they will be more than willing to accept the small risk of a numbing shot.

Oh, and don't forget to find out if the patient is on Coumadin. If they are, you may want to check an INR to make sure things are not too out-of-control prior to an injection (more on this in Chapter 26). It is very easy to forget to do this when things are busy, but a busy day is exactly when the spiteful Retina Gods will make you try to remember how to decompress an orbital hemorrhage in an anticoagulated patient...

Hey, sorry *to throw in two text boxes that are only two paragraphs apart, but it is worth pointing out that if a patient has a really high INR, yet you still need to get some laser in, it is a great time to use the less invasive anesthesia techniques mentioned in the preceding blue box.*

Also, remember that people who have had Lasik or cataract surgery may now be refractively emmetropic, when in fact they still have big, pear-shaped eyes. Do not assume that an aggressive placement of your retrobulbar needle is safe just because patients are not wearing thick myopic spectacles. A needle through the retina tends to be worse than any degree of proliferative disease. Duh.

Finally, you should have appropriate resuscitation equipment available, and your staff should check on patients shortly after performing an anesthetic injection in the office. Remember that if your anesthetic gets into the brainpan, you do not want the patient to be alone when they stop breathing. Be especially alert for any patient who starts to complain of trouble swallowing or breathing within a few minutes of the injection—watch them carefully, and do not assume that they are just having a vasovagal response. Interesting fact: There has been at least one case report wherein a patient developed respiratory arrest from a retrobulbar, and when the patient recovered, he said that he was awake the whole time—he just could not talk or move during the episode.[3] So watch your language!

Whatever method you use to make your patients comfortable, your most useful tool is your clinical experience. It will not take long for you to realize that some patients do extremely well and other patients are likely to have real problems with the laser—and you will get a sense about which category a patient is in just by interacting with them well before you sit them down in the laser suite. (Insert, once again, the standard stereotype about the burly, tattooed male being unable to tolerate much of anything.) Another group that is guaranteed to be miserable are patients who take a lot of narcotics for chronic pain. Their opiate receptors are saturated, and everything you do to them can be very painful.

You will likely find that a patient's ability to tolerate the laser decreases as you put in the treatments. Some patients can do well with the first treatments, but end up needing an injection with subsequent ones. Just be flexible.

Also, recognize that there will be patients that are unable to decide between the risk of an injection and the pain of the laser. Although modern medicine emphasizes informing patients and "letting them decide for themselves," this is a situation in which you may want to gently suggest that they try an injection one time to see how they like it. They will usually choose to use an injection henceforth, once they see how easy it is, and you will have avoided a very, very long session at the laser. (Understand that this is not a situation in which saving the doctor's time is more important than the patient's safety. Instead, what you are avoiding is a long, tedious session wherein both the doctor and the patient can become toxic. This is bad for everyone, and can lead to an unhappy patient who does not return for follow up, which is the worst outcome. In this case, the overall karma allows you to revert to being a typical movie doctor from 1948 and just telling the patient what to do—not a good idea in general, but very effective when used sparingly.)

Some doctors will routinely give retrobulbar injections to everyone because they make treatment faster. Although this does rev up the assembly line, the sheer number of injections inevitably increases the risk of a bad complication. Also, you will find that patients who have been in such a practice are often very grateful if they end up going to a doc who gives them a choice, rather than automatically giving them a retrobulbar. It is much better to take a little more time to sit the patient down and let them see what a PRP is like. This way, you can explain in advance the potential risks of regional anesthesia, and they can decide for themselves if they want to bail out and get a numbing shot. You will find that many patients can tolerate a fairly stiff dose of laser without an injection, especially given the faster settings that are available on newer lasers. It takes a little more time, but most patients appreciate being given the chance to decide (preceding paragraph notwithstanding!).

What about post-op pain?

Most of the bad pain tends to occur right at the time of the laser, and then resolves once the treatment is over. However, sometimes the pain shows up later and can be quite severe, especially if the patient was blocked and you put in a lot of treatment. First of all, you do need to see the patient if there is increasing pain. As will be discussed in the next chapter, you need to make sure the cornea, and, in particular, the intraocular pressure are OK because these things can cause pain that needs to be treated with something other than "take two aspirin and call me in the morning."

Most of the time the eye itself will be doing well, but the person attached to the eye will be miserable. If you do a lot of laser at one session, you may want to give them a topical steroid and cycloplegics to head this off. You can also try oral pain medicine, although many diabetics are not allowed to have nonsteroidals due to possible effects on kidney function. Diabetics can also get violently nauseated from narcotics due to GI motility problems combined with the tendency of eye pain to produce nausea. Sometimes simple things like a cool or warm compress can help, and on rare occasion the most merciful thing to do is to re-block the patient using a long-acting anesthetic. Usually, time is your best friend.

Rarely, patients can get so sick from pain that they throw themselves into diabetic ketoacidosis, so have a low threshold of referral to their internist if they are telling you that they are having trouble keeping their food down or controlling their sugar. This type of severe problem seems more likely in younger patients with brittle disease, and fortunately the kind of post-op pain covered in this section is not common with modern techniques.

In any event, if you do run into problems with post-op pain, be sure to note it in the chart; such patients benefit from doing the laser in smaller increments over longer intervals if at all possible. Plus, monitor the patient to be sure they continue to return for follow-up. Patients who have a bad experience are more likely to blow off the whole thing and end up in real trouble.

References

1.	Muraly P, Limbad P, Srinivasan K, Ramasamy K. Single session of Pascal versus multiple sessions of conventional laser for panretinal photocoagulation in proliferative diabetic retinopathy: a comparitive study. *Retina*. Jul-Aug 2011;31(7):1359-1365.

2.	Al-Hussainy S, Dodson PM, Gibson JM. Pain response and follow-up of patients undergoing panretinal laser photocoagulation with reduced exposure times. *Eye*. Jan 2008;22(1):96-99.

3.	Simon MA, Cosgrove G, Zwillich CW, Chan ED. Respiratory arrest in the eye clinic. *Chest*. Jun 2001;119(6):1953-1955.

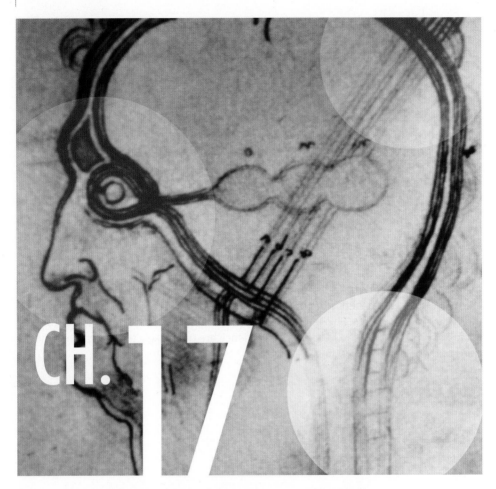

You Should Not Do Magic You Do Not Understand: Complications of Laser Treatment

Wise men learn by others' harms; fools by their own. Ben Franklin

Although each chapter covers some of the complications related to using laser to treat diabetic retinopathy, it is probably a good idea to gather all the potential complications together in one place so you can be reminded why you spent years learning how to do this.

ANTERIOR SEGMENT COMPLICATIONS

Probably the most common problem is scruffing up the corneal epithelium. Diabetics, especially by the time they have retinopathy, tend to have a bad combination of decreased corneal sensation and anterior basement membrane abnormalities. This can predispose them to punctate epithelial erosions or even full-thickness epithelial defects from the use of the contact lens. Fortunately this is not very common, and if there are symptoms they tend to be mild and self-limited—meaning that they are a perfect indication for all those artificial tear samples that keep building up in your cabinets. It also helps to rinse out the methylcellulose after treatment, both to increase the patient's comfort and because sometimes the methylcellulose can thicken and make the eye very irritated once the topical anesthetic has worn off. Don't forget to remind the patient to avoid rubbing their eye while it is numb, as well.

If there are a lot of pre-existing anterior basement membrane changes, or if the patient has a history of recurrent erosions or epithelial defects after a laser, you want to be very careful with their epithelium. You can consider adding copious ointment to the eye or even patching it temporarily to protect the epithelium while the anesthetic wears off. And take any epithelial defects seriously—don't become epithelial complacent. All it takes is one patient with a non-healing abrasion that turns into a scar because you didn't follow them closely, and you will feel really bad. This warning is perhaps more for those choosing to specialize in retina—we can get cavalier about the replaceable parts of the visual axis...

Really fragile corneas may need "no touch" techniques, such as using a 90-diopter lens to deliver the laser without using a contact lens. It is a bit of a hassle because you don't have as much control over the eye and you have to keep the lids open with your other fingers, but it is a technique that comes in handy at times. It has also been suggested that you can use a bandage contact lens underneath your laser contact lens if necessary.[1] Another option would be to deliver the laser using an indirect ophthalmoscope—although most general ophthalmologists' offices do not have one of these. If you are interested in doing this, there is an excellent reference at the end of Chapter 14.

Occasional patients may even get surface problems with the fellow eye—the eye you aren't treating. These patients are so busy trying to keep their fellow eye open and to fixate properly that they can dry it out, creating a lot of post-laser pain in an eye you never touched. Always encourage patients to periodically close their fixating eye, so as not to run into this problem. (By the way, this is particularly likely if you are treating both eyes at the same session. If they keep the eye you first treated wide open while you treat the second eye, they can really dry out the cornea because they are numb— especially if any methylcellulose is holding the anesthetic on the epithelium. You definitely need to remind them to close their first eye in this situation.)

It is also possible to cause corneal or lens burns with the laser, especially if you are using high powers. As mentioned in the chapter on contact lenses, the wide-field indirect lenses can result in high irradiance at the plane of the cornea or lens, especially with very large spot sizes. This becomes important if there are any opacities that might take up the laser on its way to the retina—such as eyelashes or bits of mascara stuck under the contact lens, or corneal pigmentation near the limbus.

A problem that was more common in the past was the occurrence of burns in the lens. This would happen if there was significant nuclear sclerosis: The yellowed lens would take up the laser (especially the blue-green wavelength that was more common back then). Patients would end up with very characteristic lenticular burns (see Figure 1).

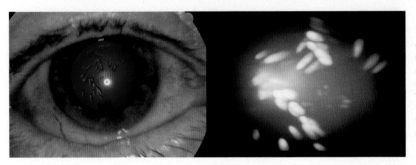

Figure 1: Lens burns seen with the red reflex and up close with direct illumination. With conservative powers and spot sizes, you will likely never see this, but be careful if you are using an indirect contact lens with large powers and spot sizes of 500 microns or more.

Other anterior segment complications include a dilated pupil, which can result from very heavy laser, especially anterior to the equator where the short ciliary nerves branch out to reach the ciliary body and iris. This probably will not have any significant visual consequences, but patients may get very fussy if they feel you have changed their appearance—not everyone wants to look like David Bowie. Try not to use heavy burns unless absolutely necessary, especially when treating over the long ciliary nerves in the horizontal meridian or when treating anterior to the equator. Some recommend not placing any spots directly on the horizontal meridian where the nerves are clearly visible due to the subtle pigment defining their borders.

You can bet that if your laser can affect iris function, it can also affect ciliary body function—and this can be far more annoying. A heavy PRP can definitely decrease accommodation. This is particularly important in a patient who is in the pre-presbyopic or early presbyopic age range. Remember that diabetics can have autonomic neuropathy to begin with, and if you tip them into more pronounced presbyopia, you can end up with a very unhappy patient, even if your superb laser has spared them from total blindness. Again, you have to do what you have to do, but it is important to both

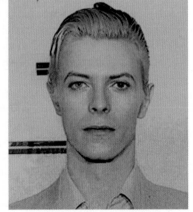

Figure 2: David Bowie's eyes.

warn patients about this possibility so they are not surprised, and to try to go easy when treating over the nerves if possible.

There are also patients that can develop rather severe iritis after a laser.[2] This is more likely with hot and heavy treatment, and sometimes it can even result in synechiae formation—something to be avoided in patients that need to be dilated a lot to see the back of their eye. (Synechiae can also occur of you are clipping the pupil margin with your treatment. This is more likely with an indirect ophthalmoscope delivery system, but it can happen with a slit lamp laser, too.) Consider using a topical steroid and cycloplegic if you put in a lot of laser or if you have a patient with a history of uveitis. Beginning a topical NSAID a few days before the PRP is not a bad idea either.

Patients can also have problems related to elevated intraocular pressure.[3] Heavy panretinal photocoagulation can cause diminished outflow because of swelling of the ciliary body. Occasionally this swelling can even rotate the iris enough to cause angle-closure glaucoma. This is more likely in patients who already have narrow angles, and you may want to avoid very heavy treatment in one session with such patients. This is also something to keep in mind if you have a patient with longstanding glaucoma and fragile nerves. Even if they don't get angle closure they can have a transient rise in pressure that can threaten their nerve, and you should adjust your treatment accordingly.

The important thing is that if a patient calls you because of pain subsequent to panretinal photocoagulation, do not assume that they are a wimp and phone in some narcotics. You really should look at them to determine if they have developed an abrasion, uveitis, elevated pressure or even angle closure. By the way, these problems tended to be more common in the old days when patients were pounded with confluent white-hot laser burns or, worse, were treated with xenon photocoagulation. Doing a modern, careful PRP is much less likely to result in trouble, but it is still important to be aware of all the things that can go wrong.

Speaking of Glaucoma

Here is another item that goes into the "It's always something" file. Although the past literature is variable on whether diabetes predisposes people to glaucoma, there is a growing sense that diabetics are more likely to get it.[4] Plus, patients may be getting steroid shots or anti-VEGF shots, both of which can raise the pressure acutely and chronically—and this problem is more likely to occur in patients with pre-existing glaucoma or ocular hypertension (this was covered in Chapter 11). Also remember that any patient that has had a vitrectomy is at increased risk for glaucoma, especially in pseudophakic patients (perhaps because the increased oxygenation causes damage to the trabecular meshwork).[5] Finally, retina specialists can be rather lame about diagnosing glaucoma; they might start to think of it by the time they can see the brainstem through the cupped-out nerve. So as a comprehensive ophthalmologist you have to be responsible and monitor for the possibility of glaucoma.

And it gets trickier because doing a PRP can mess up your ability to catch early glaucoma. Both the PRP and the peripheral retinal ischemia that prompted the treatment will whittle away at the nerve fiber layer.[6] This can make the cup bigger and also make the nerve look paler.[7] Plus, between the peripheral capillary drop out and the laser, the patients will have visual fields that are hard to interpret. It can be easy to miss early glaucomatous changes if you assume everything is due to the diabetes and its treatment. So be extra careful in patients that you think might end up with glaucoma— don't blow off changes in the nerve as simply being from the retinopathy and/or laser.

POSTERIOR SEGMENT

Most posterior segment issues have already been discussed in the preceding chapters— but a little repetition is good, because you want to make it through your whole career without gaining personal experience with any of these problems. The first thing, of course, is to be sure you treat the correct eye. You should have already received tons of advice about this. One handy thing is to put a piece of tape over the eye that you, your tech and the patient all agree is the correct one (especially if you will see other patients prior to getting back to someone that has been moved to the laser room).

Perhaps the most disastrous mistake is to create an inadvertent foveal burn. Follow all the advice about constantly checking your location in the fundus and *always* know for sure where you are. Remember that you are far more likely to do something like this when you start to feel very comfortable with your laser skills, and that it is especially likely to occur when you are frantically trying to stay above water on a busy clinic day. Don't ever get overconfident, and don't ever let yourself feel rushed when you are guiding coherent light into a fellow human being's eye. You don't want your handiwork to turn into a treasured slide in some retina specialist's talk on laser complications.

If you forget which eye you are treating, or if you mix up which side of the eye you are treating while using an indirect lens, you can easily get lost. This is especially likely when treating in the temporal aspect of the posterior pole, where there is no optic disc or vascular arcade to warn you that you are crossing into no man's land. This can happen more readily if your view is limited by a small pupil, or if media opacities interfere with your ability to sweep around and orient yourself. Also, remember that if you are using the large mirror in a Goldmann three mirror lens, it is possible to get deep into the macula without realizing it, especially if the patient is looking toward this mirror (Figure 2 in Chapter 7). Sometimes patients will have large vessels running across the posterior pole that can simulate the appearance of nasal retina, and this can really confuse you if you are not careful. If you come across such a patient, be *very* careful about where you are treating (Figure 3).

Almost all of these problems can be overcome by simply checking where you are at all times so that you do not get a chance to get lost. As mentioned before, it is good to set landmarks in your head so that if you see them, you know you are in a danger zone. Another

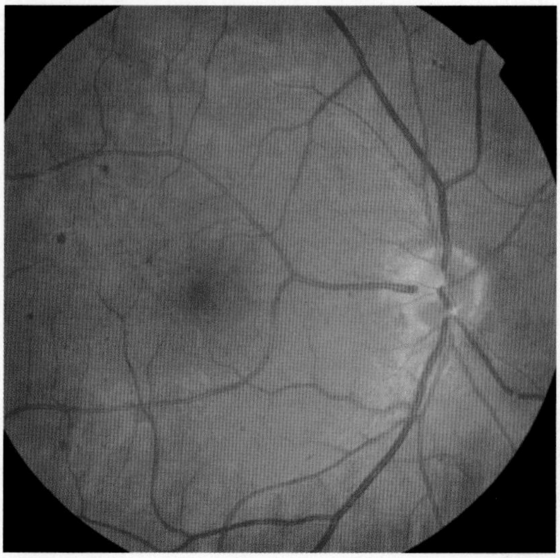

Figure 3: An example of a large vessel heading toward the fovea. If you get lost in this eye you can mistake the macula for nasal retina and end up with something really unpleasant to remember whenever you can't sleep at 3 a.m.

option, especially when performing PRPs, is to put a line of laser spots at the posterior edge of your planned treatment pattern and then treat outward from this line—always moving from the back of the eye to the front—so at all times you are moving away from the posterior pole as you place spots.

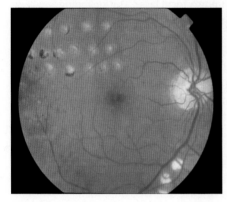

Figure 4: (Left) Whew, just in time. Five out of five doctors recommend not putting your PRP here...

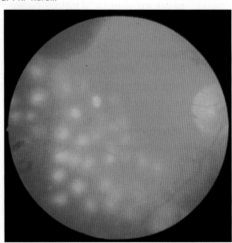

Figure 5: (Right) This should make you cringe. But you can see how easy it could be to do this, given the hazy view, the hemorrhage that obscures retinal vessels and the nearby laser scars. All of these things can make you think you are where you are not.

There are also a host of complications related to poor power management with your spot size and intensity. If you remember all of the variables that can get you into trouble, you can stay out of trouble. For instance, if you decrease the spot size, or if your aiming beam suddenly becomes smaller and brighter, you know you need to cut back on the power.

A hot spot can create any number of problems, all of which are bad. A hot spot can cause a vitreous hemorrhage, intraretinal hemorrhage, subretinal hemorrhage, and even choroidal hemorrhage if you manage to burn down deeply. Remember, too, that if you have actually done any of these things, then you should keep pressure on the eye with the contact lens until any bleeding stops. What if the bleeding does not stop? Double the duration and ¼ the power – long slow burns have excellent coagulation properties.

Also remember that if you burned something bad enough to cause a hemorrhage, you have probably also created a full-thickness retinal hole. You want to make sure you treat around the offending area enough to tack the retina down so you don't get a detachment. This is one of the reasons why you need to be really careful around traction retinal detachments. Sometimes the edge of these areas will have darker pigmentation and take up laser really fast. If you manage to poke a hole in the retina right next to a place where scar tissue is trying to pull off the retina you can precipitate a full-blown detachment.

A severe burn in the peripheral retina can also result in a late complication known as a choroidal-vitreal anastomosis. In this case a hot burn gets so deep that choroidal vessels are induced to anastomose with retinal vessels and then the ensuing network grows up into the vitreous, creating very aggressive, destructive neovascularization. This problem was more likely in the bad old days, and often occurred when people were using very heavy treatment with laser or xenon arc in an attempt to directly shut down NVE. It is something that is useful to know about in the abstract, but you should never come close to causing it.

You can also poke holes in things without a hemorrhage, and this is particularly noticeable if you burn through Bruch's membrane while doing a focal laser. The sickening sight and sound of this, as mentioned in Chapter 9, is something you should strive to never experience. If it does happen, remember that such a spot may be a nidus for the development of a choroidal neovascular membrane, and you will want to watch for any unusual subretinal hemorrhage or localized macular edema that heralds the development of a new vessel. Also, recall that you do not necessarily have to break Bruch's membrane to get a neovascular membrane; it can also occur around less intense laser treatment. All of this is why you should strive to do the least amount of laser necessary to treat macular edema.

Also remember that there are occasional patients who are extremely good observers and will notice each and every focal spot that you apply. These are more likely to be younger, type-A patients who do not have a lot of diabetic disease and who are much more likely to notice the punctate changes in their perifoveal vision. As mentioned in the chapter on informed consent for treating diabetic macular edema, you want to make sure patients are aware of this possibility and you should always treat as lightly as you can—but if they need treatment, they need treatment.

There are also a few things that can happen when treating proliferative disease that are not really complications, but your patient may be likely to feel that they are— for instance, the occurrence of a vitreous hemorrhage shortly after a PRP due to the shrinkage of the blood vessels. There is really no way to avoid this, and it may actually represent a good response to treatment. However, you do need to warn the patient about this possibility, especially if they are presenting with asymptomatic proliferative disease.

The other "complication" is that the patient may develop more significant traction, perhaps even a retinal detachment, as the neovascular tissue responds to your treatment. This can be very frustrating because you can see the new vessels retract nicely thanks to your treatment, but the patient is rewarded with blurred vision and metamorphopsia that wasn't present prior to your laser. If you think something like this might happen, you want to warn the patient, especially if they are presenting late in their proliferative career with extensive disease that should never have been allowed to develop in the first place. If you are worried that this could be a big problem, you might want to refer the patient to your friendly neighborhood retina specialist.

Sometimes a very aggressive PRP can result in an exudative retinal detachment and/ or choroidal effusions, which can even simulate a rhegmatogenous retinal detachment. Usually this problem is evidence of a very sick eye, and it is more likely to occur in patients who get lots of hot spots in one sitting. If you actually manage to do something like this to a patient, you should give them topical steroids and cycloplegics to help things settle down, and then try to be gentle with any additional treatment.

There are other, stranger things that have been reported. For instance, patients have developed thermal optic neuritis from excessive treatment near the nerve, or retinal vasculitis and even vascular occlusion from hot burns on vessels. You should never, ever have any experience with entities such as this; they are included simply for completeness.

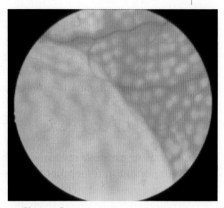

A more common problem associated with panretinal photocoagulation is peripheral field loss, and this was especially likely in the olden days when large amounts of laser were applied rapidly. Measurable changes can occur in up to 50% of patients, although milder treatment seems to have less of an effect.[8,9] Of course, patients are receiving

Figure 6: Intense PRP resulting in a peripheral serous retinal detachment. (**Figures 1, 4, 5**, and **6** courtesy of James C. Folk, M.D. [the images—not the techniques]).

the treatment because the bulk of their peripheral retina is either dead or dying off— the difference being that if they choose to have field loss from their disease alone, they have to accept the risk of total vision loss from untreated retinopathy. In other words, whether peripheral field loss is related to the disease or your treatment is largely academic; the patient really has no choice. Hopefully you, with your newly gleaned knowledge, will be able to put in a gentle yet effective PRP with less risk of dramatic visual field loss than was seen in the old days. Still, this can be a real problem—especially in terms of driving—and hopefully a time will come when patients won't have to risk this additional insult to their vision as new treatments come online. For instance, recall that anti-VEGF drugs can to some extent reverse retinopathy. If studies show that combining partial PRPs with anti-VEGF agents has the long-term safety and efficacy of a full PRP, it may allow control of proliferative disease with much less treatment.

Panretinal photocoagulation can also cause problems with dark adaptation, nyctalopia and color vision, all of which seem more likely with heavier treatments. However, it is again hard to know to what degree these can be attributed to the laser versus the severity of the underlying retinopathy. Even diabetics who do not need PRP complain of problems along these lines as they get older and experience the general deterioration of retinal function that occurs with the disease. Nevertheless, if significant problems occur right after a laser, then it probably was the laser and patients need to be warned about this possibility.

A related problem is that diabetics will complain of increased sensitivity to light, which usually represents generalized deterioration due to diabetes. However, it may also be possible that the loss of peripheral pigmentation and RPE absorption that accompanies extensive scarring from laser treatment allows light to bounce around in the eye, so the remaining retina has even more problems in bright light situations. Whether it is from the laser or just a sick eye, you will often hear this complaint.

Of course, one of the main complications of both macular treatment and PRP is decreased central visual acuity. This is usually due to exacerbation of preexisting macular edema, and ways to avoid this are specifically covered in the chapters on performing these treatments—especially with the increasing use of pharmacologic agents to pre-treat both the edema and proliferative disease.

ONE LAST COMPLICATION

After having carefully reviewed all the different ways you can screw up with lasers, it is important to remember that perhaps one of the most worrisome complications is to have your treatment fail because it was inadequate. Generally, a "less is more" technique is the best way to go, because the fewer spots you need to place—for any treatment—the more vision your patient gets to keep. Unfortunately, if you don't put in enough spots to control the disease, then you for sure haven't done the patient any favors. Plus, if you are using anti-VEGF agents, you need to remember that the effect of those drugs wears off. Macular edema, and especially proliferative disease, can recur once patients are no longer getting injections, especially if the injections have lulled you into a false sense that the disease is well controlled. An incomplete PRP in this setting can allow aggressive recurrence of the proliferative disease.

Ultimately, decisions about how aggressive to be with laser will become easier with time and experience, but if you do end up going light with any treatment, watch the patient closely and do not allow them to be lost to follow up for any reason.

OK. THE REALLY LAST COMPLICATION

This is covered in other chapters, but worth repeating. PRP can be very unpleasant, and, depending on your situation, very expensive. And it definitely isn't Hollywood—patients don't suddenly see a lot better and are forever grateful. Instead, they tend to really hate the whole thing. And it is very easy for them to decide to never come back, which is the worst complication because they will return much later with really bad disease that may not be possible to control. So make sure they understand what is going on and that you do everything you can to be sure they are following up appropriately.

References

1.   Folk JC, Pulido JS. *Laser photocoagulation of the retina and choroid*. San Francisco: American
        Academy of Ophthalmology; 1997.

2.   Sinha MK, Narayanan R, Chhablani JK. Hypopyon uveitis following panretinal photocoagulation in a
        diabetic patient. *Seminars in ophthalmology*. May 2014;29(3):166-168.

3.   Blondeau P, Pavan PR, Phelps CD. Acute pressure elevation following panretinal photocoagulation.
        Archives of ophthalmology. Jul 1981;99(7):1239-1241.

4.   Zhao D, Cho J, Kim MH, Friedman DS, Guallar E. Diabetes, Fasting Glucose, and the Risk of
        Glaucoma: A Meta-analysis. *Ophthalmology*. Oct 2 2014.

5.   Wu L, Berrocal MH, Rodriguez FJ, et al. Intraocular Pressure Elevation After Uncomplicated Pars
        Plana Vitrectomy: Results of the Pan American Collaborative Retina Study Group. *Retina*. Oct
        2014;34(10):1985-1989.

6.   Kim J, Woo SJ, Ahn J, Park KH, Chung H, Park KH. Long-term temporal changes of peripapillary
        retinal nerve fiber layer thickness before and after panretinal photocoagulation in severe diabetic
        retinopathy. *Retina*. Nov-Dec 2012;32(10):2052-2060.

7.   Singh H, Garg S, Sharma R, Venkatesh P, Saxena R, Dada T. Evaluation of the effect of pan retinal
        photocoagulation on optic nerve head parameters using HRT3. *Journal of glaucoma*. Sep
        2014;23(7):467-470.

8.   Fong DS, Girach A, Boney A. Visual side effects of successful scatter laser photocoagulation surgery
        for proliferative diabetic retinopathy: a literature review. *Retina*. Sep 2007;27(7):816-824.

9.   Tsilimbaris MK, Kontadakis GA, Tsika C, Papageorgiou D, Charoniti M. Effect of panretinal
        photocoagulation treatment on vision-related quality of life of patients with proliferative diabetic
        retinopathy. *Retina*. Apr 2013;33(4):756-761.

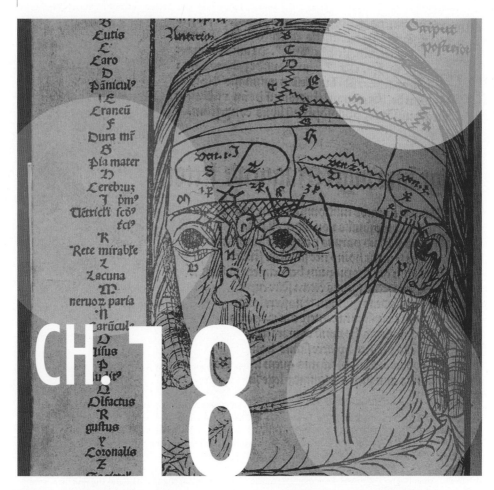

Now What? Following up a PRP and All Those Little Hemorrhages

All bleeding eventually stops. Jeffrey M. Goller M.D.

One of the most difficult aspects of treating proliferative diabetic retinopathy is deciding whether further laser treatment is warranted. About two-thirds to three-fourths of treated eyes will demonstrate regression, and sometimes this can begin as early as a few days after treatment. It usually takes a bit longer to see the full effect of the laser, so it is common to check patients at about six to eight weeks after the last laser session to get a sense their response. If you were treating mild neovascularization or severe NPDR you can wait longer, perhaps a few months. If there is a potential for significant traction, or if the patient is particularly worrisome, it makes sense to see them sooner. (Remember, this refers to PDR being treated only with laser. If you are using anti-VEGF agents the new vessels will disappear really fast—in days—but then you need to check in about a month to be sure they are staying away and then decide how often they need to be reinjected.)

The ideal response to laser is complete and permanent resolution of the neovascularization, period. Unfortunately, this ideal is not as common as one would wish, especially in younger patients, and often there are persistent vessels of some sort. If there is any sense that the vessels are growing, or if there is evidence of vitreous hemorrhaging (even small amounts of blood in the far periphery that are otherwise asymptomatic), then it is very reasonable to put in more laser. Although there are no controlled studies defining the amount of laser, there is a sense that if the first treatment does not work, a rather substantial amount of laser is necessary to generate any sort of useful response the second time around. For instance, it probably does not help to put in 200 to 300 spots in a patient with persistent disease—instead, it seems that such patients usually need an additional critical mass of perhaps 500 to 1,000 spots.[1] The exception to this would be if there is an area of the fundus that has less treatment, and especially if the new vessels are clearly growing in the direction of the untreated area. In this case, a smaller amount of treatment directed to the ischemic area may be all you need.

As mentioned before, you can squeeze in over 6,000 spots to control the disease, but such patients may benefit from referral for intravitreal therapy and/or a vitrectomy, rather than dribbling in more and more laser over several months and slowly eliminating all their visual field. Anti-VEGF agents can definitely decrease persistent neovascularization, although the treatment may need to be repeated.[2] And sometimes bad vessels need to be cleared out with a vitrectomy, which eliminates the vitreous scaffolding. Chapter 19 discusses when to consider referral in more depth.

If the blood vessels seem to have shrunk back somewhat, but have not disappeared, the decision to treat can be more difficult. Some patients may simply have persistent neovascularization that doesn't cause trouble for years, and for these patients additional laser is a waste of time and peripheral vision. If the residual vessels are small in size and have really shrunk down—and if they are not widespread—it makes sense to watch them a bit. Another pattern that suggests quiescence is if the tips of the vessels have receded into thick, club-like endings (Figure 1).

If the vessels are becoming more fibrotic in nature it suggests that the retinopathy is leaving the proliferative phase and laser may not be needed (but do watch for progressive traction). On the other hand, if the tips of the vessels consist of fine, sprouting buds, then treatment should be added. Sometimes a fluorescein angiogram can be helpful—active vessels can be very leaky, whereas quiescent, involuted vessels will leak much less (Figure 2).

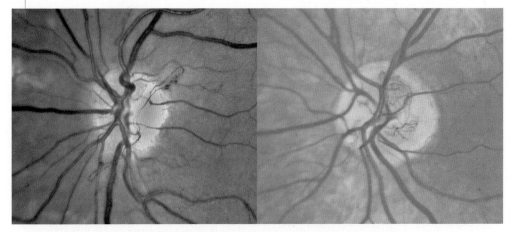

Figure 1: Old and new neovascularization. The photo on the left shows the kind of thready, ropy appearance of regressed neo after PRP. Note the clumpy, grape-like appearance of the ends of the vessels; they have shriveled up in failure. The photo on the right shows active vessels. Note how they are spread out and arborized with fine vessels at the tips growing in all directions. (Right photo courtesy of the Early Treatment Diabetic Retinopathy Study Group.)

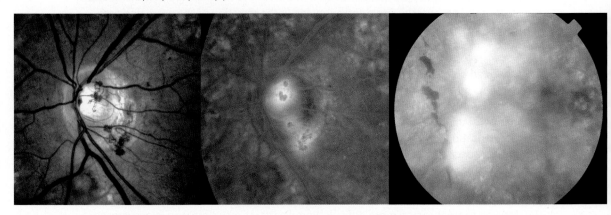

Figure 2: Another example of regressed neovascularization, showing the shriveled appearance of the old vessels. Note the relative lack of staining in the later phases of the angiogram (middle). Such vessels are often nicely backlit by the small amount of fluorescein that does leak out. Compare this to the figure on the right, which shows the florid leakage seen with new, active vessels. There is no view whatsoever of the actual vessels themselves because they are obscured by all of the fluorescence.

Another important variable is the density of your PRP. If you were trying to go lightly and the vessels don't seem to be regressing, then you should consider filling in the PRP pattern. An angiogram may be helpful here because it may demonstrate areas of non-perfusion that are not obvious clinically and you can see whether your initial laser covered such areas. Wide-field angiography can be really valuable to determine where treatment is needed if you have access to that technique (see Figure 2 in Chapter 13).

If you do decide to add treatment, you can fill in between spots and extend your treatment further into the periphery. You can also extend the treatment closer to the center of the macula, but if you really think you need to laser valuable real estate, you may want to get a second opinion beforehand. Also, if you need to treat over previously treated retina you need to be very careful about where you place your spots. Treatment that hits previous laser scars may be painful for the patient, and more importantly, the cicatricial pigmentation can dramatically increase the laser uptake and cause a hemorrhage or hole.

Other factors that may help you decide about how hard to treat residual vessels were discussed in preceding chapters. They include the patient's age, the course of the fellow eye, the degree of compliance and control, and whether the patient is anticoagulated.

*A **conundrum** that occasionally comes up is when a patient had the first stage of a PRP performed, but either never returned for follow up or the treating physician was happy with the initial results and did no further treatment. You may see these patients years later with partially treated neovascularization, no symptoms, and laser treatment in only one sector of the fundus. If they have been stable for quite some time, and if they have good systemic control, it is reasonable to observe them. There is a risk of progression of their proliferative disease if they are left untreated, but there is also a risk of converting a happy asymptomatic patient into a bitterly symptomatic patient from problems related to a full dose of PRP. You just have to use your clinical judgment, and if the patient does elect observation it is important that they understand the risks and the need for continuous follow up.*

The converse occurs when a previously untreated patient needs treatment and has only a single clump of neovascularization in one part of the fundus.* It may seem that doing laser in only that area is all that is needed. This is not a good idea. A localized area of neovascularization does not mean that only one part of the retina is ischemic—especially as the vessels grow closer to the nerve. You may be able to get away with a milder PRP in such a patient, but once a patient crosses the line into needing laser, it is a good idea to treat all around the fundus rather than in one local area.

*By the way, make sure you have the correct diagnosis in a patient with a localized area of neovascularization. For instance, they could have the entity mentioned in Chapter 27 that begins with a "B".

In addition to figuring out how to manage residual neovascularization, there can also be problems deciding what to do about patients who have recurrent vitreous hemorrhages. It is not uncommon for diabetics with persistent neovascularization to have intermittent hemorrhages over the years. If the vessels are growing or appear succulent, and there are significant areas of untreated retina, then adding more PRP is the simplest thing to do.

Sometimes, however, hemorrhages may be due to intrinsic vascular fragility; an eye that is full of beat-up old blood vessels will have an occasional spontaneous hemorrhage, just like people can have spontaneous bruises on their legs. More laser is unlikely to make any difference in such patients, and if you feel their proliferative disease is burned out and their PRP pattern is adequate, then observation is all that is needed.

A more common problem is age-related vitreous contraction that begins to tug at old neovascularization. In fact, patients may go years with nicely controlled disease, and then suddenly start to get hemorrhages simply because they have survived long enough for their vitreous to shrink and start pulling on the regressed vessels. Adding more laser may be irrelevant for such patients, because now a mechanical problem is being imposed on their otherwise quiescent proliferative disease. On the other hand, it may be reasonable to fill in with more laser if there are large areas of untreated retina in the periphery. The assumption would be that vasoproliferative factors released by the untreated retina are keeping the vessels a bit more swollen than they might otherwise be, and they are therefore more likely to hemorrhage with even a little traction. Usually, however, such patients will need a vitrectomy if the hemorrhages are recurrent and do not clear quickly.

A variation on this theme is if the patient begins to develop vitreous contraction, and then is fortunate enough to get a complete vitreous separation from the retina. If this happens, patients almost always get a vitreous hemorrhage, but the process also eliminates all the traction. These patients may have very little in the way of subsequent hemorrhaging, and there is no role for more laser. (And just because nothing is simple, sometimes these patients with light laser, vitreous detachments—and often poor control—will start to get anterior segment neovascularization instead of retinal neovascularization. It is almost as if the vessels can't find anything to grow on in the back so they start sprouting all over the front. So don't forget to look at the iris and even the angle in such patients—see Chapter 20.)

And once again: Although complete vitreous separation is usually a cause for celebration in the setting of diabetic retinopathy, don't forget to look carefully for retinal breaks or tears.

However, a total vitreous detachment is a lucky event that does not happen too often; usually the vitreous is only partially separated, and it then applies even greater traction wherever it remains attached. If there are areas where the PRP pattern is light, then more laser may help to shrink down the vessels that are now being tugged on more aggressively. Usually a vitrectomy is required if the hemorrhaging is persistent.

If there is one patch of neovascularization that keeps bleeding in spite of good laser, some doctors advocate attempting to directly close the offending vessels with localized laser. This may be worth trying if the vessels are small and flat and the retina is relatively healthy—but this is something that is much easier said than done even in the best of circumstances. In general, use a very large spot size and low power laser to shrink the vessels slowly and systematically. However, if the vessels are big or elevated, or if the retina is thin and on stretch, you can end up creating a hole which will cause a detachment. This is a big disaster. If you really want to try this technique, consider getting some help before you do—nowadays a vitrectomy is probably safer.

If you have a bunch of diabetics with proliferative disease in your practice, it can be easy to assume that if they call with vision loss they must have a hemorrhage. It gets weird if they come in with profound vision loss and—voila—there is no hemorrhage (or other immediately obvious cause). Well, there is another sneaky thing that eyes with proliferative disease can do: they can develop a branch or central retinal *artery occlusion with minimal findings (**Figure 3**). This occurs because the retina is thinned out from both ischemia and your lasers, so it doesn't dramatically swell up and turn white, or demonstrate a nice cherry red spot, compared to patients with normal retinas. You need to look for subtler thickening and may also need to do an FA to identify the vascular occlusion. Increased inner retinal thickness and reflectivity on OCT is another typical finding (as well as the inner retinal atrophy that occurs over time). Unfortunately, these eyes are also more likely to get anterior segment neovascularization in spite of a robust PRP, so they need to be followed for this more closely than a typical patient with an artery occlusion.[3]*

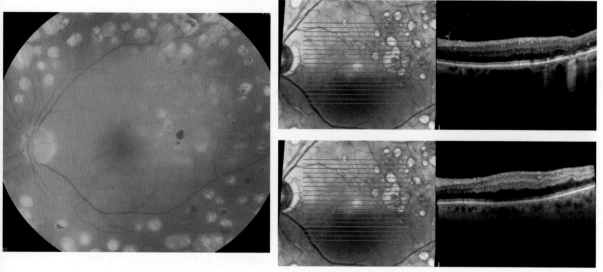

Figure 3: This patient presented with acute vision loss but no hemorrhage. You can get a sense that there may be some whitening of the retina below the fovea, but it is not really obvious that there was an acute branch retinal artery occlusion (note the obstruction in the inferior branch artery—this is another image best viewed in the online version of the book). OCT testing, however, shows the typical thickening of the inner retinal layers that occurs with an artery occlusion—see the difference between the inner retinal layers in the cut above the fovea (upper OCT) and the cut through the ischemic area (lower OCT). Note also how the infrared imaging of the OCT photo enhances the ischemic area—it appears darker below the fovea.

ODDS & ENDS

How soon do you bring in a diabetic with symptoms from a hemorrhage?

Traditionally, any patient with a sudden change in floaters needs same-day service to rule out a retinal tear. Because diabetics may have off-and-on hemorrhaging for years, and because such symptoms rarely indicate an acute problem like a retinal tear or detachment, there is a tendency to bend this rule.

In an ideal world, it would be best to get everyone in quickly just to be safe. It will relieve the patient's anxiety, and you may occasionally have a chance to get some laser in before a hemorrhage spreads around, or you may rarely find something unexpected like a retinal tear. Practically speaking, however, if you have a lot of diabetic patients you could bring your practice to a standstill trying to get everyone in immediately—something that is usually not necessary for patients who have already had occasional hemorrhages and who have longstanding disease that is otherwise well controlled. You will even find that diabetics who have intermittent hemorrhages will ask you if it is okay to *not* call when they have a hemorrhage so they don't have to keep coming in all the time.*

All these symptomatic patients can create a rather difficult dilemma that is not fully addressed in the literature. Although the safest approach is to get everyone in as soon as they call, at times doctors will compromise by bringing them in within a few days. This allows the hemorrhage to clear a bit and also prevents a totally overbooked schedule—something that can lead to a different set of quality-of-care problems. You must understand, however, that although this is a rationalization retina doctors feel comfortable with, there is always a chance of missing something acute.

Ultimately, deciding whether to get a diabetic with vitreous hemorrhage symptoms in immediately is a function of several variables. One important factor is the level of panic on the part of the patient (you should always try to get a freaked-out patient in quickly, even if you don't think anything is going on—it is both nicer and safer). Other factors include whether this is their first hemorrhage or one of many, how well you know the patient's retinopathy and whether they have a complete PRP and are therefore less likely to develop a detachment. Another variable is the patient's ability to accurately convey the symptoms over the phone. For instance, is their vision diffusely hazy but intact—implying a hemorrhage—or do they have a dense black shadow in one area, suggesting a detachment? A final factor is how much sleep you will lose if you postpone the evaluation for a day or so. The choice will be yours.

What about the effect of physical activity on hemorrhages?

Almost all patients assume that any sort of lifting or straining just has to make the little blood vessels in their eyes burst open. It turns out that it is very unusual for a diabetic patient to routinely hemorrhage due to physical activity; usually, hemorrhages occur during sleep or rest.[4,5] As a result, patients are not normally given any sort of restrictions. This is important because it allows them to pursue a normal life that includes vigorous exercise and other activities that are beneficial to their diabetic control and overall health. You may want to mention this specifically, even if they don't ask, because some patients will simply assume they should restrict their activity (or their family members may restrict it for them).

You may come across rare patients in whom straining will contribute to hemorrhaging, and usually these patients will be able to give a very consistent history indicating an association. These patients may need more laser or even a vitrectomy, although sometimes simply waiting it out allows the vessels to become fibrotic and the problem goes away.

Even though it is reasonable for a patient with well controlled disease and a history of intermittent hemorrhages to "wait it out and call only if it gets worse," it is probably not a good idea for you to actually suggest this. If the patient turns out to be the rare one who has a "routine" hemorrhage and then has their retina fall off because they waited before calling, you will feel very bad and their attorney will feel very good. It may be best to simply tell them the risk of not calling—small though it may be—and then let them decide what they want to do. It turns out that most diabetic patients who are used to having occasional hemorrhages will wait them out anyway.

Finally, there are times when a patient with old, quiescent proliferative disease will hemorrhage after an episode of coughing or vomiting, or perhaps after some sort of trauma. At times a hemorrhage can even occur after an insulin reaction. If the retinopathy is stable, these events tend to be self-limited and are unlikely to require additional treatment.

Here is one other useful tip when caring for patients with proliferative disease—or for patients with any form of retinopathy, for that matter. You should always point out at the end of your exam that retinopathy can be very unpredictable, and that although a patient may appear stable in the office they need to understand that something unexpected could happen anytime—even that evening. If you take care of enough diabetics you will have one or two of them call back with a hemorrhage within a day of an exam wherein you pronounced them "clean." It is quite easy for them to think that you missed something when, in fact, there was nothing to treat and the blame lies with unpredictable changes in their vitreoretinal interface. Once again, it is always better if you warn a patient about something before it happens. (Of course, if you did miss something, this can be a great way to cover yourself—but hopefully this will never be your primary reason for mentioning this.)

References

1.   Davis M, Blodi B. Proliferative Diabetic Retinopathy. In: Ryan SJ. Retina, 4th ed. Philadelphia: Elsevier, 2006: v 2, pp 1285-1322.

2.   Cintra LP, Costa RA, Ribeiro JA, et al. Intravitreal bevacizumab (Avastin) for persistent new vessels in diabetic retinopathy (IBEPE study): 1-year results. *Retina*. Jun 2013;33(6):1109-1116.

3.   Chen SN, Chao CC, Hwang JF, Yang CM. Clinical manifestations of central retinal artery occlusion in eyes of proliferative diabetic retinopathy with previous vitrectomy and panretinal photocoagulation. *Retina*. Sep 2014;34(9):1861-1866.

4.   Sheth BP, Mieler WF. Ocular complications of pregnancy. *Curr Opin Ophthalmol*. Dec 2001;12(6):455-463.

5.   Anderson B, Jr. Activity and diabetic vitreous hemorrhages. *Ophthalmology*. Mar 1980;87(3):173-175.

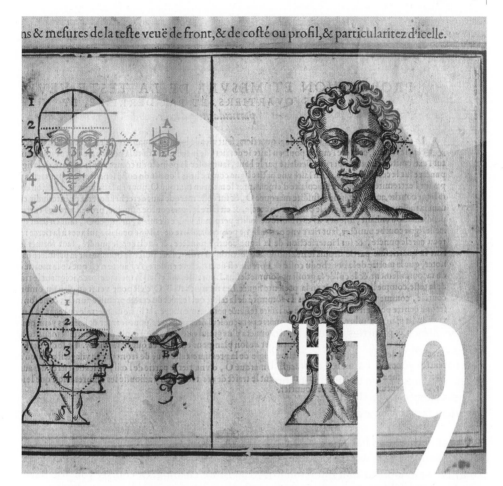

When to Bail Out, Give Up, Drop Off the Key, Lee, and Refer for Vitrectomy

Smooth seas do not make skillful sailors. African Proverb

Vitrectomy has dramatically changed the prognosis for many patients with severe proliferative diabetic retinopathy. But it can't fix everything—the level of expectation that goes along with cataract surgery does not apply to vitrectomies. Although patients with routine non-clearing vitreous hemorrhages tend to do very well, patients with more aggressive neovascular traction can be disappointed with the results of even very successful surgery. It is also important to remember that vitrectomy can have significant complications, and these complications are more likely in sicker eyes. A nicely reattached retina may just not work because it is dead, or an ischemic diabetic eye may unavoidably fold up into neovascular glaucoma after perfect surgery. You cannot have patients thinking that a quick trip to the vitrectomy shop will solve things lickety-split.

One never quite knows which diabetic eye will be the one that will fall apart after surgery, and it is this ever-present risk that tends to make retina surgeons a bit conservative. This is a very different mindset from cataract surgery or Lasik, which are performed more readily because they carry a smaller risk of complications and because experience tells you that the patient is likely to be happy with the result. In fact, the best way to do a vitrectomy is to avoid it altogether with aggressive control of the patient's systemic vascular risk factors and aggressive treatment of their retinopathy. Unfortunately, in spite of all the king's horses, etc., there are patients who cannot be controlled with injections and laser alone, and it is great that many heroic pioneers developed vitrectomy surgery so that we can save these downward-spiraling eyes. You just have to know when the time is right to refer.

Non-clearing Vitreous Hemorrhages

The traditional indication for vitrectomy is a non-clearing vitreous hemorrhage. The exact timing of surgery is variable. It would be great if you could just memorize one number, but there is no "automatic" time to operate. There are guaranteed risks with surgery; vitrectomy carries about a 2% to 5% complication rate, and that number goes up in eyes that are sicker or out of control. On the other hand, doing nothing can also be risky because you can't see the retina to be sure it is safe from problems such as macular edema or a progressive traction detachment. The real issue is deciding at what time the risks of observation become worse than the risk of intervention. Perhaps the most important factor is how aggressive the patient's retinopathy happens to be.

Older patients tend to have more quiescent disease, and they may have longstanding vitreous hemorrhages without developing any irreversible problems. For these patients, it may be reasonable to wait three months to allow for clearing. Of course, you also have to factor in the risk of a few months of poor depth perception and the chance for a hip-breaking fall or car accident. This may hasten the need for surgery in a patient's mind. On the other hand, for some elderly patients the thought of having surgery is way worse than a blurry eye, and so they may want to wait much longer than a few months.

However, most retina folks start to get a little itchy when no one has seen the retina after about three to four months—even for these relatively calm eyes—because there is always a chance that edema or traction not seen with a B-scan could be sneaking up on the fovea. In other words, even if the patient is content to wait they need to understand that the three- to four-month time frame is about when the progressive risk of unobserved retinal damage gradually begins to outweigh the fixed risk of surgery. This does not mean they have to have surgery; it just means that you need to convey the shifting of the risk-to-benefit scales. Note that some patients will not give you the chance to wait things out like this—having all that junk sloshing around in their vision is very disturbing, and you might as well refer them earlier because they are unlikely to listen to you anyway.

By the way, if you are going to observe these patients on your own, you really need to have access to a B-scan to be certain that everything is OK while you wait. It is risky to follow patients if you cannot be reasonably certain that the retina is where it is supposed to be. How often should they be checked? There is no definite answer, but most of the time it is safe to monitor patients about once a month. This does not give the eye a lot of time to mess itself up between visits. (Remember that the patient may not be able to tell if they are getting a retinal detachment because they don't have enough vision to notice a change.) The monthly visit will also assure you that the patient has not developed a slow IOP rise from red blood cells jamming up the angle. If the hemorrhage is mild or clearing, the patient may not need to be seen as often. Patients should also be reminded to call immediately if they think their vision is getting noticeably worse or if the eye is getting red and painful (i.e., neovascular or hemolytic glaucoma).

Although the two- to three-month rule can work for benign hemorrhages in otherwise calm eyes, there are other patients who may need to be encouraged to move more rapidly towards surgery. This is especially true in younger patients with more aggressive disease, and trebly true if the patient has an eye full of blood but has not had a chance to get a full laser treatment. These patients should be considered for early vitrectomy, perhaps within a month of presenting, in order to avoid tractional problems that arise as the blood vessels continue to slowly grow unobserved beneath the hemorrhage. Sometimes, these patients will have dense premacular hemorrhages, such that the blood is loculated in front of the posterior pole. Although you can still see a lot of the peripheral retina in such an eye, it is felt that there is a significant risk of progressive fibrovascular growth and traction and that early vitrectomy is warranted. (FYI: Sometimes these patients can benefit from YAG puncture of the loculated hemorrhage in order to allow it to spread out and dissolve. This is not done commonly—and the technique is well beyond the scope of this book—but it does come in handy on occasion.)

A brief pep talk for you and the patient you are referring:

Sometimes patients think that if you are referring them out it is a sure indication that all those lasers that you hammered in (and billed them for) didn't do anything. Actually, sending the patient off to the retina world is a clear-cut sign that the lasers have saved the eye—without the laser to reverse the eye's suicidal tendencies, the retina would have crumpled up a long time ago and there would be no vision whatsoever to save. What the laser cannot do, however, is to reverse vitreous traction on the patient's blood vessels. Emphasize that the patient now has a largely mechanical problem that needs steel, not more of Planck's constant, and that the laser has worked well enough to get them safely to the point of referral. A good retina specialist will make this point for you when the patient is first seen—but it helps for the patient to hear it on both ends of the consultation.

Another factor that may influence the decision to operate is whether the patient has specific visual needs that require rapid recovery. Some patients are willing to take the risk of surgery quickly, just to try to get better faster for professional or personal reasons. Such patients need to be reminded, however, that the recovery from a vitrectomy can be much more unpredictable than the recovery from anterior segment surgery. For instance, if the patient needs a gas bubble for any reason, or if there is a post-op hemorrhage, their visual recovery can be rather slow. Although your friendly neighborhood retina specialist will go over this fully with the patient, you should not promise your patients a fast, easy recovery when you refer them because you will jinx them for sure.

A final "hemorrhagic" reason to have surgery can occur in patients who have well-controlled proliferative disease, yet continue to have recurrent mild hemorrhages from involuted vessels. Such hemorrhages can drive a patient nuts as they come and go, even if the hemorrhages clear and the vision is good between episodes. There is no definite number of hemorrhages that merits surgery; some patients will put up with only a few, while others will have a hemorrhage every few months for years before asking for surgery. Because these patients are more "elective" than the typical diabetic who needs a vitrectomy it is especially important that they understand the risks and benefits.

Can't I just give them an anti-VEGF shot?

We covered this a bit in Chapter 14. We know that anti-VEGF agents can help shut down the neovascularization, but we don't know for sure if those drugs can actually help get rid of the hemorrhage. There is some data that suggests that injecting something will speed up the clearance of the hemorrhage.[1] And there are some patients, especially after having had a vitrectomy, that seem to need a periodic shot of an anti-VEGF agent to minimize recurrent hemorrhages.[2] But then there is the DRCR.net trial that showed that although ranibizumab had a mild effect on clearing, it was by no means dramatic.[3] (In the study, those getting saline injections also saw an almost equally fast clearing of hemorrhage.) We do know that vitreous hemorrhages will often clear on their own, especially at first, so maybe we are fooling ourselves that injecting anti-VEGF drugs really speeds things up. And remember that you can mess up an eye with a shot if the neovascularization contracts and pulls the retina off. So there really is no defined approach to this. There may be some patients that can avoid a vitrectomy with an occasional shot, but you may want to consider referring such patients anyway. A vitrectomy may solve a lot of problems and minimize the need for recurrent injections; your friendly retina specialist can give you some guidance based on the latest data and the patient's specific situation.

Other Indications

There are some other indications for vitrectomy besides a non-clearing vitreous hemorrhage, and most of these are fairly obvious. For instance, referral is mandatory if the patient appears to be developing progressive traction that is threatening the macula, or if the macula has just been yanked off. Sometimes, however, making this call is not as easy as one would think. The traction can build up very slowly, often simulating refractory macular edema as the retina is slowly thickened—like a peanut butter and jelly sandwich being pulled open. This is where an OCT is crucial.

Don't depend entirely on technology, though. You can always resort to ancient and primitive methods, such as actually talking to the patient about their symptoms. Slowly progressive traction can cause metamorphopsia or changes in peripheral vision that patients can detect, and you should take complaints along these lines very seriously, even if you cannot see any clinically apparent changes. Sometimes it helps to provide patients with an Amsler grid to help them monitor for progression. If there is any doubt, a referral is in order. This is because the results of surgery in this situation tend to be much better if the problem is fixed before the fovea pops off.

On the other hand, sometimes ominous-looking traction can be quite stable. In fact, the majority of patients with localized areas of traction do not progress. At times the retina can even look like a campground full of hammocks and pup tents, yet the patient never needs surgery. A very creepy pattern can occasionally develop because many so-called diabetic traction retinal detachments are, in fact, areas of tractional retinoschisis—there is still an outer layer of retina stuck to the RPE. These eyes can sometimes get nasty-looking inner-layer holes that resemble Swiss cheese draped over clotheslines, leaving one wondering how on earth the retina is remaining attached at all. (It remains in place, of course, because there are no true full-thickness holes.) Monitoring, and especially lasering, eyes filled with traction can be a bit nuanced and usually such eyes are referred to specialists until they are known to be stable. If you are watching eyes like this, make sure the patients know when to call.

Retinas can become so atrophic, however, that they do develop full-thickness holes, and then patients get a rhegmatogenous detachment in addition to any traction that is present. The rather dramatic downturn in their vision and the floppy, bullous appearance of the retina usually make the need for referral obvious. Putting an atrophic, lasered-out retina back on the RPE and getting it to stay there can be difficult, to say the least, and the visual outcomes—although better than nothing—do not tend to be great. Please don't pat such a patient on the back and say that they will be as good as new after surgery.

Another indication for vitrectomy is the presence of progressive rubeosis in the setting of a vitreous hemorrhage that precludes laser treatment. In the old days, people would try to put in panretinal cryotherapy without visualizing the retina, trying to kill off enough retina to stop the neovascularization and give the eye a chance to clear the hemorrhage. This approach may still be used if a patient is too sick for surgery or if you do not have access to a vitreoretinal specialist. If there is a chance of useful vision being obtained from the eye, however, it is best to do a vitrectomy rather than "blind" cryotherapy; cryo can really stir up pain, inflammation and scarring, and is more of a last-resort approach. Intravitreal anti-VEGF treatment can be invaluable in this situation, as well—check the next chapter for more info on this. Basically, patients who have progressive anterior segment neovascularization and a vitreous hemorrhage should receive a prompt referral.

Another less common reason for performing a vitrectomy is elevated intraocular pressure secondary to the presence of vitreous blood coming into the anterior chamber and clogging up the trabecular meshwork. This process can actually occur in three ways:

> *1. Fresh erythrocytes accumulating in the meshwork*
>
> *2. Hemolytic glaucoma, wherein hemosiderin-filled macrophages obstruct the meshwork*
>
> *3. Ghost cell glaucoma, wherein erythrocytes lose their hemoglobin and block the meshwork because they are less pliable than normal erythrocytes. Such cells are khaki-colored and are usually seen with old, yellowish vitreous blood.*

Whatever the pathology, the pressure can get quite high, and if it does not respond to medical management a vitrectomy is required to wash the eye out.

There is another group of patients that would likely benefit from early referral: the ones who respond poorly to PRP—even if a hemorrhage has not yet occurred. These tend to be younger Type 1 diabetics with a history of non-compliance, and it is hard to specify the exact level of disease that merits referral. Like the line about knowing the difference between art and pornography, however, you will recognize such patients when you see them. Anytime vascular fronds fail to respond to a solid PRP, you can assume you are dealing with an eye that is hell-bent on destroying itself and you generally do not want your name to be the last one on the chart.

One option for these patients is to keep hammering in laser from the arcade to the ora, but this may just destroy peripheral visual field without controlling the problem—recall that the vessels are locked onto the vitreous and supping on the vasoproliferative substances that reside there because the eye is diffusely ischemic. Anti-VEGF agents may tip the balance in your favor, but then you have to watch closely for recurrence, and these are exactly the type of aggressively neovascularized eyes that can get a traction detachment from the injection.

The decision whether or not to operate on these sick eyes is complicated; they tend to have relatively preserved vision, and the risks are not small. The point is that if your laser is not slowing down the growth of new vessels, it is better to get an early consult than to wait for multiple lasers and/or injections to not work and then refer in a patient with big vessels, traction detachments and a totally atrophic peripheral retina, all of which carry a more guarded prognosis with surgery.

Refractory macular edema due to traction is another indication that may respond to a vitrectomy. Obvious cases usually have an epiretinal membrane that is tugging on the fovea and keeping the retina swollen. Sometimes the cortical vitreous can remain diffusely attached to the entire posterior pole, causing edema as it contracts without the presence of a distinct epiretinal membrane. This can sometimes appear as glistening sheen on the surface of the retina. OCT has really helped to identify situations where traction is contributing to the edema—this was discussed in earlier chapters.

Warning. We just spent a lot of time talking about recognizing patients whose edema is more related to traction at the vitreoretinal interface rather than intraretinal vascular leakage, and how such patients should be referred for consideration of vitrectomy. But, as mentioned in the beginning of the chapter, even though you have carefully identified such patients, neither you nor the patient should expect that surgery should automatically make a huge improvement in vision. The DRCR. net looked at this, and even though most patients will do better overall with surgery, the results were not stellar.

In a group of patients with vitreomacular traction and macular

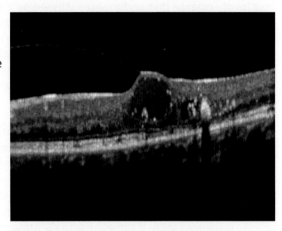

Figure 1: OCT demonstrating very subtle traction contributing to cystoid macular edema. Also note how the inner/outer segment line (ellipsoid zone) is starting to break down. Finally, for Master of Retina Points, note the hyperreflective dots lining the inside of the cysts. This is known as the pearl necklace sign, and carries a guarded visual prognosis.[4] Think about referring such a patient sooner than later.

thickening, most had a decrease in retinal thickening, but less than half of the eyes had visual improvement, and up to 30% had worsening vision.[5] This was a real WTF moment for the retina world—in our brains we figured that our awesome surgery would for sure make everyone better, but that wasn't always the case. The point is that diabetic eyes don't come with a guarantee—you can't have patients thinking that they will be OK, even though you may be very proud of your ability to diagnose tractional disease with your OCT.

The data from the study doesn't mean that all patients have such a guarded prognosis— the study didn't use adjuvant injections or prompt laser; they may have done better with more aggressive use of additional modalities. Plus, retina specialists feel that the results of surgery are better if you get to the eye sooner. This means you shouldn't play around with patients if you think that traction has a role. Doing treatments that don't work simply allows more time for the retina to degenerate under traction. And diabetic retinas tend to degenerate faster, probably because of the shoddy vascular supply. So if you are worried that the patient may need a vitrectomy, send them in for a consult sooner than later. The inner/outer segment line (ellipsoid zone) seems to be really useful here—if it is breaking down the prognosis for visual recovery gets worse and worse. Don't let that happen on your watch. (Refer back to Chapter 3 for the details.)

The role of vitrectomy for macular edema is less defined if there is no obvious epiretinal membrane or vitreous traction. Some people feel that getting in there and removing the vitreous, often combined with removal of the internal limiting membrane, can deturgess the retinal nicely. Unfortunately, the literature is conflicting, and there does not seem to be a lot of evidence that performing a vitrectomy in this setting is consistently effective. It gets complicated because this type of surgery is done on patients whose edema is refractory to all the other modalities, and it is often done as a last ditch attempt to control the problem. Would an earlier vitrectomy have restored vision? That is the million-dollar question that is still without an answer. But, as mentioned in Chapter 4, if an early vitrectomy is proven to safely reverse DME you can bet you will be hearing about it from your retina colleagues muy pronto.

Proponents of vitrectomy and ILM peeling in patients without traction suggest that this tendency to delay intervention is why the results are so variable. They suggest that it would be better to operate on such patients long before the retina has had a chance to degenerate, and that surgery may actually be safer and more cost effective than years of injections and lasers, even if the vision doesn't get a lot better.[6,7] Studies are under way to try to define the role of vitrectomy in this situation, so hopefully there will be specific guidelines soon. If someone actually proves that vitrectomy beats all the other treatments, you can be sure that your local retina specialists will be kicking your door down with the news, and you can unload all your DME patients on them.

However, given all the potential treatments, anyone with bad macular edema should be referred to a retinologist whether it is for a vitrectomy or not. Remember that you can make two people happy with cataract surgery in the time it takes to explain treatments for refractory macular edema to one patient. Your unfixable problem is the retina person's reason for being, and retina specialists actually like doing it.

A more obscure reason to consider vitrectomy is the presence of vitreopapillary traction.[8] Sometimes the vitreous can be freed from the posterior pole but can still exert traction at the nerve. This is a fairly common configuration; many diabetics with burned-out proliferative disease will have sclerotic vascular fronds that emanate from the nerve and are tugged up into the vitreous. Occasionally there is actually enough traction that the nerve fiber layer is slowly choked and vision is lost. These patients have progressive visual field defects and worsening central vision without any obvious cause such as a hemorrhage or direct foveal traction. This problem is relatively uncommon, but it should at least be kept in mind with patients who have decreasing vision and a lot of traction yanking on the nerve.

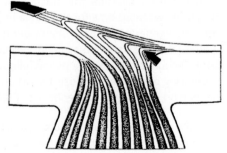

Figure 2: Schematic drawing of how traction at the nerve can damage the axons. Not a very common cause at all, but a good reminder of all the ways things can go wrong inside an eye. (Used with permission from Kroll P, Wiegand W, Schmidt J. Vitreopapillary traction in proliferative diabetic vitreoretinopathy. Br J Ophthalmol. Mar 1999;83(3):261-264.)

Finally, when it comes to performing a vitrectomy, whether for proliferative disease or macular edema, the path taken by the patient's fellow eye may help decide the issue. For instance, one would be much more inclined to do a vitrectomy if the fellow eye developed vision loss because a vitrectomy was not done soon enough. Conversely, a failed vitrectomy in one eye will make a patient very reluctant to have any surgery in the remaining eye—although this is usually the retina specialist's problem and not yours. Your job is to get the patient's disease as controlled as you can, and if things are not looking good then get them to a specialist at the appropriate time, and ideally a bit sooner, so that surgery can be considered when it can do the most good.

References

1.   Salam A, Mathew R, Sivaprasad S. Treatment of proliferative diabetic retinopathy with anti-VEGF agents. *Acta Ophthalmol.* Aug 2011;89(5):405-411.

2.   Ferenchak K, Duval R, Cohen JA, MacCumber MW. Intravitreal bevacizumab for postoperative recurrent vitreous hemorrhage after vitrectomy for proliferative diabetic retinopathy. *Retina.* Jun 2014;34(6):1177-1181.

3.   DRCR.net. Randomized clinical trial evaluating intravitreal ranibizumab or saline for vitreous hemorrhage from proliferative diabetic retinopathy. *JAMA Ophthalmol.* Mar 1 2013;131(3):283-293.

4.   Gelman SK, Freund KB, Shah VP, Sarraf D. THE PEARL NECKLACE SIGN: A Novel Spectral Domain Optical Coherence Tomography Finding in Exudative Macular Disease. *Retina.* Oct 2014;34(10):2088-2095.

5.   Haller JA, Qin H, Apte RS, et al. Vitrectomy outcomes in eyes with diabetic macular edema and vitreomacular traction. *Ophthalmology.* Jun 2010;117(6):1087-1093 e1083.

6.   Doi N, Sakamoto T, Sonoda Y, et al. Comparative study of vitrectomy versus intravitreous triamcinolone for diabetic macular edema on randomized paired-eyes. *Graefes Arch Clin Exp Ophthalmol.* Jan 2012;250(1):71-78.

7.   Hoerauf H, Bruggemann A, Muecke M, et al. Pars plana vitrectomy for diabetic macular edema. Internal limiting membrane delamination vs posterior hyaloid removal. A prospective randomized trial. *Graefes Arch Clin Exp Ophthalmol.* Jul 2011;249(7):997-1008.

8.   Kroll P, Wiegand W, Schmidt J. Vitreopapillary traction in proliferative diabetic vitreoretinopathy *The British journal of ophthalmology.* Mar 1999;83(3):261-264.

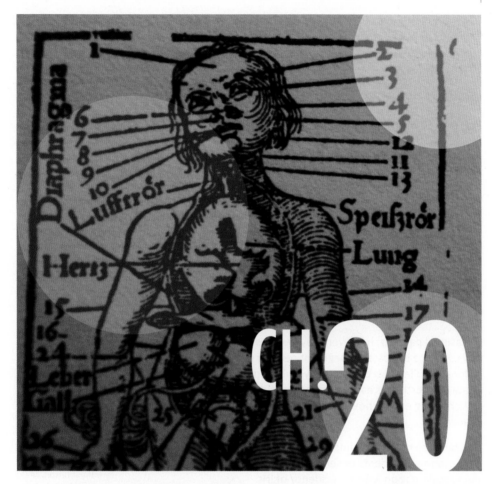

Front End Trouble—Iris Neovascularization

When sorrows come, they come not single spies, but in battalions. Hamlet—Act IV

Iris neovascularization is another form of proliferative diabetic retinopathy, and it usually indicates a very sick eye. First of all, though, do not be fooled by findings that may mimic true neovascularization. For instance, if you look carefully, you will often see tiny, reddish globular vessels on the pupil margin, especially if you study the iris prior to dilation in older diabetics. These vascular tufts may increase in number over time, but they do not usually cause any of the problems associated with true anterior segment neovascularization.

Another process that can simulate neovascularization is the development of iris atrophy, which can occur in patients with long-standing diabetes. This results in increased visibility of normal iris vessels, especially in light-colored irides. The fact that such vessels are within the substance of the iris, and that they follow the normal iris architecture, will distinguish them from true neovascularization.

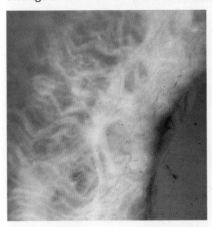

Figure 1: An example of iris neovascularization. The arrow points to a dilated yet normal vessel coursing within the iris stroma. This can simulate neovascularization, but is visible simply due to stromal atrophy. The rest of the vessels are arborizing over the surface of the iris, and are clearly abnormal. Note the puddle of blood loculated in an iris crypt (arrowhead). (Courtesy of Wallace L.M. Alward, M.D.)

However, if you see vessels arborizing on the surface of the iris—or if there is any neovascularization of the angle—then you are dealing with the real thing. This type of anterior segment proliferative retinopathy is usually an end-stage phenomenon that shows up well after problems have already occurred in the back of the eye. Diabetics start with proliferative diabetic retinopathy in the posterior segment and as the eye becomes progressively ischemic, vessels develop in the anterior segment, often in spite of previously adequate laser treatment.

Occasional patients, however, may develop anterior segment neovascularization without any evidence of posterior segment neovascularization—so always look at the iris closely before it is dilated. It can be really awkward if you tell a patient they are fine, yet they show up shortly thereafter with neovascular glaucoma—and then everyone in the clinic is wondering exactly how carefully you looked at the iris before diving into your 90-D exam.

Just because nothing is simple, there are even case reports of patients developing angle neovascularization without evidence of iris neovascularization.[1] Does this mean that you should be doing screening gonioscopy on every diabetic at every visit? In a perfect world, the answer to this question might be yes, but as a practical matter there is little chance that one could do this. The odds of finding something are very small, and the time involved (and the risk of scruffing up a bunch of diabetic epithelial cells) makes this approach impractical. Or, at least that is one possible rationalization--you are free to develop your own approach.

Figure 2: (below) Florid iris neovascularization. (Courtesy of Timothy Johnson, M.D.)

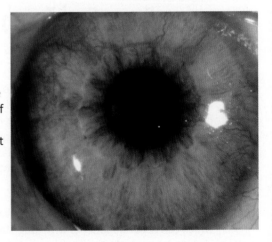

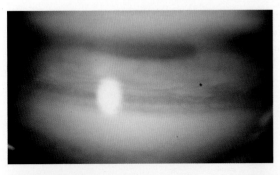

Figure 3: Angle neovascularization—you can see how the vessels arise from deep in the angle and arborize over the scleral spur and up to Schwalbe's line. (Courtesy of Wallace L.M. Alward, M.D.)

If you end up being like most folks, who do not automatically gonio everyone, you should still remember that isolated angle neovascularization is a possibility. It will serve to remind you that everything we do is a compromise on some level; by choosing not to do gonioscopy on all diabetics, someone, somewhere may get burned. But definitely think of this if a diabetic shows up with a pressure that is higher than their usual range.

A related issue is the way retina specialists often dilate patients without examining the iris first. This is also a compromise, but as a conscientious, comprehensive ophthalmologist, you are above this because you actually look at your patients before they are dilated. If you are worried about something in the anterior segment that may not be seen after dilation, you need to make sure you let your retina specialist know in advance.

If a patient has vessels growing in the front part of the eye you should consider obtaining carotid Dopplers. The concern is that such patients may be developing global ocular ischemia from carotid disease superimposed on typical diabetic small-vessel disease. Dopplers are particularly important in a patient who develops anterior segment neovascularization without any posterior neovascularization—these patients may be more likely to have large-vessel disease. Finally, you should try to remember that there are other things that can cause new vessels to sprout in the anterior segment, such as uveitis or venous occlusive disease hiding behind diabetic retinopathy. These entities require very different diagnostic and therapeutic interventions. Never trust a diabetic eye to do anything predictably.

If you do pick up a case of diabetic anterior segment neovascularization, it is reassuring to know that it tends to evolve into neovascular glaucoma more slowly than neovascularization associated with, for instance, central retinal vein occlusions or ocular ischemia. In fact, not all diabetic anterior segment neovascularization will automatically turn into neovascular glaucoma; occasional patients can go for some time without getting a pressure rise.[2] However, it is generally considered risky to do nothing when faced with vessels on the iris—best to assume the worst and treat.

Speaking of treatment...

Remember the chapters on treating DME and PDR, and how there was all this vague verbiage about combining laser and intravitreal anti-VEGF agents because no one knows for sure what to do? Well, there is no such ambiguity here. Anterior segment neovascularization is a great indication for intravitreal anti-VEGF therapy if you have access to it. Although aggressive laser is the mainstay of treatment—injections are transient but the laser is permanent—intravitreal treatment can stop the disease cold, giving you time to treat the patient gradually (for instance if there is a vitreous hemorrhage or dense cataract that makes laser difficult). Anti-VEGF drugs can also help protect the macula—these eyes can be very sensitive and fast and furious laser can blow out a delicate fovea. Finally, some patients will never completely respond to laser, and chronic intravitreal treatment is the only way to save the eye.

The injection is usually given when the diagnosis is made, and bevacizumab is the most commonly used agent—it is hard to get either an insurance company or the patient to pay for one of the high priced drugs for such an off-label indication. Be very aware that the dramatic response to the drug will be transient—the vessels come back usually within a month as the drug wears off, so you have to be ready to get more definitive treatment in.

By the way, *if all that stuff in Chapter 11 made you reticent to stick needles through the pars plana—and it should—there is a growing literature about the use of intracameral bevacizumab for this problem.[3] If you feel uncomfortable poking holes in the eye in places where you do not routinely operate, you can look into this approach. Heck, there is even a study that suggests it works if the drug is injected subconjunctivally—something to keep in mind if the pressure is so high that you are worried about infracting the nerve by raising the pressure with an intraocular injection.[4]*

And speaking of definitive treatment...

Doing a PRP for anterior segment neo has its own concerns. First, recall that diabetic anterior segment neo does tend to be a bit more indolent relative to neo from other causes. Plus if you have injected bevacizumab, you have some real flexibility as far as how you treat the patient. Rather than firing in 2,000 fast spots, as you might do for progressive angle neovascularization from a central retinal vein occlusion, you can often do the laser in a divided dose. This can be important because these can be frail eyes—you can run into complications more easily than in a typical diabetic eye. These patients will still need a faster and more aggressive PRP than typical posterior segment proliferative disease; one can often prevail by putting in 1,000 spots at first, and then repeating the treatment in a week. More aggressive disease calls for more aggressive treatment with even higher numbers, especially if the pressure is elevated. Sometimes these patients may need four to six thousand spots to get control of the neovascular stimulus—real arcade to ora type treatment—and that may be the case even if you also use anti-VEGF drugs. It is important to get good control of the vessels, especially if the patient may need glaucoma surgery; you don't want a lot of bleeding or neovascular invasion of your favorite seton. As an aside, some docs feel that a functioning tube shunt actually washes out much of the VEGF protein. As a result, anterior segment neovascularization becomes less aggressive for some patients once a seton is placed.

Things get tricky if you identify the neovascularization, but the patient does not have any symptoms. Things get really tricky if they also have a fragile macula. Under these circumstances, it is good to know that the neovascularization tends to progress slowly and you can try to start out with a slower PRP to spare the macula (along with anti-VEGF agents).

If the patient already has a fairly full PRP, you need to pull out all the stops and squeeze in treatment anywhere you can—such patients need dead retina, and lots of it. You should aggressively try to fill in between spots, and also try to get out to the ora. This almost always involves fancier techniques, such as indirect laser or even cryotherapy, especially if the view is poor. As mentioned, there are even some eyes that won't respond and will end up needing periodic anti-VEGF injections to fully control the disease. (This may be due to the fact that the ciliary epithelium is perfectly capable of generating plenty of VEGF even after you have eliminated most of the retina.[5])

If there is no view due to vitreous hemorrhage or cataract, the patient needs to be referred for whatever surgery is necessary to get to the retina and treat it. If a cataract is obscuring the view, avoid just popping it out and waiting for the eye heal before moving on to the laser. Cataract surgery can stimulate the new vessels to go berserk without anti-VEGF treatment, so get the PRP in quickly before everything falls apart.

If you can't visualize the back of the eye and are trying to buy time with anti-VEGF injections, don't forget that warning from Chapter 14. If there is extensive proliferative disease back there, your injections may stop the anterior segment neovascularization but you may also be pulling the retina off as the posterior vessels contract. Patients like that should be referred so everything can be cleaned out with a vitrectomy.

Note that some patients with anterior segment neovascularization may have an additional problem above and beyond diabetic retinopathy known as ocular ischemic syndrome (OIS), which means that the perfusion to the entire eye is very poor (this entity is covered in Chapter 27). It is worth mentioning here, however, that patients with OIS may be more likely to get a permanent central retinal artery occlusion after an injection, and the problem seems to not be entirely related to raising the ocular pressure with the injection—the artery just conks out. If patients have a lot of aggressive anterior neo, though, you really don't have much choice; this is just another thing to be aware of if you are trying to tackle such sick eyes.[6]

Also, keep in mind that patients in this situation need a fairly intense informed consent—and this is really true if they aren't yet symptomatic. They need to know that you are dealing with an eye that in the old days would often end up blind and painful and in a jar. Your treatments will likely prevent that, but they cannot expect to have a fun time or a great visual outcome. They may need multiple injections with no obvious visual benefit, and the heavy laser and possible glaucoma surgery will take a toll on their vision. Patients also need to understand that although there are potential complications, the biggest danger is that the treatments may not work. And if that happens, they will get worse as they are being treated, and if things really go south they may even end up enucleated. And, to repeat for the second time in one paragraph, if they don't have a lot of symptoms, they are going to really be unhappy with you and your crazy treatments because they were just fine before you started in on them. So take some time to explain how desperate the situation is.

Speaking of enucleation, have you ever had a patient tell you that some doctor wanted to take their eye out, and the patient made it sound like the doctor was going to do it just because he or she could? Patients can really misinterpret what you are saying when you talk about enucleations. It is hard to imagine how anyone could think that we would sit around and just decide to pry someone's eye out for fun, but this thinking is not uncommon, especially in unsophisticated patients. Here's a tip: If you are dealing with a disease whose outcome might include enucleation—like endophthalmitis or neovascular glaucoma—phrase the possibility as something that the patient will ask for, rather than simply stating that it might occur. In other words, say "The eye can become so painful that you will beg us to take it out of your head." rather than "If we don't stop this, we may need to remove the eye."

References

1.   Browning DJ. Risk of missing angle neovascularization by omitting screening gonioscopy in patients with diabetes mellitus. *American journal of ophthalmology.* Aug 15 1991;112(2):212.

2.   Fernandez-Vigo J, Castro J, Macarro A. Diabetic iris neovascularization. Natural history and treatment. *Acta Ophthalmol Scand.* Feb 1997;75(1):89-93.

3.   Chalam KV, Gupta SK, Grover S, Brar VS, Agarwal S. Intracameral Avastin dramatically resolves iris neovascularization and reverses neovascular glaucoma. *European journal of ophthalmology.* Mar-Apr 2008;18(2):255-262.

4.   Ryoo NK, Lee EJ, Kim TW. Regression of iris neovascularization after subconjunctival injection of bevacizumab. *Korean journal of ophthalmology* : KJO. Aug 2013;27(4):299-303.

5.   Chalam KV, Brar VS, Murthy RK. Human Ciliary Epithelium as a Source of Synthesis and Secretion of Vascular Endothelial Growth Factor in Neovascular Glaucoma. *JAMA ophthalmology.* Jul 31 2014.

6.   Higashide T, Murotani E, Saito Y, Ohkubo S, Sugiyama K. Adverse events associated with intraocular injections of bevacizumab in eyes with neovascular glaucoma. *Graefes Arch Clin Exp Ophthalmol.* Apr 2012;250(4):603-610.

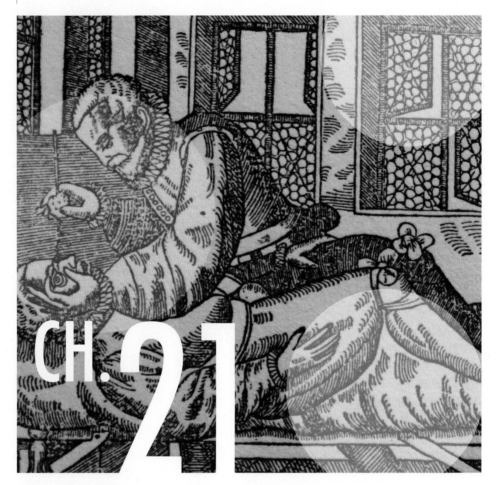

The Big Bucks

Always do what is right. It will gratify half of mankind and astound the other. Mark Twain

Unless you are reading this as you lug your laser to the nearest free clinic, it is likely that you will be involved in some sort of economic transaction when you treat a patient. If you are in a developed country that has first-dollar universal coverage, you can stop reading this right now because this section does not apply to you. If you are in a developing country, then you do need to worry about this stuff because there are insufficient healthcare resources available to cover the population. There are some suggestions about what to do at the end of this chapter (and at the end of Chapter 5).

If you are living in America, reportedly the richest country on earth, you really need to read this because you will inevitably have patients with no way to afford the care they need. Go figure.

At the beginning of your career there is a tendency to focus on the difficult task of being the best doctor you can be, and it is therefore easy to be unaware of the economic ramifications of what you are doing. There is an inclination to surrender your control in this area to whatever large bureaucratic structure you happen to be a part of—this way some other functionary has to fuss with droll matters like billing and collections while you concentrate on the noble task of being a physician. Try not to think like this—it can result in your patients making extremely bad decisions. Here's how:

Many of your diabetic patients will not have insurance. Being diabetic, it is hard to get a job with good insurance, and individual insurance can be very expensive. Many diabetics learn to survive without insurance by paying for their medical care on an intermittent basis and/or with the help of charity clinics. This is not ideal, and this approach usually breaks down when they start to develop complications and need more expensive care (which is where you come in).

But even if they do have insurance, recent developments in the marketplace have made many types of "insurance" almost useless. The classic example is a high-deductible plan, where the patient may be responsible for the first several thousand dollars of their care. If one is healthy and well off, these plans are no big deal, but if you have a chronic disease then it is almost the same as being uninsured as people struggle to pay off huge accumulated debt.

So imagine you are an otherwise healthy diabetic, but now you are getting proliferative disease. Some doctor is telling you that even though you don't have any symptoms, you need to sit down and get pounded with a laser that will hurt, maybe blur your vision, and certainly won't help you see any better. Then you go talk to the billing person, and they tell you that all of this bliss is going to cost thousands of dollars that you don't have. And then throw in the cost of OCTs and injections—especially if they hear about the insanely priced anti-VEGF drugs.

You may be totally caring and empathetic, but a relatively disinterested bean counter can completely undo things by making patients visualize eating cat food in order to pay for something that they don't want to do anyway. Some of these patients will walk away and not get treatment. They will then return in one to two years with severe proliferative disease and tractional detachments that may not be fixable. It turns out that this works out well for the accounts receivable department, because now the patient is blind and they are at least eligible for Medicaid—some blood can finally be squeezed out of their particular turnip. You—and the Great Ophthalmologic Court in the Sky judging our actions—should be somewhat less than sanguine about how the system allows this to happen.

This scenario simply should not occur, but it does, due to the nature of human beings and the nature of the healthcare system. You are in a position to stop this from happening, given that only you know how desperately such a patient needs treatment. If you don't consider the patient's worries about money, you won't be providing the best care possible.

Take a moment to look at the patient's chart to see if they have insurance, and what kind of insurance it is—does it really cover their care? Do a little bit of ACLU-proscribed profiling. If you think money might be an issue, then you should consider bringing it up. And you need to do it carefully. Most patients, especially patients in this situation, will immediately assume that any time a doctor talks about money, it means that the doctor is simply performing a wallet biopsy prior to putting on the big squeeze. It behooves you to quickly explain why you are exploring this issue. Remind them that they need the treatment to avoid blindness, and you want to make sure that they get treated properly whether they can pay or not.

The alternatives available to you depend on how much control you have over your billing. It is likely that if you are reading this book you are in training or just starting your career and you may not have much control over how patients are billed. If cost is an issue for the patient you should try to take a moment to explain to the billing person the severity of the situation, making sure they know to go as easy as possible on the patient. (Depending on the situation, one can even consider doing the laser without circling the laser code on the billing sheet. This could be dangerous ground—for instance, Medicare considers doing a procedure without billing for it to be fraud, no matter how noble the cause.* Still, if you are trying to keep a patient from going blind you need to at least think about all your options. Hopefully someone somewhere will realize how utterly illogical all of this is and the system will be fixed.)

If you have more control over your situation, you can tell the patient they can set up some sort of payment plan, or you can even bargain over the price if you are so inclined. Probably the simplest thing is to offer to do the treatment gratis. This eliminates any financial stress, and offering to do something regardless of payment is a very powerful way to demonstrate to a patient the importance of the treatment. And if you need to do injections, you may well be able to get free drugs from the makers of Lucentis and Eylea. You may actually find that such a patient will remain quite devoted to you, and you may find that the whole process is rather rewarding on a number of warm and fuzzy levels that are beyond the scope of this book.

If such an approach does not fit into your worldview, consider a more cynical argument for this policy: if you can keep them functioning in society, they will certainly think of you when they do eventually get insurance and may need elective procedures. They will also speak very highly of you to all of their friends, family, and other doctors and, yes, there may be a risk of inundating your office with their equally uninsured acquaintances—but it is far more likely that the long-term goodwill you acquire in the community is going to transcend any short-term irregularities in your cash flow. On an even grander note, it is a little-known fact that Dante's Inferno mentions that there is a spot reserved for American ophthalmologists somewhere in the Fourth Circle of Hell. (Dante said it had something to do with taking drug

I am Waiting for You

---

*Of course, you can write off Medicare copays and deductibles, but patients have to sign a waiver documenting financial hardship.

company swag.) It is likely that doing the right thing for patients like this will get you a few weekends of vacation up in Purgatory. Everybody wins.

The bottom line on the bottom line is that it is hard enough to convince diabetics to show up for evaluation and treatment without adding financial impediments. Although it is technically not part of your job description, try to be aware of economic hurdles that your patients may be facing—try not to let the billing department define your patient's treatment options.

This chapter really applies only to doctors in situations where patients may have a significant financial burden when undergoing treatment. As mentioned at the beginning of this section, doctors in developing countries have a related problem, and it has to do with the fact that there are tons of patients in need of help, but there are no resources to help with paying for their care. If you are in this situation, it turns out that there are a lot of organizations out there that are interested in helping—you just have to start making the effort to contact them. It is very likely that someone, somewhere has already faced the problems you are having, and has figured out a way to deal with it—and often quite successfully. The world is full of places that have skillfully combined capitalism and altruism to create very effective, self-sustaining programs that reward both the population and the doctors who take the time to go beyond their borders and ask for help. Appendix 2 goes into this in more detail.

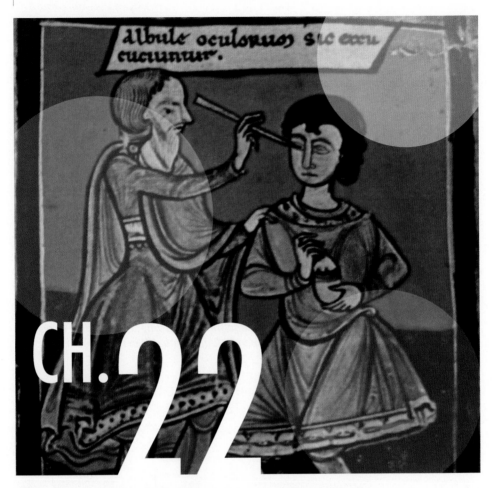

albule oculonuos sic exu cuciuntur.

CH.22

The Most Useful Chapter in the Book

(But You Wouldn't Read It If It Had an Informative Title)

Co-author: Taniya de Silva, M.D.

To get back my youth I would do anything in the world, except take exercise, get up early, or be respectable. Oscar Wilde

Don't blow off this chapter because you think you know it already. You will be amazed at how you are largely wasting your time if your patient is noncompliant. The converse is also true. When you see how a set of eyes can improve when a patient gets religious about control, and how your treatments work way better in such patients, you will realize that it is definitely worth the time to rag on your patients about their systemic status. You can give the sweetest intravitreal injections and do the finest lasers, but if you don't emphasize systemic control with both patients and their physicians you are functioning at the Epsilon-Minus Semi-Moron level of doctorness.

For that matter, you could do a lot better for your patients if you threw this book under a bus and devoted your efforts entirely to filling your community with endocrinologists.[1] But it is fun to spend all day keeping people from going blind, so do keep the book, but also internalize the info in this chapter. There is a lot more useful stuff here than you think.

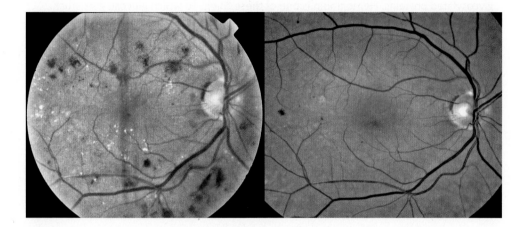

Figure 1: This patient had some mild grid laser to the center, but most importantly she really began to take care of herself once she realized that the writing was on the wall. Note the almost total resolution of the multiple hemorrhages and the overall healthier appearance of the fundus after several years of better systemic control. No laser-slinger can do this by treating microaneurysms alone. As mentioned in earlier chapters, anti-VEGF injections can sometimes reverse retinopathy like this, but these photos predate the anti-VEGF era.

There are only a few risk factors that need to be covered. The most obvious one is glucose control, and the quickest way to assess this is to ask the patient what their hemoglobin A1c is. Almost all patients will check their sugars periodically, and they may even remember some of their results (especially the best ones), but a sporadic sampling of glucose levels does not convey the overall level of control. In developed countries there is no reason why a patient should not be aware of their hemoglobin A1c level, although sometimes it helps if you call it the "three-month glucose test" if a patient does not recognize the test by name. Simply finding out whether they have heard of the test is useful—if they do not know what you are talking about you know you have a really big problem. Such a patient needs to be educated about the test and you need to express your concerns to their primary care physician. You can even order the test yourself to be sure it is done and to motivate both the patient and their doctor. Do not accept an answer like "My sugar is good." This isn't 1984.

Most patients will know the about the test, and even if they do not know their actual number, they can tell you whether their doctor was happy with the results. Knowing the actual number is best, though. A good number means that your treatment juju is strong. A bad number may completely change your ophthalmic management. What is a good number? A quick review may be in order...

RAPID REVIEW OF THE HEMOGLOBIN A1C TEST

Glucose in blood sticks to all kinds of proteins like barnacles on a pier; the technical term for this is glycosylation. The higher the glucose level, the higher the amount of glycosylated proteins. Hemoglobin is one of these things to which glucose gets stuck. Red blood cells last two to three months, and because they do not manufacture fresh hemoglobin, measuring the fraction of hemoglobin that has been glycosylated offers an idea of the average glucose level over that time period. The test is basically a variation of the hemoglobin electrophoresis that one might do to evaluate for sickle cell disease, but one is looking for the hemoglobin fraction that has the glucose moiety, rather than hemoglobin S. The result is expressed as a percentage of the total hemoglobin. The translation of the A1c value into the corresponding glucose value varies with the testing method, and the actual result implies a range of values. For instance, a hemoglobin A1c of 6% implies a glucose value between 100-152. Table 1 shows the "average" glucose value that can be inferred from the hemoglobin A1c. Normal is less than 6%. Most diabetologists like to shoot for less than 7%. This has to be individualized however. A general rule of thumb is to shoot for a hemoglobin A1c as close to normal as possible without inducing excess hypoglycemia.

Note *that there is some controversy about how aggressive to be in patients with Type 2 diabetes. Recent studies suggest that intensive control can help slow down retinal and renal disease, but there was an overall increase risk of mortality in the intensive control group.[2] This means that some of these patients may do better with control that is not quite as tight. The point is that you—as an ophthalmologist—should not dictate a specific A1c level to the patient. That is a decision for the patient's internist. Your job is to encourage them to follow their doctor's advice and strive for the hemoglobin A1c that is best for them.*

Table 1: Hemoglobin A1c Values and Corresponding Average Glucose Level

Note that even the "good" value of 7% corresponds to a consistently elevated glucose.

(Data from: Nathan DM, et al. Translating the A1c assay into estimated average glucose values. Diabetes Care. 2008 8:1473-8.)

A1c (%)	Mean Blood Sugar (mg/dl)
6	126
7	154
8	183
9	212
10	240
11	269
12	298

The risk of complications starts to go up almost asymptotically as the hemoglobin A1c increases. The classic paper on the subject is the Diabetes Control and Complications Trial (DCCT).[3] Data from the study was used to create Figure 2, and this figure should be burned into your brain—it shows how poor control can undo the results produced by your treatments. If you know a patient has bad systemic control, then your ophthalmic management may need to change.

For instance, a patient with poor control should be checked more frequently because they are very likely to progress faster. You may also need to be more aggressive about treatment decisions when patients have borderline ophthalmic disease. A patient with severe nonproliferative retinopathy and good control may simply need to be watched, whereas a patient with the same level of retinopathy but with very poor control may need to be treated with an early PRP to stay out of trouble. Of greatest significance is the fact that a bad hemoglobin A1c means that you really have to make sure the patient has appropriate expectations with any treatment that you do, whether it be laser, injections or cataract surgery. Patients with poor control have a worse prognosis for everything, and they must understand that although your interventions will slow things down, the odds are they will tend to worsen, even with perfect treatment.

Two things:

1. If you have a lot of patients that do not know their A1c level, you can buy or lease your own machine to get immediate results. The test only requires a finger stick, and the machine does not require sophisticated training.

2. Be careful how you harangue the patient about improving their control. Make sure they work with their internist before they start to do anything. The last thing you need is for the patient to bottom out their glucose on their own because you scared them so much.

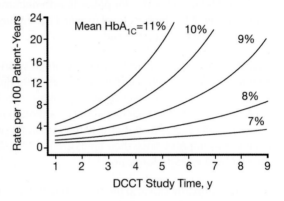

Figure 2: Rate of retinopathy progression relative to mean hemoglobin A1c. (From The relationship of glycemic exposure (HbA1c) to the risk of development and progression of retinopathy in the Diabetes Control and Complications Trial. Diabetes. 1995; 44: 968-983. Used with permission.)

Other Factors to Consider

There are other systemic factors that can play a role in progression of retinopathy. Four significant ones are hypertension, renal failure, lipid abnormalities and anemia. In fact, these factors can cause acute deterioration of a patient's retinopathy in a far worse way than poor glucose control alone. For instance, it is not unusual to see patients who present with progressive renal failure and macular edema, only to have the edema resolve without treatment as soon as the renal failure is treated.

Hypertension is particularly well studied—the sine qua non coming from the United Kingdom Prospective Diabetes Study Group.[4] Elevated blood pressure can be as important as glucose control—both in terms of contributing to chronic damage and causing acute problems in the setting of accelerated hypertension.[5] It makes sense to routinely check the blood pressure on diabetic patients, especially if it is not clear how good the patient is with their medical follow up. Yes, you might end up writing more letters, and you might actually have to check some blood pressures yourself, and you may even need to do general medical things like putting the patient in a room to calm down and then rechecking their blood pressure. Also, do not write off a high blood pressure as being due to "white coat syndrome." Such patients are more likely to get into trouble in the long run and should be monitored closely.

All this is worth it, though, because you will be surprised at the number of patients who are not as well controlled as they tell your technicians. It also helps to encourage patients to talk to their doctors about home blood pressure monitoring in the same way they monitor their glucose—automatic blood pressure cuffs are effective and cheap. By the way, the current recommendation for blood pressure control in diabetics is less than 140/90. It used to be 130/80, but the data for the lower level wasn't solid (although a goal of 130/80 may be better for patients with nephropathy and proteinuria). Ultimately, like hemoglobin A1c, the best level for each patient needs to be individualized and the internist should be making the call.

Dyslipidemia also seems to accelerate the progression of retinopathy. Although there have not been many studies looking at the effect of lipid control on retinopathy progression, it is felt that lowering serum lipids is another important way to decrease the risk of vision loss for diabetic patients—although not all authors agree on this.[6,29,30] You will certainly see some patients with excessive amounts of hard exudates who will noticeably improve once their lipids are treated. (Chapter 5 shows an example of exuberant hard exudate formation.)

Diabetic nephropathy can also be associated with retinopathy progression.[7] This is particularly true if the patient has rapidly progressive renal failure, and this is always something to assess in a patient with aggressive retinopathy. Remember that the converse also applies: By the time patients have retinopathy, they may also be developing renal disease. And marked retinal capillary non-perfusion is clearly associated with progression of renal disease.[8] Make sure you remind the primary care physician to monitor renal function and look for microalbuminuria* in a patient who is beginning to get retinopathy. You should always include the patient's endocrinologist and nephrologist in your communications. Although it is easier to just send a letter to the primary care physician, these medical subspecialists are in a good position to use the information you provide to get the patient as tuned-up as possible.

Anemia also seems to play a role in retinopathy progression. Treating anemia in diabetes is known to have beneficial effects such as slowing progression of nephropathy, enhancing cognitive function and improving exercise capacity. Although there are no large randomized trials on this issue, it is felt that treatment of significant anemia may help slow retinopathy progression, especially if the anemia is secondary to kidney disease.[9]

*Recall that the typical urine dipstick is not sensitive enough to detect the small amount of protein that can indicate the presence of early nephropathy. The older term for this was microalbuminuria—now it is referred to as "moderately increased albuminuria." Whatever you call it, special testing is required.

All of the above factors—glucose control, hypertension, renal failure, dyslipidemia and anemia—are important when it comes to both the patient's overall health and their response to your treatment. You should consider them inseparable when counseling patients and their doctors, and you should always stress the need to monitor all of them. Have your transcriptionist create a macro so you can easily throw in a comment about all of these in every letter you write. For instance:

"The patient understands how important it is to work with their physician to optimize not only their glucose control, but also any element of hypertension, elevated cholesterol, early renal failure and anemia."

See how easy that was?

> **By the way,** if the patient improves thanks to the efforts of their medical doctors, you should definitely communicate this in your letters. It is a good feeling to snatch someone from the jaws of blindness, and most of the time we in ophthalmology get to take all the credit. In the setting of diabetes, however, nothing we do works very well if the patient is not systemically controlled. Taking the time to thank everyone for their help and to let them know they helped avoid blindness will likely juice up their day. It may also encourage them to keep trying with all their other patients, and because the best treatment for retinopathy is to avoid it in the first place, one can create a nice ripple effect by providing the positive feedback.

Some More Factors

Smoking is a factor that one would assume to be a real problem when it comes to exacerbating retinopathy. However, there is not as strong an association as one would think, although it may play a role in vision loss in Type 1 patients.[10,11] However, smoking clearly worsens other problems, such as large-vessel disease and renal failure, and these in turn can exacerbate retinopathy. Besides, smoking can aggravate other ophthalmic problems such as cataracts and macular degeneration, so you should feel free to nag patients about their smoking whether they have diabetes or not. The American Academy of Ophthalmology has a nice handout on the effects of smoking on the eye. Sometimes, though, patients will be more worried about their eyes than lung cancer or emphysema, and by taking the time to warn them about smoking on the basis of your retinal exam you may get more mileage than their medical doctors.

Additional factors that may play a role in retinopathy progression include obstructive sleep apnea, obesity, physical inactivity and, yes, yang deficiency.[12,13,28] Family history can also be important—patients who have a lot of relatives with bad retinopathy, and especially proliferative retinopathy, may need very aggressive care.[14] Perhaps the strongest risk factor is duration of the disease, but this is not particularly modifiable without time travel. Finally, don't forget the potential effect of pregnancy on retinopathy (which is so important that it gets Chapter 24 all to itself).

OBSTRUCTIVE SLEEP APNEA

Risk Factors

Obesity

Large neck size

Enlarged tonsils in children

Small airway due to nasal congestion or bony structure

Family history of sleep apnea

Increasing age

Male gender

African-American, Hispanic, or Pacific Islander ethnicity

Signs and Symptoms

Loud snoring

Gasping or choking while asleep

Frequent nighttime urination

Morning headaches, dry mouth, or sore throat

Lack of energy or excessive daytime sleepiness

Hypertension

Memory, learning, or concentration problems

Depression, irritability, or mood swings

Let's take a moment to dwell on the association with sleep apnea. More and more evidence is suggesting that obstructive sleep apnea (OSA) is associated with progression of diabetic retinopathy and diabetic macular edema. Some people feel that the presence of multiple cotton-wool spots superimposed on diabetic retinopathy is suggestive of OSA. Plus, OSA may be related to other ocular problems such as floppy eyelid syndrome, non-arteritic ischemic optic neuropathy, increased intracranial pressure, and even glaucoma. Patients whose DME seems less responsive to anti-VEGF treatment may even have an increased risk of OSA.[15] And real doctors know that patients with sleep apnea have higher incidences of hypertension, stroke, myocardial infarction, dysrhythmias, diabetes and dementia. As a result, it makes a lot of sense to be aware of the risk factors and symptoms of OSA. Check the box to the side for the full scoop, and consider recommending sleep studies on worrisome patients.[16,17]

CAN CERTAIN DRUGS SLOW RETINOPATHY?

There are studies that suggest that some drugs may be better at controlling retinopathy, above and beyond their ability to treat risk factors such as hypertension and dyslipidemia. For instance, certain angiotensin inhibitors have been proposed to be better for slowing retinopathy progression. There has also been research suggesting that the lipid-lowering agent fenofibrate may slow progression, although the effect may be limited to males.[18] However, a recent review of the topic did not find that there was enough data to recommend any specific agent over another.[19] It is best to control these risk factors as much as possible with whatever means necessary, rather than focus on using a single drug or class of drugs because they might have an effect on retinopathy progression.

There have been other drugs specifically designed to target retinopathy; the protein kinase C inhibitor ruboxistaurin is an example. Preliminary studies suggested it might slow the development of macular edema, and several years ago there was even an advertising surge in anticipation of its approval. Eli Lilly has since stopped clinical testing as a large trail failed to reach statistical significance. A different approach involves the off-label use of doxycycline. It has anti-inflammatory effects that may help preserve inner retinal function in diabetics.[20] This approach is only investigational right now, but it suggests that retinopathy-specific treatments are very likely to be in our future.

The bottom line is that there doesn't seem to be a specific anti-retinopathy drug at this point in time. There are a lot of potential avenues being explored, and the section at the end of the chapter will address the subject a bit more. There may be a time when ophthalmologists can make specific drug recommendations based on a patient's level of retinopathy.

On a more cynical note, it is worth pointing out that—given the number of diabetics in the world—a drug that stops retinopathy will be both a very good thing and will make someone some serious coin. That kind of cash can make it tempting to draw overly enthusiastic conclusions from ho-hum results. Perhaps one of the most worrisome papers ever published showed how this plays out regarding glaucoma therapy, another lucrative field. They found that while 90% of corporate-sponsored papers had abstract conclusions favoring the sponsor's product, the data presented in the body of the text showed a significant outcome measure only 24% of the time![21] And the editorial accompanying the paper indicated that this problem extends across all of medicine.[22] So learn how to read publications critically before plying your patients with new drugs.

NUANCES TO CONSIDER WHEN ADDRESSING SYSTEMIC CONTROL:

Nuance Number 1: Rapid Institution of Tight Control in Patients Who Have Been Poorly Controlled

The rapid institution of tight control can result in temporary worsening of diabetic retinopathy in some patients. This effect was best demonstrated in the DCCT, wherein motivated study patients were treated very aggressively and brought under control very quickly. The problem tends to be transient and the long-term benefits of good control by far outweigh any temporary problems. It is more likely to occur in patients who have a history of very poor control and active retinopathy, and it has therefore been suggested that such patients should be brought under control slowly. For instance, an older study suggested that the HbA1c should be improved no faster than one percentage point a quarter.[23] This approach has never been proven, however.

In the real world, patients who have had poor control tend to be incapable of improving things as rapidly as patients in the study, so this potential problem is usually not an issue. Still, you need to be aware of this possibility and watch for it in the appropriate setting. For instance, as we will see in the next chapter, there is a concern that rapid improvement in control may be a factor in the development of diabetic papillopathy. Patients whose control rapidly improves after bariatric surgery may also be at risk for transient retinopathy progression.[24]

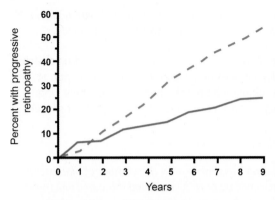

Figure 3: The effect of intensive control on progression of retinopathy. You can see the initial blip in the progression of retinopathy with rapid initiation of intensive control in the setting of this study (the red line). Note that even if this occurs, there is a huge long-term benefit for maintaining good control. (Data from the Diabetes Control and Complications Trial Research Group, N Engl J Med 1993; 329: 977.)

If you do think you have a patient who has this problem, you have to be cautious about how you discuss it. First of all, it is never clear in a particular patient whether worsening is due to this phenomenon or whether it is just their natural history given their prior poor control. Second, you have to carefully explain that the long-term benefits of good control always trump any temporary short-term changes, because patients may mistakenly think that good control is now their enemy. By the way, there is no study that shows that you can undo this transient worsening by letting the patient go back to poor control, so don't let them even think about doing that.

Caveats:

There are two specific situations in which the rapid institution of tight control can influence your ophthalmic management:

1. Pregnant diabetics have to be rapidly controlled to protect the fetus, and this phenomenon may be part of the reason why retinopathy can progress during pregnancy. See Chapter 24.

2. There is a concern that rapid institution of tight control may be especially problematic if it is done around the time of cataract surgery. See Chapter 25.

Nuance Number 2. Lack of Immediate Gratification with Institution of Good Control

Although the preceding section discussed the transient effect of rapidly instituting tight control, a far more common problem from the standpoint of the patient is that once they actually manage to improve their control, they are almost never rewarded with total reversal of their diabetic complications.

This is the usual scenario: Around the time that you need to start treating them they also begin to get other systemic complications. They finally understand how important it is to control the risk factors discussed in this chapter, and for probably the first time ever they start to take better care of themselves. Unfortunately, there is a certain inertia to diabetic complications and things tend to worsen in spite of their new control. They can easily draw the incorrect conclusion that it does not make any difference whether they maintain good control because they keep getting worse no matter how they live.

There is also the concept of metabolic memory.[31] Studies like the DCCT showed that if a patient has a hemoglobin A1c of 9 for 10 years and then lowers it to 7, the risk of microvascular and macrovascular complications is much worse than if the HbA1c started at 7 for the first 10 years and then went up to 9. It is almost as though the kidneys, eyes and heart "remember" all those years of poor control and therefore have more complications. This is why you need to bug your patients to do their best as soon as they are diagnosed. It also helps to explain why, even though they may be taking better care of themselves, they are still having problems with diabetic complications.

But you have to discuss all this very carefully. If you quickly say, "You have to pay for all your bad control in the past," what your patient may think is, "I have been trying my best and it sounds like I am going to get worse no matter what, so I might as well eat whatever I want."

Instead, you should point out that they are dealing with damage that began years ago, and that they cannot make this old damage suddenly disappear with good control. They need to understand that their eye disease is like a moving freight train: It takes time to bring things to a halt. Fortunately, it always pays off to have better control—but it just takes a while for the patient to appreciate it. As you treat diabetics over time, you will have the opportunity to see patients who persevere with excellent control and actually reverse the level of their disease. Such experiences will make you a much better advocate for the importance of good control, because you will believe.

EVEN MORE COMPLICATED ISSUES

Warning: Touchy-feely stuff coming up. Just shut up and read it.

As you review the importance of control, there may be certain patients who become overwhelmed with feelings of guilt about past indiscretions, i.e., they are going blind and it is totally their own fault. (Or they are made to feel this way by especially malignant family dynamics.) You do want them to be inspired to do better, but be aware that this type of guilt can make some patients so depressed that they are incapable of caring for themselves properly—especially if they are afraid that they are going blind, too.

And it doesn't stop there...

Remember that, for some patients, the fact that you are treating them—or even just telling them that they have background retinopathy—may force them to face something they have been denying up until now: that diabetes will make the rest of their life very different from everyone else's. It could be that for the first time they have to confront their fears of ending up blind, amputated and dead at an early age. This is a huge issue to drop into someone's life, and you can totally miss the impact of this if you blast through the office visit in order to get on to the next patient. You can end up being utterly clueless about their inner life, and this is not a good way to be.

Try to listen beyond their questions and comments for signs of anxiety or depression. Don't hesitate to ask about these issues, or about symptoms of depression, and to inform the patient's other doctors if you are worried. It is possible that a few carefully chosen words about how diabetic complications are not inevitable may really ease their pain. The bulk of this book is about making sure that patients have appropriate expectations about our treatments. However, if you think your patient is mentally nose-diving, you definitely want to make it clear that although there are never any guarantees, it is rare for someone to go hopelessly blind from diabetes if they take care of themselves and are compliant with follow up (and they don't have horrible retinopathy).

There is a sense of balance to be struck here, as usual. If they are leaving Doritos crumbs in your laser room while they brag that their hemoglobin A1c of 10 is way better than it used to be, then you should throw the book at 'em. But if they are depressed and guilty, give them some reassurance—and get them help.

There is a reason why you are doing this work and not some laser/injection robot that could do a better job of treating the retina than any of us anyway. Ophthalmologists tend to be spared the sturm und drang of mental health issues, but diabetics are more likely to be depressed and you can be far more helpful to your patients if you remain sensitive to this.[25]

Diabetics often have another source of stress that may require your attention: problems at work caused by fluctuating vision. They may have transient difficulties, for instance with a vitreous hemorrhage, or they may have more chronic problems such as trouble with lighting or with using a computer. You may need to call or write to their employer to explain any special needs to help them keep their job. You may need to educate them about any vocational rehabilitation services that may be available. Of course, if there is too much fuss they can get fired—nothing is simple. It gets even more complicated for some patients because at times their vision may be bad enough to keep them from working but not bad enough to qualify for disability. This can put tremendous financial strain on the patient and their family. Finally, remember that if they can't work they will likely be unable to afford insurance, and this can literally be a matter of life and death for a diabetic. All of this means that you need to be aware of any employment-related issues and be ready to help in any way you can.

If things are really bad, they may even have trouble functioning at home. You should be able to provide recommendations about low vision, vocational rehabilitation and resources to assist with daily living. And you may need to be proactive about this—giving them a brochure for the closest low vision provider is not sufficient. Patients in this situation are often stressed-out and depressed, and that can limit the mental energy they can bring to bear on figuring out what to do. So something that seems obvious to you, like Googling for local resources, may never occur to them.

Get to know those local resources, such as government agencies and non-profits that can help with social services, transportation, etc. Ask patients and family members that have gone through this for any advice that you can pass on. The American Academy of Ophthalmology has some good information under the SmartSight section of their website. You may be awesome in the operating room, but you can do even more good if you can help someone figure out how to get to the grocery store.

SUMMING UP

Everything in this chapter sounds like it could be a lot of work, and it seems to go way beyond the call of duty for the average ophtho-mechanic. It doesn't take more than a few moments, though, to ask about the various systemic risk factors and to listen for any indications that that patient may be getting frustrated or dangerously depressed. It is crucial to recognize that treating diabetic retinopathy involves acknowledging that the patient exists in a matrix far more complex than what you see on your OCT. The matrix includes things like their socioeconomic status, their degree of sophistication and their emotional state, as well as whether or not they have hard exudates within 500 microns of the fovea. If all of these issues are not addressed it is impossible to get the best results with your treatments.

ONE MORE THING...DIPLOMACY IN ACTION...IS IT THE DOCTOR OR THE PATIENT?

As you delve into a patient's medical care you need to get some idea about how aggressive their medical doctor is when it comes to controlling all of their risk factors. Sometimes the patient will tell you that their doctor doesn't do very much for them. If this happens, try to avoid riding any excessively high horses until you have learned all the facts. It is far more likely that the patient is poorly motivated, and their otherwise-busy healthcare providers have recognized this and therefore do not pour a lot of effort into the patient's management. A high-handed letter from the ophthalmologist demanding to know why no one has checked the HbA1c and insisting that everything be fixed straight away will not accomplish much, especially if the medical team has, in fact, been trying to do this for years. It is best to start slowly by communicating your findings and concerns—taking the time to call the patient's doctor may also be invaluable to get the full story. It is all too easy for a patient to blame a doctor rather than accept their own responsibility.

If, after all this, the patient still isn't getting the kind of care you think they need, then there may be a problem with the caregivers. A recent study looking at quality of care for adult diabetics showed that only 7.3% attained recommended goals of an HbA1c level less than 7%, a blood pressure less than 130/80 mm Hg, and a total cholesterol level less than 200 mg/dL. In fact, two in five had poor LDL cholesterol control, one in three had poor blood pressure control, and one in five had a hemoglobin A1c that was over 9%.[26]

You may need to be the one that nudges both the patient and their doctor in the right direction—and you may even need to start by being the one that checks the blood pressure and gets all the various tests such as hemoglobin A1c and renal function studies. Another approach would be to suggest to the patient that they discuss with their doctor the option of getting an endocrinology consult if they are having problems getting their glucose under control. If you really feel that no progress is being made, you may even have to make a referral to a diabetologist on your own.

All this involves treading a fine line between being helpful and ticking off your medical colleagues—but ultimately the best interest of the patient has to prevail. Knowing your medical community, and knowing each doctor's abilities, can be helpful here. Whatever you do, don't abrogate your role in the patient's care by whining that "it's someone else's job." It has to be your job because your outcomes depend on it.

Look at it this way: Systemic control is fundamental to the success of your ophthalmic interventions in the same way that implanting the proper IOL is important to your surgical results. You would never let a patient haphazardly pull their own IOL out of the pile. You should consider the treatment of diabetic retinopathy in the same way—never allow a patient to screw up your fine work with poor control if there is anything at all you can do to help.

> **One last blue box thought:** *If patients actually listen to you and their other doctors and improve their glucose control, recognize that a visit to your office may now represent a real threat to their health. If you get backed up with emergencies, and they have to wait a long time to be seen, they can easily become hypoglycemic. Always keep some orange juice or some other form of glucose around the office so that patients can be readily treated if this happens.*

LOOKING TO THE FUTURE

This chapter covered a lot, but you can't ignore the patient that is attached to the eyes you are treating. However, even if everyone is doing the best they can, patients still can get into trouble. It is fortunate that researchers are constantly expanding our understanding of the pathophysiology of diabetic retinopathy and other diabetic complications. Diabetes clearly increases the toxic effects of metabolic abnormalities such as hyperglycemia, dyslipidemia and hypertension. This occurs through a number of mechanisms including oxidative stress, activating protein kinase C, the formation of toxic advanced glycosylation end products (AGEs) and increased sorbitol (the latter being the mechanism of increased myopia associated with hyperglycemia). However, it is becoming apparent that diabetes also interferes with the regenerative effects of protective factors such as insulin, platelet derived growth factor, nitric oxide and antioxidant enzymes. Figure 4 demonstrates this one-two punch: diabetes damages tissues and then prevents the body from making repairs.[27]

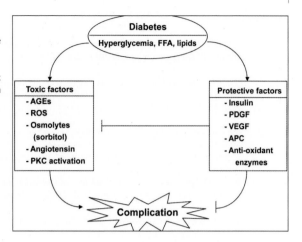

Figure 4: Diabetes induces an imbalance between toxic and protective factors to cause complications. FFA, free fatty acid; AGE, advanced glycosylated end products; ROS, reactive oxygen species; PKC, protein kinase C; PDGF, platelet-derived growth factor; VEGF, vascular endothelial growth factor; APC, activated protein C. From Jeong IK, King GL. New perspectives on diabetic vascular complications: the loss of endogenous protective factors induced by hyperglycemia. Diabetes Metab J. Feb 2011;35(1):8-11 (Creative Commons license).

The exciting thing about this is that it may lead to ways of preventing diabetic complication beyond controlling the usual risk factors such as glucose control and hypertension. In other words, we may be able to avoid damage, and perhaps even repair injured tissue, without being as dependent on the patient's ability to be compliant with their medical care. This can be especially important in the developing world, where the number of diabetic patients is increasing and the ability of healthcare systems to treat them is limited. Hopefully someday we will have treatments that will make this book obsolete.

References

1. Beck RW. The burgeoning public health impact of diabetes: the role of the ophthalmologist. *Archives of ophthalmology.* Feb 2011;129(2):225-229.

2. Riddle MC, Karl DM. Individualizing targets and tactics for high-risk patients with type 2 diabetes: practical lessons from ACCORD and other cardiovascular trials. *Diabetes care.* Oct 2012;35(10):2100-2107.

3. The effect of intensive treatment of diabetes on the development and progression of long-term complications in insulin-dependent diabetes mellitus. The Diabetes Control and Complications Trial Research Group. *The New England journal of medicine.* Sep 30 1993;329(14):977-986.

4. Tight blood pressure control and risk of macrovascular and microvascular complications in type 2 diabetes: UKPDS 38. UK Prospective Diabetes Study Group. *Bmj.* Sep 12 1998;317(7160):703-713.

5. Arauz-Pacheco C, Parrott MA, Raskin P. The treatment of hypertension in adult patients with diabetes. *Diabetes care.* Jan 2002;25(1):134-147.

6. Leiter LA. The prevention of diabetic microvascular complications of diabetes: is there a role for lipid lowering? *Diabetes Res Clin Pract.* Jun 2005;68 Suppl 2:S3-14.

7. Cruickshanks KJ, Ritter LL, Klein R, Moss SE. The association of microalbuminuria with diabetic retinopathy. The Wisconsin Epidemiologic Study of Diabetic Retinopathy. *Ophthalmology.* Jun 1993;100(6):862-867.

8. Lee WJ, Sobrin L, Kang MH, et al. Ischemic diabetic retinopathy as a possible prognostic factor for chronic kidney disease progression. *Eye (Lond).* Sep 2014;28(9):1119-1125.

9. Sinclair SH, Malamut R, Delvecchio C, Li W. Diabetic retinopathy: treating systemic conditions aggressively can save sight. *Cleve Clin J Med.* May 2005;72(5):447-454.

10. Aiello LP, Cahill MT, Wong JS. Systemic considerations in the management of diabetic retinopathy. *American journal of ophthalmology.* Nov 2001;132(5):760-776.

11. Klein R, Lee KE, Gangnon RE, Klein BE. The 25-year incidence of visual impairment in type 1 diabetes mellitus the wisconsin epidemiologic study of diabetic retinopathy. *Ophthalmology.* Jan 2010 117(1):63-70.

12. Mohamed Q, Gillies MC, Wong TY. Management of diabetic retinopathy: a systematic review. *JAMA : the journal of the American Medical Association.* Aug 22 2007;298(8):902-916.

13. Loprinzi PD, Brodowicz GR, Sengupta S, Solomon SD, Ramulu PY. Accelerometer-assessed physical activity and diabetic retinopathy in the United States. *JAMA ophthalmology.* Aug 1 2014;132(8):1017-1019.

14. Cho H, Sobrin L. Genetics of diabetic retinopathy. *Curr Diab Rep.* Aug 2014;14(8):515.

15. Nesmith BL, Ihnen M, Schaal S. Poor responders to bevacizumab pharmacotherapy in age-related macular degeneration and in diabetic macular edema demonstrate increased risk for obstructive sleep apnea. *Retina.* Dec 2014;34(12):2423-2430.

16. Mason RH, West SD, Kiire CA, et al. High prevalence of sleep disordered breathing in patients with diabetic macular edema. *Retina.* Oct 2012;32(9):1791-1798.

17. Stuart A. Obstructive Sleep Apnea and the Eye: The Ophthalmologist's Role. *EyeNet.* February 2013 2013:33-35.

18.   Chew EY, Davis MD, Danis RP, et al. The Effects of Medical Management on the Progression of Diabetic Retinopathy in Persons with Type 2 Diabetes: The Action to Control Cardiovascular Risk in Diabetes Eye Study. *Ophthalmology.* Aug 26 2014.

19.   Frasier CE, D'Amico DJ. Prevention and treatment of diabetic retinopathy. *UpToDate.com.* 2013:Accessed 3/2014.

20.   Scott IU, Jackson GR, Quillen DA, et al. Effect of Doxycycline vs Placebo on Retinal Function and Diabetic Retinopathy Progression in Patients With Severe Nonproliferative or Non-High-Risk Proliferative Diabetic Retinopathy: A Randomized Clinical Trial. *JAMA ophthalmology.* Mar 6 2014.

21.   Alasbali T, Smith M, Geffen N, et al. Discrepancy between results and abstract conclusions in industry- vs nonindustry-funded studies comparing topical prostaglandins. *American journal of ophthalmology.* Jan 2009;147(1):33-38 e32.

22.   Alward WL. How I choose a prostaglandin analogue. *American journal of ophthalmology.* Jan 2009;147(1):1-2.

23.   Funatsu H, Yamashita H, Ohashi Y, Ishigaki T. Effect of rapid glycemic control on progression of diabetic retinopathy. *Jpn J Ophthalmol.* 1992;36(3):356-367.

24.   Murphy R, Jiang Y, Booth M, et al. Progression of diabetic retinopathy after bariatric surgery. *Diabetic medicine : a journal of the British Diabetic Association.* Feb 16 2015.

25.   Ducat L, Philipson LH, Anderson BJ. The mental health comorbidities of diabetes. *JAMA : the journal of the American Medical Association.* Aug 20 2014;312(7):691-692.

26.   Saydah SH, Fradkin J, Cowie CC. Poor control of risk factors for vascular disease among adults with previously diagnosed diabetes. *JAMA : the journal of the American Medical Association.* Jan 21 2004;291(3):335-342.

27.   Jeong IK, King GL. New perspectives on diabetic vascular complications: the loss of endogenous protective factors induced by hyperglycemia. *Diabetes Metab J.* Feb 2011;35(1):8-11.

28.   Lee CH, Li TC, Tsai CI, et al. Yang Deficiency Body Constitution Acts as a Predictor of Diabetic Retinopathy in Patients with Type 2 Diabetes: Taichung Diabetic Body Constitution Study. Evid Based Complement Alternat Med. 2015;2015:940898.

29.   Klein BE, Myers CE, Howard KP, Klein R. Serum Lipids and Proliferative Diabetic Retinopathy and Macular Edema in Persons With Long-term Type 1 Diabetes Mellitus: The Wisconsin Epidemiologic Study of Diabetic Retinopathy. JAMA ophthalmology. 2015;133(5):503-510.

30.   Das R, Kerr R, Chakravarthy U, Hogg RE. Dyslipidemia and Diabetic Macular Edema: A Systematic Review and Meta-Analysis. Ophthalmology. 2015;122(9):1820-1827.

31.   Rand LI, Ferris FL, 3rd. Long-term Contributions From the Diabetes Control and Complications Trial Cohort. JAMA ophthalmology. Aug 2015, epub ahead of print.

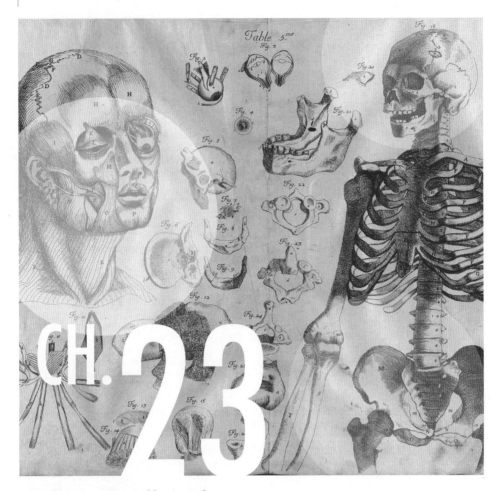

Diabetic Papillopathy.

Or Non-Arteritic Ischemic Optic Neuropathy That Happens to Occur in Diabetics. Or Whatever...

A mind is like a parachute. It doesn't work if it is not open. Frank Zappa

This is an entity that does not quite fit into the categories of non-proliferative or proliferative disease. It is traditionally considered a relatively mild problem, but on occasion it can be a real pain because it may create both a diagnostic and therapeutic challenge. It can also be easy to miss, especially if the patient has a lot of widespread macular edema that masks subtle swelling on the temporal aspect of the optic nerve. You do not want to miss it, though, because it adds a potential wild card to the patient's visual prognosis. It is far better to recognize the problem and educate the patient in advance, rather than be surprised and go back and look at the fundus photos and realize you missed it.

Diabetic papillopathy was originally described in juvenile (Type 1) diabetic patients, but since then it has been described in older, Type 2 patients as well.[1,2] The problem is most likely related to capillary damage that results in chronic ischemia and secondary nerve swelling, which, for reasons known only to the gods of diabetes, does not tip the nerve into full-blown ischemic optic neuropathy (usually). Perhaps the nerve doesn't lapse into full-fledged visual loss because the vascular system isn't that bad—which may go along with it occurring in younger patients. It may also represent some other form of metabolic insufficiency in the optic disc—for example, tissue anoxia due to poor glucose utilization or build-up of toxic substances related to diabetes.

Recent papers have focused on the fact that rapid institution of better control is a risk factor for this entity.[3] Recall from the last chapter that this same factor can cause transient worsening of diabetic retinopathy in general, so it seems reasonable that the same thing can occur at the nerve. Another risk factor is the structure of the nerve; patients are more likely to have small cup to disc diameters (not unlike non-arteritic anterior ischemic optic neuropathy—NAION).

Now, pundits wonder whether diabetic papillopathy is truly different from NAION, or whether it is just an extremely benign form of NAION causing disc ischemia (reversible) without frank infarction (permanent). It really does not make any difference, because you will still be biting your fingernails and hoping that it just goes away without causing any problems. Fortunately, this is indeed what happens to most patients, which is a good thing given the utter lack of proven treatments.

Many patients have no symptoms, and the problem is identified incidentally upon clinical examination. Patients who do have symptoms tend to have non-specific blurring that is mild and intermittent, but patients with more severe disease may have marked visual changes. The vision tends to be only mildly affected, with most patients having better than 20/50 vision initially. There is usually little, if any, afferent pupillary defect unless there is significant and asymmetric loss of optic nerve function—although if there is significant visual loss as evidenced by a large afferent papillary defect and visual field loss, one would tend to diagnose NAION rather than diabetic papillopathy. The disc edema tends to be mild to moderate, with dilated capillaries in the superficial layers of the nerve, and often some splinter hemorrhages. Occasionally, patients may have little or no associated diabetic retinopathy, but most patients will have some degree of background diabetic retinopathy that may vary from mild disease to significant macular edema and even proliferative disease. About half of the time the disease is bilateral, although not always simultaneously.

An angiogram can be very helpful, because it will light up the nerve in a characteristic way, which may help you avoid the embarrassment of missing the diagnosis in subtle cases. There are usually very obvious swollen vessels within the nerve substance that cause late staining that can mimic the appearance of proliferative disease if you don't look carefully. Studying the nerve, though, shows that the staining is limited to the nerve and that there are no overlying new vessels causing the leakage.

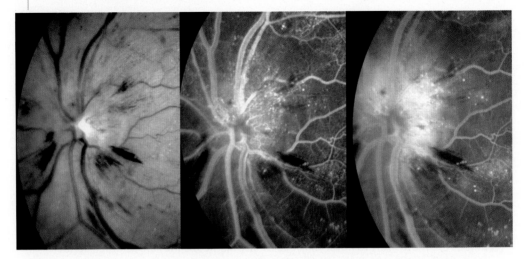

Figure 1: Diabetic papillopathy. The red free photo shows swelling of the nerve fiber layer with loss of the disc margins. There are also nerve fiber layer hemorrhages. The early phase of the angiogram shows typical dilated vessels and the late phase shows staining within the substance of the nerve which nicely backlights the overlying nerve fiber layer hemorrhages.

The visual field usually demonstrates enlargement of the physiologic blind spot, even in asymptomatic patients, although more pronounced constriction or altitudinal changes occur in more severe disease (and again, some would just call this type of vision loss NAION). Overall, the visual prognosis is relatively good, with most patients ending up 20/50 or better unless other aspects of their diabetic retinopathy intervene. There is a subset, perhaps 5 to 15%, who end up with significantly worse vision, and this may be the result of progression to frank NAION or from associated macular edema (which can be very treatable, so don't forget to look for it while you stare at the nerve). As a general rule, the patients who are younger and who present with minimal symptoms and findings tend to do best. Older patients with long-standing systemic vascular disease are more likely to end up with poor vision.

A notable thing about this entity is that it takes many months for the edema to resolve, which is different from the relatively rapid resolution that occurs with ischemic optic neuropathy. The swelling usually begins to diminish by three to six months, although some patients have persistent swelling for a year or so. There is usually not a lot of pallor in the involved nerve once the swelling resolves unless there has been significant nerve fiber damage. There are some patients, however, for whom the presence of diabetic papillopathy heralds the onset of more progressive problems, such as proliferative disease or worsening macular edema. As a result, even if the nerve swelling subsides nicely, patients with this entity need continued close monitoring.

Aspects of Diabetic Papillopathy That Can Be Problematic...

Although diabetic papillopathy is fairly benign most of the time, it has the potential to make trouble for two reasons: (1) the clinical findings can be quite similar to other conditions in which the outcome is not necessarily benign, and (2) it can be an unpredictable time bomb in terms of visual acuity.

DIFFERENTIAL DIAGNOSIS Issues

Unfortunately, when it comes to the differential diagnosis, there is nothing about the clinical exam that can definitively distinguish diabetic papillopathy from more ominous causes of optic nerve swelling. Some authors suggest that the diagnosis of diabetic papillopathy can be made if the patient is in the appropriate demographic and the vision and visual field are relatively preserved. This sounds reasonable, but the optic disc appearance is non-specific and diabetic papillopathy is really a diagnosis of exclusion. Although the differential diagnosis of optic nerve swelling is legion, here are some things to at least consider before simply deciding a patient has diabetic papillopathy:

A mild central retinal vein occlusion can have associated disc edema, especially in younger patients. The associated venous tortuosity and engorgement, and characteristic hemorrhages, should suggest venous occlusive disease. (Fluorescein angiography with timing sequences is a good way to evaluate for central retinal vein occlusion.) Optic neuritis can also cause disc swelling, but there are usually more pronounced effects on vision, and patients generally have the typical pain on movement associated with this entity. Compressive optic neuropathy (as from an optic nerve glioma or meningioma) typically causes optic disc edema with variable loss of optic nerve function. In the early stages, the changes in disc appearance can pre-date any change in vision. In most cases, careful examination will show proptosis but it is reasonable to obtain an MRI to more fully rule out a structural lesion.

Inflammatory or infectious disc swelling usually has an associated cellular infiltrate of the retina and/or vitreous, which suggests something more than plain old diabetic papillopathy. Examples include disc swelling in association with anterior or intermediate uveitis, or infectious causes such as cat-scratch disease or toxoplasmosis. Other more obscure entities such as orbital tumors, congenital abnormalities, or infiltrative lesions may need to be considered in the appropriate setting, but this all begins to get into very different clinical presentations. If you are really worried about this kind of stuff, you need to be reading a textbook with the word "neuro" in the title.

Finally, there are occasional patients who may develop vitreous traction on the nerve, and this can simulate the swelling caused by diabetic papillopathy[4]. It is important to distinguish traction from papillopathy, because traction on the nerve can sometimes benefit from vitrectomy in order to avoid visual field loss (see Chapter 19).

The real problem with patients with unilateral disease is deciding whether they have ischemic optic neuropathy, which, in turn, is all about deciding whether they need an evaluation for giant cell arteritis. The best way to tell diabetic papillopathy from either arteritic or non-arteritic ischemic optic neuropathy is simply observation over time. Diabetic papillopathy usually resolves with little sequelae, unlike ischemic optic neuropathy, which usually leaves more pronounced pallor of the nerve and permanent visual field loss. Also, as mentioned, the swelling caused by diabetic papillopathy may last much longer than that caused by ischemic optic neuropathy. Unfortunately, once the specter of giant cell arteritis is raised, the concept of "observation over time" becomes an unaffordable luxury—waiting to see if the fellow eye goes irreversibly blind is no way to make a diagnosis.

For younger patients with presumed diabetic papillopathy and minimal visual changes, this is much less of an issue and observation is warranted (assuming you have ruled out the entities mentioned above). For older diabetics (>55 years old), you are obligated to perform an evaluation for temporal arteritis—especially if there is significant loss of function. This becomes even more problematic because the usual tests (erythrocyte sedimentation rate and C-reactive protein) tend to be a bit abnormal in older diabetic patients, and you may be forced to consider invasive maneuvers such as temporal artery biopsies and prednisone treatment. The perils of missing a diagnosis of giant cell arteritis are great, but so are the risks of putting an elderly diabetic on prednisone. Whichever way you go, please make sure you have documented your rationale, and strongly consider obtaining other opinions to support your gut feelings, especially if you decide the patient simply has diabetic papillopathy and you are going to observe them. (A full discussion regarding the diagnosis of temporal arteritis is beyond the scope of this book—you know where to look.)

Making the diagnosis of diabetic papillopathy becomes problematic for a different reason if the patient presents with bilateral disease. One then needs to consider increased intracranial pressure as well as all the other causes of disc swelling. It is very risky to simply attribute bilateral disc swelling to diabetic papillopathy because of the rather grave consequences for the patient if you happen to be wrong. Also, remember that if you decide to forego a neurologic evaluation, those swollen nerves will be staring you down for many months to come; although an MRI and LP are not without risk and cost, it is usually better to get the more worrisome aspects of the differential diagnosis out of the way first.

There may be times when you feel fairly certain that a patient has diabetic papillopathy and not bilateral papilledema from an intracranial process. An example would be a younger patient with no symptoms of elevated intracranial pressure and no reason in their medical history or general exam to indicate that they are predisposed to developing increased intracranial pressure. In this situation, some feel that a spinal tap can be deferred. This begins to resemble the kind of thing that neuro-ophthalmologists are clearly best at; you should consider getting another opinion before you do nothing but observe the patient.

Also, never forget that one of the most important things to do with bilateral swollen nerves is to dust off your blood pressure cuff and check for severe hypertension. One would want to be the first in line to diagnose this problem and not wait for the ER to make the diagnosis two days later.

If you have easy access to the various ophthalmic specialties (i.e., if you are in training at a program where you can actually talk to the staff), you can get a sense for just how much variability there can be when it comes to making this diagnosis. If you show a case that looks like diabetic papillopathy to a retina specialist, they will probably feel comfortable with simple observation, but if you show the same case to a neuro-ophthalmologist, you will likely be spending more time ruling out giant cell arteritis and/ or elevated intracranial pressure. As a general rule, the neuro-ophthalmologist wins and you should consider diabetic papillopathy a diagnosis of last resort.

As an aside: Don't ever succumb to the illusory comfort that you are off the hook if you can get a retina specialist to make the easy diagnosis of diabetic papillopathy—especially if you are worried about something else in your heart of hearts. At times retina specialists don't know what they don't know when it comes to optic nerves, so just do what you think is the right thing.

A final point in the differential is that, sometimes, the dilated capillaries seen on the nerve with this entity can simulate neovascularization of the disc. In general, the vascular changes associated with papillopathy tend to be more radially oriented and are within the substance of the disc, whereas true neovascularization forms an irregular network above the surface of the disc. Also, true neovascularization tends to leak more on a fluorescein angiogram. However, because this entity can occasionally evolve into frank neovascularization you cannot just ignore the appearance of the vessels once you have decided the patient has diabetic papillopathy; instead, you need to watch them carefully to make sure that they do not sprout high-risk proliferative disease.

VISUAL ACUITY and Treatment Issues

OK. Having worked through the above diagnostic process, let's assume the patient actually has diabetic papillopathy. Fortunately most patients end up doing well, but there are occasional patients who develop severe vision loss, and this may occur at any point in time. It is particularly frustrating if it occurs around the time you have performed a laser or injection to treat their retinopathy, because the patient will think their vision loss is your fault. Even if the patient does not have marked worsening of their vision, diabetic papillopathy can still limit visual recovery from interventions such as cataract surgery. Finally, they need to know there is a chance this could evolve into high-risk neovascularization, bringing with it all the joys of panretinal photocoagulation. In essence, you have to be able to recognize this entity and, once it is recognized, you have to spend some time educating the patient about the potential problems it can cause—even if most patients do fine.

In terms of treatment, there is no proven approach. Like any other diabetic manifestation, the patient should be urged to control all of the usual vascular risk factors, as outlined in Chapter 22. However, the fact that this entity can be associated with rapid improvement of glucose control has led some to argue that patients with a cup to disc ratio of less than 0.18 might benefit from more gradual improvement of their control, with a specific suggestion of lowering the HbA1c no faster than 1.5 percentage points a quarter.[3] There is no prospective data to prove this, though, and there probably never will be. (But keep in mind the data from Chapter 22 suggesting that even with transient worsening, the overall benefit from improved control is tremendous.) By the way, once the papillopathy shows up, you can't make it go away by having the patient slack off on their control—that doesn't seem to work.

Of course, the fact that there are no proven treatments means that, inevitably, you will find someone who is willing to inject something into the eye. As of this writing there is no definitive study, but there are case reports suggesting that steroids, bevacizumab, and/or ranibizumab can be helpful.[5-8] If the patient has marked vision loss, it may be worth considering one of these. The patient really needs to understand the potential risks, though, and understand that such treatment is undertaken in desperation—without a lot of support from the literature (for instance, no one knows what might happen to an ischemic nerve if it is exposed to a pressure in the 40s from steroid-induced ocular hypertension). Moreover, the effect of the transient intraocular pressure rise at the time of injection has not been studied in diabetic papillopathy (and those small optic disks). Some feel that it would be prudent to check the IOP right after injection, and more readily consider an anterior chamber tap.

Ultimately, diabetic papillopathy is an entity that spans other specialties. There are additional references at the end of the chapter, but neither the list of references nor this chapter is meant to be exhaustive. If you have a patient with diabetic papillopathy, you may want to run the case by your friendly neighborhood neuro-ophthalmologist to be sure you have a handle on the latest thoughts on this condition.

References and Suggested Reading

1.   Lubow M, Makley TA, Jr. Pseudopapilledema of juvenile diabetes mellitus. *Arch Ophthalmol.* Apr 1971;85(4):417-422.

2.   Bayraktar Z, Alacali N, Bayraktar S. Diabetic papillopathy in type II diabetic patients. *Retina.* Dec 2002;22(6):752-758.

3.   Ostri C, Lund-Andersen H, Sander B, Hvidt-Nielsen D, Larsen M. Bilateral diabetic papillopathy and metabolic control. *Ophthalmology.* Nov 2010;117(11):2214-2217.

4.   Saito Y, Ueki N, Hamanaka N, Shiotani Y, Nakae K, Kiuchi Y. Transient optic disc edema by vitreous traction in a quiescent eye with proliferative diabetic retinopathy mimicking diabetic papillopathy. *Retina.* Jan 2005;25(1):83-84.

5.   Giuliari GP, Sadaka A, Chang PY, Cortez RT. Diabetic papillopathy: current and new treatment options. *Current diabetes reviews.* May 2011;7(3):171-175.

6.   Feng J, Qu JF, Jiang YR. Resolution of diabetic papillopathy with a single intravitreal injection of bevacizumab combined with triamcinolone acetonide. *Graefes Arch Clin Exp Ophthalmol.* Nov 2013;251(11):2651-2652.

7.   Kim M, Lee JH, Lee SJ. Diabetic papillopathy with macular edema treated with intravitreal ranibizumab. *Clin Ophthalmol.* 2013;7:2257-2260.

8.   Mansour AM, El-Dairi MA, Shehab MA, Shahin HK, Shaaban JA, Antonios SR. Periocular corticosteroids in diabetic papillopathy. *Eye (Lond).* Jan 2005;19(1):45-51.

Regillo CD, Brown GC, Savino PJ, et al. Diabetic papillopathy. Patient characteristics and fundus findings. Arch Ophthalmol 1995;113:889-95.

Hayreh SS. Diabetic papillopathy and nonarteritic anterior ischemic optic neuropathy. Surv Ophthalmol 2002;47:600-2; author reply 602.

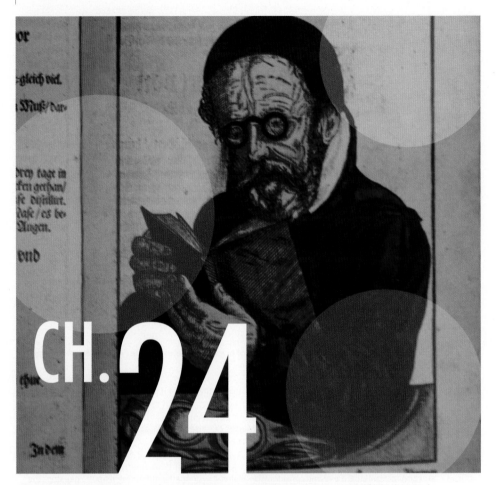

Proliferating While Proliferating: Diabetic Retinopathy During Pregnancy

Life is always a rich and steady time when you are waiting for something to happen or to hatch.
E.B. White, *Charlotte's Web*

There is no question that diabetic retinopathy can worsen during pregnancy, but there is also a chance that this progression may spontaneously regress during the postpartum period. This means that treating retinopathy during pregnancy may require a little more flair than treating "standard" diabetics. There are four main variables that are important in determining a patient's risk for progression during pregnancy: (1) the degree of retinopathy present at the onset of pregnancy; (2) the duration of the patient's diabetes; (3) the level of control prior to the pregnancy; and (4) problems with hypertension during the pregnancy.

All patients should be examined during their first trimester. It makes sense to see patients with little or no retinopathy about every three months. If there is any significant retinopathy, then the intervals should be decreased, especially if the patient has a history of poor control that is suddenly improving in the setting of aggressive perinatal care. Patients presenting with moderate to severe disease may even need to be checked every month to monitor for progression.

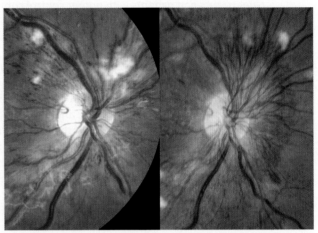

The most important exam, however, should occur well before a patient becomes pregnant. Ideally, a diabetic woman who is considering pregnancy should be informed about the status of her retinopathy and given some sort of idea about the potential risk that pregnancy poses to her vision. This also gives you a chance to treat any worrisome disease before the patient becomes pregnant. Fortunately, the risk is minimal in a conscientious patient with a history of good control, good follow up, and mild retinopathy.

Figure 1: This patient went from no neovascularization on the left to the huge frond on the right over a two-month period in the second trimester. The irregular truncated capillaries and cotton-wool spots around the nerve in the left photo suggest significant ischemia, and are a portent of real trouble. (Courtesy of William A. Argus, M.D.)

It is also helpful if the patient can be evaluated by an endocrinologist (and nephrologist if necessary). These specialists can give the patient an idea of her systemic risk. For instance, pregnancy can accelerate nephropathy, which in turn is associated with an increased risk of fetal complications. If the patient is trying to decide whether to get pregnant and is not being followed by such specialists, it may be incumbent on you to insist. If there is enough eye disease to get you involved in the decision, then the patient may need a specialist evaluation to get the best possible advice about other potential problems. Plus, getting the patient to adopt good control well before becoming pregnant is a really good idea.

As an aside, *there appears to be little or no risk of developing retinopathy in patients who are diagnosed with gestational diabetes and have no prior history of diabetes. Such patients are at increased risk for developing frank diabetes down the road, but routine eye exams during pregnancy are probably not necessary.[1] If there is any question about prior diabetes, though, an exam is warranted.*

In terms of determining a given patient's risk of progression, the easiest thing to do from an ophthalmic standpoint is to categorize patients based on their pre-existing retinopathy. If there is no retinopathy present at the beginning of pregnancy, the odds are good that the patient will not develop any significant problems during the pregnancy. The patient still needs to be examined; there are studies suggesting it is possible for patients to develop problems such as macular edema or proliferative disease even if they have little or no pre-existing retinopathy at the start of pregnancy. Problems, once again, are more likely to develop in patients with a history of long-standing diabetes and poor control.

If the patient does have pre-existing retinopathy, it is hard to be very specific about her risk for progression because the literature is quite variable. Furthermore, many of the older papers had patients with poorer control compared to the average patient in the modern era, and bad control automatically worsens the prognosis. In general, the more severe the retinopathy, the more likely the progression.

One commonly quoted paper is the Diabetes in Early Pregnancy Study.[2] This showed that patients with no retinopathy, microaneurysms only, mild nonproliferative retinopathy, and moderate to severe nonproliferative retinopathy at baseline had progression of their retinopathy in 10.3, 21.1, 18.8, and 54.8% of patients, respectively. In this case, progression referred to worsening of their nonproliferative findings or the development of proliferative disease. (Significant progression of nonproliferative disease was defined as "two-step" progression. This means that the patient moved two steps along the scale of nonproliferative disease, i.e., from mild—past moderate—to severe disease.) The percentage of patients who developed proliferative disease was smaller, but still significant: Proliferative retinopathy developed in 6.3% of patients with mild disease at the onset of pregnancy, but it developed in as many as 29% of patients who began with moderate to severe retinopathy. Note, however, that there may be less risk nowadays. This data was published in 1995—a paper published six years later looking at patients with better control had an across-the-board progression rate to proliferative disease of only 2.2%.[3]

All this data refers to patients with active disease. It turns out that if patients present with old proliferative disease that has been well controlled with previous treatment, they are much less likely to develop progression of their retinopathy during the pregnancy. There are, of course, no guarantees, but this demographic tends to be stable.

It is not clear why retinopathy progresses during pregnancy. It has been speculated to be caused by changes in cardiac output that "strain" the retinal circulation. There may also be hormonal influences. One additional factor is the effect of taking a patient whose control may have been marginal and rapidly improving her control. As mentioned in Chapter 22, the rapid institution of tight control can cause temporary worsening of retinopathy. This phenomenon doesn't make much difference in non-pregnant patients, because the long-term results clearly favor tight control and because most patients can't come under control quickly anyway. In the setting of pregnancy, however, there is a need to rapidly institute tight control in order to avoid complications such as congenital malformations and miscarriage. As a result, even if the rapid tightening of control is problematic for the retinas of pregnant patients, there really is no choice.

However, retinopathy progression is not entirely related to the institution of tight control. The fact that simply being pregnant contributes to progression is demonstrated by the observation that some patients who develop proliferative disease during pregnancy will experience spontaneous regression of the neovascularization in the postpartum period. This is not something to depend on, though, and it makes sense to treat proliferative disease during pregnancy rather than to watch it. For instance, if the patient is developing proliferative disease, treatment should be considered even if she does not have high-risk features in order to avoid problems later in the pregnancy.

It is always bad if a pregnant patient somehow manages to present with brand new proliferative disease at her first visit. It is likely that such patients had very poor control, and they need to be treated immediately and followed closely. Another bad sign is if the patient has a history of treatment but begins to develop recurrent disease during pregnancy—one should aggressively fill in any pre-existing panretinal photocoagulation pattern to try and regain control of the disease. You may be interested to know that in the bad old days, the presence of aggressive retinopathy was considered an indication to abort the pregnancy—hopefully your laser can avoid such an outcome. On the other hand, if patients develop mild proliferative disease and have a history of good control, you can make a case for treating relatively lightly, because under these circumstances you may simply need to get them through their pregnancy in hopes that the neovascular stimulus will resolve postpartum. On the third hand, given the potential consequences of untreated PDR, at least one author suggests treating even severe nonproliferative disease with PRP to avoid progression.[4] It would be great if we could just give an anti-VEGF injection to get temporary control of any proliferative disease, but the use of those drugs during pregnancy is problematic for obvious reasons—the macular edema section will discuss this a bit more.

Basically, you need to assess each patient on a case-by-case basis—you can titrate the treatment depending on how aggressive their disease is and how precarious their medical situation is. If you are not sure how to proceed, a retinal consultation is in order.

Whatever you do, all pregnant patients with proliferative disease require much more frequent monitoring than a non-pregnant patient—perhaps every two to four weeks—in order to be sure that the process is not worsening. You do not want such patients heading into the perinatal period with uncontrolled proliferative retinopathy. If they have any complications related to the delivery—or even if they are just figuring out how to get some sleep with a newborn at home—it may be weeks before you can get them into your office again.

One other thing: You have to be very careful about how you do your PRPs in this setting. Not only do you have to worry about all the usual stuff that can go wrong—like macular edema—but you also have to remember that for most people anything that causes eye pain can also induce vagal problems such as nausea. This is bad because pregnant women may be constantly on the verge of vomiting anyway, depending on where they are in their pregnancy. If you hit them with a lot of laser, and if they are particularly sensitive, you can throw them into an episode of diabetic ketoacidosis simply from pain and nausea and vomiting. This can happen even if you block them *at the time of the laser—when your block wears off, they can still be miserable. This scenario is not a good thing for someone who is pregnant, and might cause more morbidity than the proliferative disease you are trying to treat. There is no magic solution here. You can use all the tricks in Chapter 16 on pain management. You can make sure the patient is working closely with her obstetrician and endocrinologist if she does have problems, and if she needs medication to treat any nausea those specialists can choose ones that are safe in pregnancy. You may also have to do several lasers using a small number of spots over many closely spaced visits, if necessary. Whatever it takes. Fortunately, this doesn't come up often, but it is a reminder of how much you need to be ready to customize your PRPs.*

MACULAR EDEMA

Treating diabetic macular edema may also require a very different approach relative to treating non-pregnant patients. It is possible to be very conservative with these patients because treatment may not be necessary. One study suggested that as many as 88% of eyes that develop diabetic macular edema during pregnancy will undergo resolution of the edema without laser treatment.[5]

However, you need to consider treatment if the vision is markedly decreased or if there are areas of focal leakage that are allowing lipid to build up and threaten the fovea. It may also be necessary to treat patients who develop significant central thickening early in their pregnancy; it is not a good idea to leave the macula swollen for several months. As usual, there really is no definitive data that guides the approach in this situation, and you also have to look at the patient's systemic status and history of control.

What about intravitreal treatment? This is basically uncharted territory and there are no definite guidelines. One might consider intravitreal triamcinolone because it might buy these patients time to get to their delivery without putting permanent laser spots in their posterior pole. Ozurdex may be another option if you have access to it. We know from Chapter 4 that steroids don't work so well in phakic patients, but long-term control is not the issue here. But you do need to balance the risk of endophthalmitis, glaucoma and eventual cataract, none of which is a good thing during pregnancy (although those risks may be less problematic than permanent macular damage from edema).

Of course, anti-vascular endothelial growth factor drugs are unlikely to be an option given the potential effects on the baby. There are several reports of use of these medications without problems during pregnancy—usually for choroidal neovascularization—but there are other cases of possible miscarriages related to intraocular use.[6-8] Although they might be ideal for getting temporary control of retinopathy until delivery, there really is not enough data to guide us about safety. Basically, if you are thinking about any type of intravitreal treatment you should spread the risk and get some additional opinions.

Fluorescein angiography? The decision to perform a fluorescein angiogram can be difficult in the setting of pregnancy. Although there is no report of teratogenicity associated with the use of fluorescein, almost everyone tries to avoid injecting things into pregnant women. It is felt that an angiogram is reasonably safe if the results would change the treatment approach in a patient facing the risk of blindness.[9] As a comprehensive ophthalmologist, it is unlikely that you would truly find yourself in this situation; any patient this complex should probably be referred. Besides, most of the worrisome changes that occur in a diabetic retina can be identified with a careful clinical examination alone. The risk of an angiogram probably outweighs any benefits in a typical situation—even if the risk is largely theoretical.

What about the actual delivery? There have been a few cases of vitreous hemorrhage reported during labor and delivery in patients with proliferative disease. However, there is some degree of risk to performing a cesarean section, and the general feeling is that it is probably safer to go ahead and have a vaginal delivery and avoid a cesarean section if the only reason for performing a cesarean section is the fear of a vitreous hemorrhage. We can always operate on a vitreous hemorrhage, and the morbidity associated with a cesarean section is more than that associated with a vitrectomy, especially for a diabetic patient. But it is unlikely that retinopathy will be the only deciding factor as far as how the baby will be delivered. If the patient has retinopathy they probably have other, more worrisome systemic issues that may require earlier delivery. Plus, these babies tend to be large, making vaginal delivery problematic. So these mothers are more likely to have a C-section anyway. But the mother may need reassurance, and you may get a phone call from the OB team. If it looks like this will be an issue, the patient might benefit from a retina referral well before the time of delivery.

Once the patient delivers, things tend to settle down from the standpoint of retinopathy progression. The exact schedule for follow up would depend on how much trouble occurred during the pregnancy. It is important to monitor patients closely over the first year after pregnancy—even if they spontaneously improve postpartum—because one of the DCCT studies suggested that for some patients the risk of progression may last up to a year.[10] Finally, although retinopathy can worsen during pregnancy, pregnancy itself does not appear to change a woman's long-term risk of retinopathy progression.[10] This is a reassuring thing to tell patients.

SUMMING UP

It is important to realize that the ramifications of treating retinopathy during pregnancy are significant; you are caring for at least two people. This section is really just an overview of what is a rather detailed literature. If there is any question about how to approach a given patient, you should explore this subject more deeply; there are some good reviews available.[11,12] You should also have a low threshold for asking for help—if a pregnant woman's eyes are in trouble the disease may behave very differently from typical retinopathy and the stakes are high.

References

1.   Puza SW, Malee MP. Utilization of routine ophthalmologic examinations in pregnant diabetic patients. *J Matern Fetal Med.* Jan-Feb 1996;5(1):7-10.

2.   Chew EY, Mills JL, Metzger BE, et al. Metabolic control and progression of retinopathy. The Diabetes in Early Pregnancy Study. National Institute of Child Health and Human Development Diabetes in Early Pregnancy Study. *Diabetes Care.* May 1995;18(5):631-637.

3.   Temple RC, Aldridge VA, Sampson MJ, Greenwood RH, Heyburn PJ, Glenn A. Impact of pregnancy on the progression of diabetic retinopathy in Type 1 diabetes. *Diabet Med.* Jul 2001;18(7):573-577.

4.   Chan WC, Lim LT, Quinn MJ, Knox FA, McCance D, Best RM. Management and outcome of sight-threatening diabetic retinopathy in pregnancy. *Eye (Lond).* Aug 2004;18(8):826-832.

5.   Sinclair SH, Nesler C, Foxman B, Nichols CW, Gabbe S. Macular edema and pregnancy in insulin-dependent diabetes. *Am J Ophthalmol.* Feb 1984;97(2):154-167.

6.   Petrou P, Georgalas I, Giavaras G, Anastasiou E, Ntana Z, Petrou C. Early loss of pregnancy after intravitreal bevacizumab injection. *Acta Ophthalmol.* Jun 2009;88(4):e136.

7.   Tarantola RM, Folk JC, Boldt HC, Mahajan VB. Intravitreal bevacizumab during pregnancy. *Retina.* Oct 2010;30(9):1405-1411.

8.   Introini U, Casalino G, Cardani A, et al. Intravitreal bevacizumab for a subfoveal myopic choroidal neovascularization in the first trimester of pregnancy. *Journal of ocular pharmacology and therapeutics : the official journal of the Association for Ocular Pharmacology and Therapeutics.* Oct 2012;28(5):553-555.

9.   Sheth BP, Mieler WF. Ocular complications of pregnancy. *Curr Opin Ophthalmol.* Dec 2001;12(6):455-463.

10.   Effect of pregnancy on microvascular complications in the diabetes control and complications trial. The Diabetes Control and Complications Trial Research Group. *Diabetes Care.* Aug 2000;23(8):1084-1091.

11.   Brown J, Sunness JS. Pregnancy and Retinal Disease. In: SJ R, ed. *Retina, 4th ed*. Philadelphia:: Elsevier Mosby; 2006:1358-1363.

12.   Errera MH, Kohly RP, da Cruz L. Pregnancy-associated retinal diseases and their management. *Surv Ophthalmol.* Mar-Apr 2013;58(2):127-142.

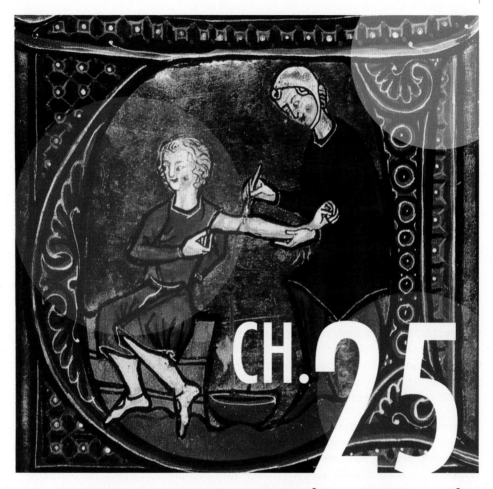

Cataract Surgery & Diabetic Retinopathy

Chose a job you love, and you will never have to work a day in your life. Confucius

Not unlike the blind men who describe an elephant based on which part they are touching, there tends to be a big difference between how a retina specialist views cataract surgery in diabetics and how a cataract surgeon views the issue. Retina people tend to be real worrywarts about this, and will be far more cautious about suggesting cataract surgery simply because of all the patients they have seen start with 20/40 glare cataracts and end up 20/200 from progression of their retinopathy after surgery. In the bad old days (a few decades ago), it was not uncommon to hold off on cataract surgery until the vision was 20/200 or worse because, if things went south, the patient would at least have a fighting chance of ending up about as bad as they were before surgery. On the other hand, most high-volume cataract surgeons will tell you that they simply do not see the type of problems that retina people fuss about. Who is right? Everyone, probably.

The older literature definitely implies that cataract surgery is far less successful in diabetics than in non-diabetics. These reports were based on rather rambunctious surgical procedures, such as intracapsular or large-incision extracapsular surgery. Doctors who have lived through this era tend to be the most conservative about suggesting cataract surgery in diabetics.

Fortunately, the results tend to be much better with modern cataract surgery. In fact, some recent papers suggest that cataract surgery may have little or no effect on retinopathy progression for patients with minimal disease. The aggressive use of laser treatment and intravitreal injections have also helped improve results. Perhaps the most important factor is the much better systemic control that patients have nowadays.

However, because studies discussing the safety of modern surgery are not large randomized trials with long-term follow up, there is no way to rule out a subtle effect on retinopathy acceleration after cataract surgery. Plus, now that we have OCT, there are lots of studies (reviewed by Giansanti et al.)[1] that suggest that even if diabetics don't develop obvious edema, they do get subtle macular thickening after surgery. And at least one population-based study suggests that even with modern techniques, there is some degree of increased retinopathy progression after phaco.[2] Something is going on back there that can cause trouble, even if most of the time things go well. Finally, remember that if you are at the top of a cataract feeding chain and you don't follow most of your patients over the long-term, you may get a skewed view of how safe the procedure is.

So proceed with an open mind—you may feel that your surgery would never make a diabetic worse, but we just don't know that such an assertion will remain true over many years. Besides, no matter how reassuring the modern literature may be, there is no doubt that some diabetic eyes will crash—even after perfect surgery. You therefore must warn all diabetics about the possible consequences, even if you think retina specialists are a bunch of overprotective weenies.

It helps to think of a diabetic's eye in terms of plumbing. A new house with shiny new pipes can handle a lot of abuse. An old house with pipes that are about to rust through will do OK if you take it really easy, but if you hammer away on them or crank up the pressure, you will blow everything out. The blood vessels in diabetic eyes can behave like rusty pipes. They seem to be very sensitive to increases in inflammatory mediators, and every effort should be made to perform surgery as smoothly and gently as possible to avoid stressing the system. Do not try out new things on your diabetic patients—they need the benefit of your best surgical technique, not the latest Suck-n-Cut that your surgical rep is dying to sell you. Anything that results in more intraocular manipulation and damage will greatly increase the risk of postoperative retinopathy progression. Repeat: If there are any problems during the surgery—even something mild like scruffing up the iris with your phaco tip—you have to watch extra carefully for retinopathy progression postoperatively.

Assuming you can provide smooth, state-of-the-art surgery for your patient, you still cannot be sure that all diabetics will do well. Your goal should be to identify those patients whose eyes may be microvascular booby-traps so that neither you nor the patient is unpleasantly surprised. Here are some things to consider:

Patients who seem to do best are usually either at the very beginning or at the very end of their retinopathy careers. In other words, patients with only minimal disease (maybe less than a few scattered microaneurysms and blot hemorrhages) tend to do well. Patients with quiescent, treated retinopathy also tend to do well. These are the patients who have taken good care of their diabetes and have a history of treatment that has stabilized their retinopathy for many years. This does not guarantee that such patients will do well—bad things can still happen to these burned-out eyes when you least expect it. As a general rule though, patients with stable treated disease have much better odds than patients with active disease.

Because patients with minimal disease tend to do better, there are occasional cataract-ists who suggest that one should be even more aggressive about doing surgery in such patients. The thinking is that one should get the incipient cataract out of there now—when the eye can tolerate it better and the odds of safe surgery are better. It is argued that if one waits years for the cataract to get worse, then the retinopathy will also be getting worse, and the chance for successful surgery is diminished. This thinking was not unreasonable in the past. Today, with multiple ways to treat retinopathy, it is hard to justify this rationale for "preemptive" cataract surgery.

Be very careful of patients whose retinopathy is in the "middle"—those who do not have very early disease or old burned-out disease. Someone with lots of microaneurysms and exudates in the posterior pole—even if there is no significant thickening—can really take off after cataract surgery. The same is true for patients with severe nonproliferative retinopathy, and it is especially true if such patients appear to be on the brink of needing treatment. If there is any doubt that the patient's retinopathy may be problematic, you may want to have the patient evaluated preoperatively by a retina specialist to cover yourself.

It goes without saying (so why is it being said?) that any pre-existing macular edema or proliferative disease should be aggressively treated prior to cataract surgery. In fact, you should have a low threshold for treating disease that you might not otherwise treat. For instance, a patient with some macular edema that is not clinically significant may benefit from treatment prior to cataract surgery. Or, you may consider doing preoperative PRP on a patient with severe NPDR whom you might otherwise just observe. It would be nice, however, if you could wait a few months after any laser before doing cataract surgery in order to let the eye settle down and to be sure that everything is really stable. There will be a blue box on this topic in a few pages.

If laser is part of your pre-op treatment plan, and the patient has a significant cataract, take special care. In order to squeak through the cataract you will be using smaller spots and higher powers, and the scattering of the beam may vary greatly from spot to spot. You need to watch your aiming beam closely, and if it suddenly snaps into tight focus, you have to turn the power down to avoid rupturing Bruch's membrane. (You can also use some of the techniques described in Chapter 10 to control the fluence without having to reach over and change the laser settings every five seconds.) This is where the ability to use an indirect contact lens can greatly facilitate treatment, allowing you to more easily work around the media opacities. Panretinal photocoagulation through a cataract tends to be less tricky than macular treatment; it is more "meatball" in nature, and you can usually work around the opacities and get at least a partial pattern in.

Hey—if you can't get laser in because of the cataract, but you think you will once the surgery is done, don't forget to think about putting a stitch in the wound. It makes it safer if you have to put a contact lens on the eye or do an intravitreal injection in the early postoperative period.

In addition to pretreatment with laser, it is reasonable to use preoperative nonsteroidals and aggressive postoperative nonsteroidals and topical steroids in these patients—and to continue such treatment a month or two longer than one would in a non-diabetic. Such treatment helps to blunt the deleterious effects of perioperative inflammation on the fragile diabetic vasculature. Don't underestimate the utility of eye drops in this situation. (But also don't forget that diabetic corneas can heal poorly so make sure your drops don't cause epithelial defects in the early postoperative period.)

Finally, when it comes to preoperative treatments, more and more specialists are considering intravitreal drugs to better control the retinopathy at the time of surgery. But there are no definitive guidelines about how to use them, or which ones to use. Do you put something in everyone to keep things from getting worse, or only those with unstable retinas? What the hell is an "unstable retina", anyway?

Let's see if the literature helps...

A recent study suggests that pre-op ranibizumab, used in patients with only background retinopathy and no macular edema, resulted in somewhat better outcomes as far as post-op macular thickening and visual acuity.[3] A study using bevacizumab found similar results, even though the patients had more advanced disease.[4] Other studies, however, suggest that pre-op bevacizumab or triamcinolone don't make much difference in the long run.[5,6]

It sounds like some patients will benefit, but it is just hard to know exactly who they are. And treating all diabetics with an injection is likely to be a waste of time; most stable patients don't need it. A recent DRCR.net study sheds some light on who might benefit from treatment: they found that patients with non-center-involving macular edema, or even those patients with a history of treatment for DME, were more likely to develop center-involving macular edema after cataract surgery.[7] But most patients didn't worsen—only about 10-12% progressed.

Soooooo, without definitive data, it is hard to be specific on whom to treat. Here is one approach. Patients with minimal disease—--some BDR but nothing close to DME or worrisome NPDR—probably don't need anything beyond more aggressive topical therapy. If there is some swelling or more pronounced NPDR, or if the patient has marginal systemic control, it makes sense to laser what you need to and add a shot of something to keep things calm in the perioperative period. That second clause is worth repeating—if they have a history of poor control, you might want to be more assertive with pre-op injections. Patients with poor control tend to do worse—we'll talk more about the relationship of systemic control on cataract surgery outcomes below.

What do you inject? If the patient has already been treated with injections, it makes sense to just use what has been working. If the patient is treatment naïve, most folks would use an anti-VEGF drug to avoid the problem of elevated IOP with triamcinolone (and the theoretical concern that the steroid might weaken the immune response and increase the risk of post-surgical endophthalmitis). That does not mean you shouldn't use triamcinolone—sometimes that drug can control things nicely because the inflammatory mediators generated by even perfect cataract surgery may be reversed by the use of steroid better than anti-VEGF agents alone. It is also sensible to consider using the dexamethasone implant (Ozurdex), which can last between three and four months (warning—it may migrate into the anterior chamber if there are unanticipated problems with a broken capsule or dislocated lens).

If you choose to start with an anti-VEGF drug, you can always move up to the steroid if things can't be controlled postoperatively. The choice of anti-VEGF drug depends on what you have and the patient's insurance. Most places end up using bevacizumab (you have to have center-involving disease to try to convince an insurance company to pay for ranibizumab or aflibercept).

An injection is much more important if the patient's disease is aggressive, i.e., if there is DME, PDR, iris neo, etc. Of course, one has to wonder why you are doing cataract surgery on such a patient; better to get control of the disease before doing surgery if you can. But sometimes you have no choice—for instance with a really dense cataract that doesn't let you see the retina well. If you are at all worried about what to do, you really should quiz your local retinal community about how to proceed. They may be able to work through the cataract more easily and get things stable before surgery.

Can you give the shot at the time of surgery? Who knows? There is a theoretical sense that giving it before surgery gets the eye "ready", but there really is no data on this. It is probably a lot easier for anterior segment surgeons to give the med at the time of surgery, and it probably would work just as well in patients that have relatively controlled retinopathy where you are using the injection to stabilize the eye for the operation. On the other hand, if the patient has active disease and has been requiring regular injections it is probably best to put the medicine in a week or so before surgery, especially if there is neovascularization that could hemorrhage at the time of cataract surgery. You definitely want those vessels as shriveled as possible before you start sticking knives into an eye.

Note: *If you only have laser available to get your patients ready for cataract surgery, there have been a couple of papers that suggest caution when doing a PRP right before the surgery. It seems that patients with a PRP right before surgery may be more likely to get DME post-op; almost as though the laser makes the eye extra sensitive to the inflammation stirred up by surgery. So if you don't have access to injections, you may want to wait a few months after getting the PRP in before operating.[8,9]*

But managing the eye is often the easiest part. Managing the patient's expectations—and yours—can be the hardest part.

Keep in mind the visual potential of the eye. If the patient has had macular problems, you cannot expect them to have excellent results, and you must really warn the patient about this. Even if they only have minimal retinopathy, remember that diabetes can affect retinal functioning in ways that aren't identified by Snellen acuity or glare testing. In other words, your experience with non-diabetic cataracts has taught you that your surgery will eliminate a host of symptoms. However, even fairly normal looking diabetic retinas have subtle problems with, for instance, decreased contrast sensitivity or dark adaptation. These subtle defects mean that taking the cataract out will not be as likely to eliminate symptoms as it would be in non-diabetics. Both you and the patient need to alter your expectations in recognition of this.

Pre-op counseling is crucial. Set the bar low, and let diabetics know that they are not like all their friends and relatives who told them they'd see better than ever before. Tell them to instead ask their friends who have had laser or shots or surgeries for diabetes—they will get a more realistic answer. Patients have a strong tendency to assume that everything will be great as soon as that cataract is popped out, and they are especially likely to think this if their vision is already a bit blurry from retinopathy. The success of cataract surgery in the general population has created such a high level of expectation that patients imagine the cataract is causing all of their problems. The patient's thinking may be wildly unrealistic in spite of careful counseling—for instance, they may think that cataract surgery will somehow eliminate all of their retinopathy. These kinds of thoughts will likely go unvoiced, so you need to anticipate them and ask about their expectations in order to make sure the two of you are thinking the same thing. And it is really important to make sure they understand that they will need continued monitoring and treatment for the retinopathy after cataract surgery. Cataract surgery is not "one-stop shopping" for diabetics. Instead, at times it may be the gift that keeps on giving.

By the same token, you should not let yourself become delusional about the visual potential of an eye or the visual significance of a cataract. It is easy to look at a mild diabetic cataract and apply the same criteria you would for a non-diabetic, ignoring the retinal pitfalls that may exist. Be sure you are familiar with the patient's vision prior to

the development of the cataract so you aren't fooled when a mildly damaged retina—
and not a mild lens opacity—is the real culprit. And definitely don't be fooled by the kind
of dramatic cortical cataracts that diabetics sometimes have—these can look terrible,
but they tend to be not very visually significant.

A wise cataractist once said, "We cataract surgeons can be the perfect surgeons and
sometimes diabetics just won't heal right. Therefore we wait way longer. Rather
disappoint them by not doing their surgery than disappoint by doing it."

*Should you perform a routine preoperative fluorescein angiogram or
OCT on diabetic patients who are being considered for cataract surgery? Most retina
specialists would answer in the affirmative, because you get a lot of information that
helps to predict the likelihood for trouble in the postoperative period. The OCT can
reveal subtle thickening, warning you that the retina is just barely handling the leakage
present. It will also demonstrate subtle epiretinal membranes that may contract
postoperatively and create the need for a vitrectomy. The angiogram will give you an
idea about pre-existing capillary dropout near the fovea, something that suggests the
eye is quite fragile—even if the vision is still good. If there is a lot of macular ischemia
on the angiogram, then it is likely that any cataract present is not visually significant at
all. An angiogram can also demonstrate subtle diffuse leakage that, even if it has not
yet caused retinal thickening, may lead to macular edema after the leakage is revved
up by post-op inflammatory mediators.*

*This is not to say that preoperative fluorescein angiography and OCT are mandatory.
You may be in a situation where such testing is not readily available, or you may
feel that the clinical exam is so good that no testing is needed. The point is that if
you have even a remote concern that occult retinopathy may be lying in wait, you
should consider these tests. This is especially true for performing an OCT—there is no
morbidity involved in doing an OCT, and you should have a very low threshold for doing
this test if you have one, even if there isn't a diagnosis you can bill for. There is just too
much valuable pre-op info available that can help set the patient's expectations.*

Another crucial preoperative factor is the degree of the patient's control. You cannot
ignore this. Your training has taught you to meticulously evaluate refractive issues,
IOL selection, and biometry with all the conscientiousness you can muster. But if you
do not ask about the patient's hemoglobin A1c and blood pressure, you are being as
irresponsible as if you were to select the IOL power by drawing numbers out of a hat.
Here's why:

There are some studies that suggest poor control is not highly correlated with
postoperative progression, at least in the short term, but there are other studies
indicating that bad control will clearly contribute to loss of vision and progressive
retinopathy after surgery. (Murtha and Cavallarano provide a nice review of all this.)[10]
Ultimately, you have to recognize that ignoring a patient's poor control will result in a
worse outcome—even if the cataract surgery had nothing to do with it.

Look at it this way—a tremendous amount of effort is devoted to preventing endophthalmitis, and rightly so. Massive editorials and reviews are written trying to identify nuances that can shave a few tenths of a percentage point off the incidence. People agonize (and drug companies battle) over which prophylactic drops to use as well as other factors, such as the surgical prep and construction of the wound. Heck, if that cataract guru in Florida said that he had eliminated endophthalmitis by having patients eat broccoli the night before surgery, you know you would try it.

All this is well and good, but go back to Figure 2 in Chapter 22 and look at how much a hemoglobin A1c of 9% can mess up the results of even perfect surgery. Even if one postulates that the level of control does not affect the surgical results per se (and it is hard to believe that it doesn't), one has to admit that in the long run patients who have cataract surgery and have good control will do far better than patients who have cataract surgery and have poor control.

Endophthalmitis is bad, of course. However, one almost never stops to realize that over time the visual results of operating on a poorly controlled diabetic's cataract can be even more problematic. Most endophthalmitis, if caught early and treated aggressively, will have a better outcome than the vision that results from a fovea ruined by macular edema. In other words, recognize that having patients take the time to get tuned-up systemically will give your diabetic patients far better surgical results compared to fussing over the latest pre-op antibiotic drop. Even orthopedic surgeons have to take some responsibility for the rest of the patient. You can, too.

There is yet another reason to make the patient's medical status as much a part of your pre-op eval as the slit lamp exam and keratometry. As mentioned in Chapter 22, patients may have temporary worsening of their retinopathy when they try to improve their control. It turns out that if a patient with poor control decides to improve their control at the same time that they have cataract surgery, they can end up with marked postoperative worsening of their retinopathy.[11] Does this mean that you should encourage any patient with bad control to continue being bad for a few months after cataract surgery? Only if you are a buccaneer trying to jack up your surgery volume at all costs. It seems far better to wait several months for the patient to get better control and then do the surgery. The point, again, is that if you are not aware of the patient's control when you recommend surgery, you have blown off a variable that may be more important than any other part of the ophthalmic exam. Remember, if you screw up an IOL, you can fix them with glasses, Lasik or an IOL exchange. If you screw up someone's macula, it is gone forever.

> *Hey—here's a useful microfact:* A group of investigators tested for diabetes in younger patients undergoing cataract surgery—patients between the ages of 45 and 60. It turns out that 34% were at high risk for developing diabetes, and 9% had undiagnosed diabetes. The authors proposed that poor glucose metabolism may underlie the development of cataracts in younger patients, and that this may be a good group to target with screening labs. So snag a hemoglobin A1c machine for your ASC—stamp out astigmatism and save lives![12]

What about patients with bilateral cataracts?

It is probably not a good idea to operate on both eyes of a patient with bilateral cataracts and worrisome retinopathy within a brief period of time, if you can possibly help it. If the patient is going to get into trouble, it may take two to three months for it to show up, and you may want to wait this long before doing the second eye. It is better to have a patient that prefers their 20/50 cataract to their nice shiny implant because their macula folded up after surgery, rather than have a patient with two shiny implants and two dead maculae. Of course, this scenario is much less likely in the modern era of good control and intravitreal drugs, but you just don't want your name on a chart like that.

What is the best IOL?

The best IOL is usually the one that you can put in best. (Bestly?) Again, your diabetic patient is not the one on whom to try some slinky new IOL from the rep; just use the tools that allow you to do your safest surgery. Some papers recommend using a lens with a large optic; this will allow better visualization in case the patient ends up needing extensive laser or a vitrectomy. It is also helpful if the patient has a larger capsulotomy, especially given the tendency for diabetic capsules to contract after surgery.[13] These are things to consider if you can do them safely, but not if you have to totally change your technique. (By the way, Dr. Tom Oetting wrote a nice review on surgery in diabetics for the ASCRS. Check it out.[14])

There has also been discussion about whether such patients should get a silicone IOL. There is no question that a silicone IOL can be a real pain during vitrectomy surgery due to the condensation that occurs when the eye is filled with air. Also, if the patient needs silicone oil to repair their retina, it pretty much guarantees that the IOL will need to be exchanged, because the oil will ruin it. However, the need to perform these maneuvers is relatively unlikely and it is hard to know which patient will get into trouble—unless the patient has horrible retinopathy that is not well controlled. As a result, if you do your best surgery with a silicone IOL, by all means, use a silicone IOL. On the other hand, if you think the patient may be heading into trouble, it might be helpful to use a more "retina-friendly" acrylic IOL—this will be less problematic if the patient does end up needing a vitrectomy. Ultimately, you know far more about IOLs than most retina doctors and you should do what you think is safest.

Multifocal IOLs are a bit more problematic. You need a perfectly functioning macula to handle a multifocal IOL, and even if your diabetic patient has no obvious retinopathy, there may be subclinical defects in retinal function that can make adjusting to such an IOL much more difficult than you might expect. (Vide supra about how diabetics can have problems with contrast sensitivity that can affect their happiness with even a monofocal IOL.) Plus, if they get any retinopathy progression at all they will have even more problems. Flexible accommodating IOLs (such as the Crystalens) may have an advantage because they do not depend on crisp macular function, but they may not provide as much near vision, and a diabetic capsule can be quirky (and don't forget that a shrunken down diabetic capsule can make future PRPs challenging). The bottom line is that there really is no data right now indicating how to use any of these lenses in patients with diabetes, although some will use them in patients with excellent control and no retinopathy. If you decide to use a presbyopia-correcting lens, both you and the patient need to be aware of the possible pitfalls.

Side note: *If you are doing cataract surgery on a patient that has already had a vitrectomy, you need to get familiar with all the extra hassles involved. Problems can include a deeper anterior chamber, zonular weakness and refractive surprises because the capsular sits more posteriorly without vitreous support. All these things are beyond the scope of this book—Google "cataract surgery after vitrectomy" for plenty of good advice. One thing to keep in mind is that if a patient develops a dense cataract shortly after a vitrectomy, the surgeon may have dinged the posterior capsule with an instrument, possibly causing a capsular tear. A good retinal surgeon will warn you that this happened—hopefully they won't be a dork and fail to mention it because they don't want to lose face. One finding that suggests a lens-strike during vitrectomy is the presence of a linear opacity that emanates from the direction of a sclerotomy. Or, if the cataract is dense, ultrasound can show a really thick lens or fluffy debris just behind the lens. You will need to really be careful in this situation because it is likely you are going in on an eye with a torn capsule—use all the tricks you have been taught to stay out of trouble.**

What about doing a YAG?

There is no clear consensus on whether performing YAG laser capsulotomy can stir up retinopathy. It probably does not have much of an effect but, as usual, there are never any guarantees. If you have to do a lot of hacking and slashing with the YAG you may cause enough inflammation to affect the retina, especially if the patient has already had complicated cataract surgery. It probably makes sense to put diabetics on some sort of anti-inflammatory drop around the time of the laser—more laser or more preexisting damage may mean more topical therapy.

Perhaps the most important thing is to not talk yourself into doing a YAG on "trace" capsular opacities when the patient is dropping to 20/50 from subtle macular edema that you are missing.

*BTW, here's another way your helpful neighborhood retina specialist may be messing you up as far as cataract surgery. A review of Medicare data suggested that patients who have had a lot of anti-VEGF injections might be at increased risk for retained lens fragments and even post-op endophthalmitis.[17] Not sure how the risk of post-op endophthalmitis is increased by multiple injections--perhaps due to resistant organisims from overuse of antibiotics. However, an accidental lens strike with the injection needle would *really* increase the risk of a capsular tear. Maybe take a minute to look carefully into the quadrant of the lens where the injections are placed for any linear opacities that might suggest a hit on the capsule.

There are a few other things to keep in mind when doing cataract surgery on diabetics.[15] First, dry eye disease is more common in diabetics, and it can be proportional to the degree of diabetic retinopathy present. Of course, they may not realize it because they also have poor corneal sensation from diabetic neuropathy, and heavy peripheral laser can also decrease corneal sensation.[19] And your surgery can make all of this worse, which in turn can compromise epithelial healing, so keep the ocular surface in mind as you do your pre-op evaluation. And don't forget that a crummy tear film can mess up your keratometry, too.*

Endothelial cell loss can also be more pronounced in diabetics, so apply plenty of your favorite viscoelastic. They may also have pupils that dilate poorly, especially if they have had a lot of PRP and/or autonomic neuropathy, so be prepared to deal with that. Finally, diabetic patients are more likely to get endophthalmitis, and if they get infected they are more likely to have worse visual outcomes compared to non-diabetics. So watch patients carefully if they have more post-op inflammation than normal.

What if, in spite of the best intentions, the macula blows out after your excellent cataract surgery?

In the past, if the macula swelled up after surgery, there was a traditional stepwise approach that is still reasonable to follow. First, continue aggressive topical therapy with non-steroidal and steroid drops to treat any pseudophakic component to the edema.[18] Rule out anything else that may be adding to the edema—left over lens chunks, vitreous strands, mild uveitis, iris capture—all that stuff you studied in cataract school. Laser any obvious retinal disease that is eccentric to the fovea, but if treating the obvious leaks does not solve the problem you need to think pharmacologically. This is particularly true if there is a lot of diffuse leakage and late staining of the optic nerve on angiography— these findings suggest that postoperative inflammation is driving the vascular leakage rather than pure diabetic disease. In such cases, it may be reasonable to try a good old-fashioned periocular steroid injection, especially if you don't do intravitreal treatment.

And that last is worth dwelling on—the difference between pseudophakic and diabetic macular edema. It is easy to assume that post-op swelling in a diabetic must be from retinopathy, but if there is no retinopathy it is likely just pseudophakic macular edema. You wouldn't want to jump in and laser such a patient, in the same way you wouldn't want to ignore retinopathy and just treat a patient with drops on the assumption that the problem is just pseudophakic edema.

If drops, appropriate laser, and a periocular shot don't fix things quickly, however, it is likely that your patient will be getting a bit frustrated. If there is center-involving disease, it is best to forgo a stepwise approach and simply initiate treatment with intravitreal drugs to get rapid control of the edema (and to get rapid control of the patient's patience). Your patient is now pseudophakic, so you have the favorable results of Protocol I to fall back on when it comes to using triamcinolone. That doesn't mean

---

*As a matter of fact, this is something that retina docs are notoriously bad about. Patients have already been given a topical anesthetic to check the pressure, and we tend to blow off surface findings that we see (assuming we remember to look for them in the first place). Yet surface problems may contribute to decreased vision a great deal in these patients, especially if they have neurotrophic corneas. So don't forget to look at the cornea if a patient has poor vision and you can't explain it with your fancy OCT and FA.

that triamcinolone is the only way to go. Remember that subjects in protocol I who were phakic and required cataract surgery after triamcinolone did not regain their lost vision after surgery. This suggests that there may be a role for combination treatment in these patients using triamcinolone followed by anti-VEGF agents to try and control the inflammation and edema.

As an aside, there is a sense that if vitreous loss occurs during cataract surgery and there is a small amount of retained cortical material, it is reasonable to wait for the cortex to resolve without the need for a vitrectomy. There may also be some reluctance on the part of the cataract surgeon to refer such patients out—it means that something went wrong that can't be fixed with time and eye drops. If the patient is diabetic, however, that kind of smoldering inflammation may cause recalcitrant macular edema (remember the section at the beginning of the chapter about how fragile diabetic vessels can be even if there is no overt retinopathy). As a result, you should consider early referral to a retina specialist in this situation. If warranted, the problem can be definitively addressed before things worsen, and it spares the cataract surgeon the need to make what may be a difficult and partially subjective decision if referral is delayed.

As always, watch out for subtle epiretinal membranes or vitreomacular traction—an OCT is crucial in this setting. Remember that cataract surgery can stimulate epiretinal membranes to contract; an unpleasant surprise indeed.[16] If traction-related pathology is present, it is very unlikely that intravitreal treatment will have a significant effect. Such patients usually need referral to a retina specialist. Hopefully you explained the potential for this prior to surgery, and the patient is not vindictively disappointed by all the extra fuss.

Don't forget that other things can happen after surgery, such as a big vitreous hemorrhage or progressive traction as the vitreous shifts forward when the crystalline lens is removed. These problems usually need referral to determine whether the patient needs surgery to protect their vision. One hopes that this will never happen to you because you will have treated everything and made sure the retina is stable before surgery—but never underestimate the ability of diabetes to scramble up your best-laid plans.

By now, you should be getting the impression that a patient with diabetes and a cataract needs to be on a totally separate track relative to a patient with just a cataract. Here are a few other things to think about:

In addition to being more aggressive with perioperative topical therapy, you should also be more aggressive with your follow up. If the macula swells it tends to do so after several weeks, and if you see the patient a couple of times in the first month and then send them off for glasses you can miss it. Also, the macula is more likely to start swelling as the drops are tapered. If you give the patient some sort of automatic tapering schedule and don't check them yourself you can miss early changes that could be easily treated—and then they will come in when they have definite symptoms with advanced disease that will be harder to control. This is especially true if you are doing the co-management thing. You must make sure that the optometrist knows how to watch for early changes in the fundus appearance that suggest trouble is brewing, and that they will follow the patient closer than a typical post-op cataract patient if you can't.

Mostly you need to remember that diabetics should not be left on the assembly-line portion of your cataract factory. They really need to be taken off the line and brought over to the custom shop for closer attention.

Finale

To review: Modern-day cataract surgery is much safer relative to older techniques, and generally does not seem to stir things up much in terms of retinopathy progression. On the other hand, there are patients who can still do very poorly, but you have a fighting chance of weeding such patients out by using your noggin. Watch out for the level of retinopathy and for the stability of the retinopathy. Have a low threshold for doing a pre-op OCT and fluorescein angiogram, and consider sending the patient out for a retina consult if necessary. Know the patient's degree of systemic control. Know the likely visual potential of the eye, and make darn sure the patient understands the limits and extra risks inherent with cataract surgery in diabetics. Do the best surgery you can, and then watch the patient closely afterwards. Don't hesitate to ask for help if problems arise. Unfortunately, the secretary will not disavow any knowledge of your actions, so be careful.

There is one other issue that doesn't quite fit in anywhere else—*and that is what happens in a patient's mind when one simply mentions that they have a "cataract." Diabetic patients may fixate on this information to a surprising degree, and this can be particularly true if the cataract is not visually significant and you have no intention of doing anything about it. The problem is that even if you tell them their cataract is insignificant, they will often assign any visual symptoms they have to the cataract whether or not this is the actual case. This means they will ignore new symptoms on the assumption that they stem from "a simple cataract," and will then assume that they can address the problem whenever they have time.*

Unfortunately, if their symptoms are from retinal disease, they may end up with irreversible vision loss while they wait to find a convenient time for an eye exam. As a result of this, many retina docs have a vague reluctance to even talk about cataracts at all unless they are definitely visually significant.* This scenario is not limited to diabetic retinopathy; it can happen with any retinal disease, and it is especially common with macular degeneration.

The real message here is that if you discuss the presence of a cataract, you need to clearly spell out to the patient that they should not diagnose themselves if their vision gets worse. If they notice a definite change they should never assume it is the cataract; they need to get back in quickly to avoid permanent vision loss.

---

*Of course, retina specialists do have to mention cataracts—even if they aren't relevant. If a patient with a visually insignificant cataract ends up going to a more anteriorly oriented doctor—who *will* mention the cataract—the patient will understandably think the retina specialist is useless for not being the first to talk about it.

References

1.   Giansanti F, Bitossi A, Giacomelli G, et al. Evaluation of macular thickness after uncomplicated cataract surgery using optical coherence tomography. *European journal of ophthalmology.* 2013;23(5):751-756.

2.   Hong T, Mitchell P, de Loryn T, Rochtchina E, Cugati S, Wang JJ. Development and progression of diabetic retinopathy 12 months after phacoemulsification cataract surgery. *Ophthalmology.* 2009;116(8):1510-1514.

3.   Chae JB, Joe SG, Yang SJ, et al. Effect of combined cataract surgery and ranibizumab injection in postoperative macular edema in nonproliferative diabetic retinopathy. *Retina.* 2014;34(1):149-156.

4.   Salehi A, Beni AN, Razmjoo H, Beni ZN. Phacoemulcification with intravitreal bevacizumab injection in patients with cataract and coexisting diabetic retinopathy: prospective randomized study. *J Ocul Pharmacol Ther.* 2012;28(3):212-218.

5.   Fard MA, Yazdanei Abyane A, Malihi M. Prophylactic intravitreal bevacizumab for diabetic macular edema (thickening) after cataract surgery: prospective randomized study. *European journal of ophthalmology.* 2011;21(3):276-281.

6.   Ahmadabadi HF, Mohammadi M, Beheshtnejad H, Mirshahi A. Effect of intravitreal triamcinolone acetonide injection on central macular thickness in diabetic patients having phacoemulsification. *J Cataract Refract Surg.* 2010;36(6):917-922.

7.   Diabetic Retinopathy Clinical Research Network Authors/Writing C, Baker CW, Almukhtar T, et al. Macular edema after cataract surgery in eyes without preoperative central-involved diabetic macular edema. *JAMA ophthalmology.* 2013;131(7):870-879.

8.   Suto C, Hori S, Kato S. Management of type 2 diabetics requiring panretinal photocoagulation and cataract surgery. *J Cataract Refract Surg.* 2008;34(6):1001-1006.

9.   Suto C, Kitano S, Hori S. Optimal timing of cataract surgery and panretinal photocoagulation for diabetic retinopathy. *Diabetes care.* 2011;34(7):e123.

10.   Murtha T, Cavallerano J. The management of diabetic eye disease in the setting of cataract surgery. *Current opinion in ophthalmology.* 2007;18(1):13-18.

11.   Suto C, Hori S, Kato S, Muraoka K, Kitano S. Effect of perioperative glycemic control in progression of diabetic retinopathy and maculopathy. *Archives of ophthalmology.* 2006;124(1):38-45.

12.   Feldman-Billard S, Sedira N, Boelle PY, Poisson F, Heron E. High prevalence of undiagnosed diabetes and high risk for diabetes using HbA1c criteria in middle-aged patients undergoing cataract surgery. *Diabetes Metab.* 2013;39(3):271-275.

13.   Takamura Y, Tomomatsu T, Arimura S, et al. Anterior capsule contraction and flare intensity in the early stages after cataract surgery in eyes with diabetic retinopathy. *J Cataract Refract Surg.* 2013;39(5):716-721.

14.   Oetting T. Cataract Surgery and Diabetes. *EyeWorld.* 2012;November:http://www.eyeworld.org/article-cataract-surgery-and-diabetes.

15.   Bikbova G, Oshitari T, Tawada A, Yamamoto S. Corneal changes in diabetes mellitus. *Curr Diabetes Rev.* 2012;8(4):294-302.

16.   Fong CS, Mitchell P, Rochtchina E, Hong T, de Loryn T, Wang JJ. Incidence and progression of epiretinal membranes in eyes after cataract surgery. *American journal of ophthalmology.* 2013;156(2):312-318 e311.

17.   Hahn P, Yashkin AP, Sloan FA. Effect of Prior Anti-VEGF Injections on the Risk of Retained Lens Fragments and Endophthalmitis after Cataract Surgery in the Elderly. Ophthalmology. 2015.

18.   Wielders LH, Lambermont VA, Schouten JS, et al. Prevention of Cystoid Macular Edema After Cataract Surgery in Nondiabetic and Diabetic Patients: A Systematic Review and Meta-analysis. American journal of ophthalmology. 2015.

19.   Bouheraoua N, Hrarat L, Parsa CF, et al. Decreased Corneal Sensation and Subbasal Nerve Density, and Thinned Corneal Epithelium as a Result of 360-Degree Laser Retinopexy. Ophthalmology. 2015;122(10):2095-2102.

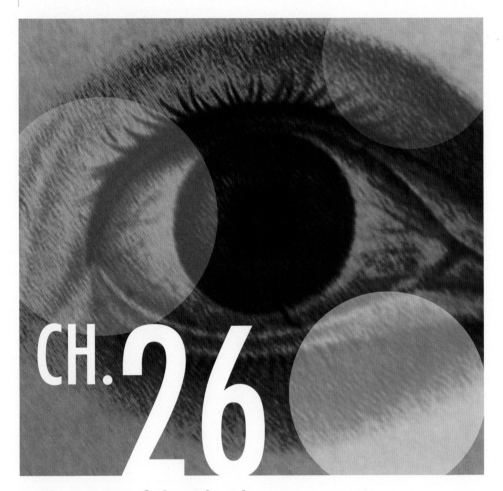

A Thinning of the Blood With James E. Schmidt, M.D., F.A.C.C

Everything in moderation, including moderation. Oscar Wilde

One issue that often arises is whether it is safe to use aspirin in the setting of proliferative diabetic retinopathy—both the patient and their internist have visions of torrents of intraocular blood. Fortunately, the Early Treatment Diabetic Retinopathy Study clearly showed that aspirin does not make any difference in any aspect of diabetic retinopathy, and in particular, does not increase the risk for vitreous hemorrhages.[1] You can reassure patients that if they need to beon aspirin for other medical problems, it really does not affect their ophthalmic disease. By the way, you are not alone if you think this result seems horribly counterintuitive. It is hard to imagine that the same patients who show you all the bruises on their forearms from taking aspirin have absolutely no increased amount of hemorrhage from the ratty vessels in their eyes. Perhaps the vitreous changes the need for functioning platelets, or perhaps the nature of the abnormal vessels is such that alterations in platelet activity aren't important. No one knows. Whatever the reason, you have one big whopping study behind you to reassure both the patient and the patient's internist that they can use aspirin with impunity.

What about other antiplatelet agents such as ticagrelor (Brilinta) and clopidogrel (Plavix)?

There are no massive studies looking at the effect of these drugs on diabetic retinopathy as there is for aspirin. However, as far as anyone can tell they don't seem to have a significant impact on diabetic retinopathy, so they are probably as benign as aspirin. "Probably" is the key word, though. Because their use isn't supported by the kind of data that supports the use of aspirin, no one can say that they are absolutely equivalent in terms of risk. In other words, you can tell patients on these other drugs that because aspirin is OK, and because these drugs are similar, it is likely that there are no ill effects— but there are no guarantees. (Check the blue box below for one other concern.) By the way, it is worth knowing the names of these drugs so you don't miss their significance on the patient's med list. Perhaps the most common is clopidogrel (Plavix); newer ones include ticagrelor (Brilinta) and prasugrel (Effient). Ticlopidine (Ticlid) is rarely used nowadays because of potential hematologic side effects.

Important safety tip:

If you grew up in the old days, you may have become used to the idea that patients are on aspirin and/or clopidogrel for "general maintenance," and that such drugs can easily be stopped on a temporary basis. It turns out that it is usually not necessary to stop such drugs for typical ophthalmic surgeries—but sometimes doctors will do it because the perceived risk of discontinuing the drug is thought to be small and they feel safer doing surgery without it on board. It may be possible to do this for brief periods under certain circumstances—but you should check with the patient's doctor if you feel you must stop it.

This is because nowadays there is a very good reason to not stop these medications at all. Patients may be on clopidogrel (or one of the others) along with aspirin because a drug-eluting stent has been placed in one or more of their coronary arteries. Discontinuing these drugs in this situation carries a definite risk of thrombosis—and death—even if the drugs are stopped for only a short period of time. (Non-drug eluting stents share this potential problem, but for a shorter period of time after placement. Drug-eluting stents take longer to endothelialize—generally about a year.) Usually patients have been warned about this and they will make a big fuss if you casually suggest stopping the drugs, but one can never depend on this. You need to specifically ask about why they are on the drugs, and you should never stop such medications without getting clearance (and in this case, you may not be allowed to stop the drugs).

The problem is that decisions about these medications are sometimes made by checking off boxes on the patient's surgical scheduling form, at a time when it is difficult to track down all the necessary information. If you really feel you need to change these medications, you must take the time to review the situation with the patient's medical specialists before making any recommendations.

What About Warfarin?

Warfarin (Coumadin) can sometimes be more difficult to sort out. Once patients on this medication hear that they could get blood in their eye from retinopathy, they (and their doctors) will become rightfully concerned about the use of this drug. This issue takes more finesse than the aspirin question. (The newer oral anticoagulants that can be used instead of warfarin are discussed below.)

If patients are placed on Coumadin, it is because they need to be on it for life-threatening problems, or at least, that is what one would assume. A tedious but conscientious step is to make sure this is indeed the case by checking with the prescribing physician. Certain medical problems mandate the use of Coumadin (i.e., atrial fibrillation, recent deep venous thrombosis, mechanical valve). Other times, patients may have been placed on Coumadin for more vague indications, and you may even find occasional patients who were left on the drug because no one took the time to decide whether they still needed it. This may be especially true if you practice in an area where non-specialists may be making decisions about anticoagulation.

If it sounds like the patient has been given Coumadin by a non-specialist for what sounds like a dodgy indication (i.e., "My doctor says my arteries are hardening and I need thinner blood"), you may want to make a quick call to learn the real scoop. Your patient may be quite grateful (and will definitely have less morbidity) if you uncover a situation in which Coumadin can be decreased or discontinued safely—and no one would have realized it unless you took the effort. You rock.

If, however, the patient is being treated appropriately and presents with some type of hemorrhage, there is another thing you should consider even though you may have sworn you would never do it again after your internship. You should have a very low threshold for actually filling out a lab slip and checking the patient's INR. With the advent of anticoagulation clinics most patients are well maintained, but sometimes a patient's INR can go up unexpectedly. If patients are being treated outside of such clinics, there is a chance that their INR may not have been monitored for some time. Either way, if their blood happens to be really thin, you might save them from a massive hemorrhage somewhere else.

You will also be called on to decide how risky it is for a patient to begin or to continue Coumadin. Many internal medicine specialists have been taught that proliferative diabetic retinopathy and/or a vitreous hemorrhage are close to absolute contraindications to Coumadin. Your patient with a vitreous hemorrhage may suddenly be taken off the drug when they need it to keep from, well, dying.

More commonly, the patient may decide to stop the drug on their own. If the patient has had relatively quiescent retinopathy, you might save their life by taking the time to explain to both the treating physician and the patient that retinopathy is at most a relative contraindication to anticoagulation.

Even if their retinal disease is problematic, it usually takes second fiddle to their systemic need for Coumadin, and the nuances of this may require a direct conversation with the anticoagulationist. You know the eye situation and the other doctor knows the patient's systemic disease, and some sort of mind-meld can usually be achieved. Moreover, the intermittent and unexpected nature of diabetic hemorrhages needs to be conveyed to the internist. They are often thinking in terms of short-term hemorrhagic problems (like a GI bleed), and they need to know that the course of diabetic retinopathy is usually unpredictable and sporadic, and not something that tends to go away after briefly stopping anticoagulation just one time.

Oh yeah, and don't forget to include the patient in all this. First of all, most patients assume that the Coumadin actually causes hemorrhages in their eye. You can use this as an opportunity to once again explain that hemorrhages are part of proliferative diabetic retinopathy and that Coumadin does not cause hemorrhages (although if a hemorrhage does occur, it may be more pronounced if the patient is on the medication). Then, you need to review with them the real issue: whether they are willing to risk their well-being by having a stroke or a pulmonary embolism, versus the theoretical risk of having more of a hemorrhage in their eye. Most of the time they understand and opt to be on Coumadin.

Some patients will not want to have anything to do with the drug, however, and this is certainly within their rights; you just have to make sure they are making the decision based on the correct information. The point is that although the overall risk-to-benefit ratio strongly favors the use of Coumadin in patients with proliferative disease, you cannot ignore the fact that the patient needs to be involved in the decision and you need to document the discussion in the same way one would document a surgical consent. Because...

...from the standpoint of a retina surgeon, patients on Coumadin can, on occasion, be problematic. Most of the time the tendency to hemorrhage to a greater degree, if present, can be handled with laser, anti-VEGFs and/or vitrectomy, and there is no problem at all with the anticoagulation. Sometimes, though, they just keep bleeding, and they need an eye full of silicone oil to be able to see. This is not common, but it is a potential outcome that, for instance, may approach the risk of a stroke in the mind of a patient who is on Coumadin because of atrial fibrillation. As a comprehensive ophthalmologist, this is not likely to be a problem you will have to face. Still, it is important to realize that some patients may feel that the risk of Coumadin to the eyes begins to equal the systemic morbidity that the Coumadin is being used to prevent.

Incidentally, as mentioned in Chapter 13, a patient's need to be on Coumadin is another factor that may lead you to be more aggressive about treating severe nonproliferative diabetic retinopathy. It can be argued that early treatment may prevent any proliferative disease and thereby really minimize the risk of recurrent hemorrhage. (Remember, even involuted neovascularization may bleed from traction—and if there was never any neo in the first place you can sidestep the whole problem.) There is no data in the literature that specifically looks at this, but it is certainly something to consider in your decision to treat. The whole reason patients come to you instead of the PRP machine at Wal-Mart is because you can individualize the treatment rather than blindly follow a rulebook. No pun intended.

What about thrombolytics?

You have no doubt been contacted by the interventional cardiologist on call about a patient who needs acute thrombolysis or heparin. Once again, the life-threatening nature of the problem trumps the eye, but the patient still deserves some sort of informed consent. It turns out that the literature suggests that most of the time patients with proliferative retinopathy will do well. For instance, the GUSTO-I trial (Global Utilization of Streptokinase and t-PA for Occluded coronary arteries – I) had no intraocular hemorrhages among 6,011 patients with diabetes, and about 300 of those patients had proliferative retinopathy.[2] Still, there is a possibility that patients could have a hemorrhage, and they deserve to be informed of the theoretical risk—but it is hard to imagine why they would not have thrombolytics if they are indicated.

What about operating on patients who are on Coumadin?

It is well accepted that it is OK to do modern cataract surgery on uncomplicated, anticoagulated patients.[3] Retina surgery—or even complicated anterior segment surgery—is more likely to have problems with bleeding and there is no definitive study that provides a solid answer. Furthermore, you can be screwed no matter what you do: If you stop the Coumadin and the patient has a pulmonary embolism or a stroke, there will always be some hired-gun "expert" to say you should have done something differently. If you don't stop the Coumadin and the patient has a choroidal hemorrhage that destroys the eye, there will always be some hired-gun "expert" to say you should have done something differently. You can't win unless you put in some thoughtful pre-op face time.

Fortunately, there is a robust literature that suggests that it is generally OK to continue Coumadin (and anti-platelet agents) when patients need retina surgery. The ocular risk is thought to be less than the systemic risk posed by stopping the drug for typical patients, and the risk of bleeding is surprisingly low.[4-6] (You still need to know the INR at the time of surgery—if it is way high, you are taking risks you shouldn't take.)

However, you can't think that one size fits all; patients can still get into trouble.[7] If you are treating a patient with a lot of hemorrhagic potential, e.g., a one-eyed smoker who has high myopia and severe proliferative disease that also needs a scleral buckle, you shouldn't stay on autopilot and leave them anticoagulated without thinking about it.

The potential risk of an intraoperative hemorrhage in the mind of such a patient may be equal to the systemic risk of being off anticoagulation. Even if they don't have such a line-up of retinal misery, they still deserve to be part of the decision making process.

One option that may come up is to switch to shorter-acting heparin derivatives, such as enoxaparin (Lovenox), and stopping it just before surgery and restarting it afterward. This involves a lot of expense and hassle, but sometimes the internist may suggest it. Another option is to stop the drug a few days before surgery so that there is still a slight anticoagulative effect but hopefully not enough to affect the case. This last approach is somewhat vague and unscientific, but it can be an acceptable compromise at times.

Although most patients can remain anticoagulated, if you have any doubts you have to use your most valuable commodity—time—and communicate with the patient and the anticoagulationist treating the patient. This is true whether you want to stop the drug or not. The patient must understand that although we think it is acceptable to do complex surgery with Coumadin on board, there are no guarantees, and they must also understand the risk of stopping the Coumadin and having a stroke (or whatever disease the Coumadin is preventing). The anticoagulationist must know what your ophthalmic concerns are—sometimes they are surprisingly content with stopping the Coumadin, and sometimes they are adamant about continuing it (or doing the Lovenox thing, for instance, if the patient has a mechanical valve).

Remember that you are the only doctor in the mix who understands what can happen to an eye, and you will be responsible. So don't play the sleazy ophthalmology game of "Well, it's the cardiologist's job, so I don't have to think about this." You have to decide what can go wrong with the eye and how much risk you are willing to balance by continuing or not continuing the Coumadin—and then you have to work with everyone to come up with a plan.

We are spoiled because we routinely get away with operating on anticoagulated patients without having any problems. It is therefore easy to become complacent about the drug and to forget that if something does go wrong, it can go very wrong, and there will be plenty of people ready to second-guess all of your actions. Even if you routinely operate on anticoagulated patients, you should review the possible concerns with the patient because you want the patient to have heard about the issues well before, heaven forbid, something bad happens.

Of all the chapters in this book, *this one is perhaps the diciest, because it involves decisions regarding systemic factors that are well beyond the expertise of even the most renaissance ophthalmologist. Please recognize that the medical doctors caring for these patients have devoted their lives to understanding the risks and benefits of anticoagulation and you should be ready to discuss problematic patients on an individual basis with them. Under no circumstances should you consider the brief overview here to represent a definitive guide about how to manage such patients.*

If you need further information there are very useful reviews found at UpToDate. com—an exhaustive database that covers all aspects of this subject as well as most of medicine. A lot of the information here is abstracted from that source. Another excellent resource comes from the American College of Chest Physicians—a very worthwhile read unless you work in a place where no one is on blood thinners.[8]

Also, recognize that there is a significant literature concerning the risks of anticoagulation relative to surgery within each subspecialty of ophthalmology itself. An approach that works for routine cataract surgery may not work for high-risk glaucoma surgery.[9] You should, of necessity, stay abreast of this information as it pertains to your own surgical practice.

What about doing a retrobulbar or peribulbar with Coumadin on board?

First, check the stuff in Chapter 16 about how to minimize pain using various laser settings, etc. If none of that works, then—surprise—there are no proven guidelines to follow. Here are some things to consider:

You can try a sub-Tenon's or subconjunctival block, also mentioned in Chapter 16. You can get pretty good anesthesia in the region you inject, and there is less chance for a globe-threatening hemorrhage. If you need to do 360 degrees of treatment, though, you can end up with a lot of tedious injections and these routes do not get as far back as you may need.

Basically, if you need to do some sort of orbital block, you have to once again use up your most valuable asset: time. You need to review with the patient the risks of a hemorrhage and the risk of delaying treatment in order to allow the Coumadin to wear off. You also need to review the risk of going off the Coumadin in terms of stroke or whatever the patient is on the stuff for. As alluded to above, it is usually not worth the risk to stop the drug for a simple retrobulbar or peribulbar injection, especially since the risk of problems is low (but not zero).[10]

Still, you should cover yourself by making sure that the INR is not way out of whack. Is there a value that is known to be safe for doing a retrobulbar? Of course not. No one has any "for sure" data. There is data from other specialties, however, that can be used to extrapolate the risk. You are probably safe if it is 2.0 or less. Indeed, you may want to let the anticoagulationist know because this may mean the patient is sub-therapeutic.

If the patient is in the therapeutic range (usually 2.0 to 3.0), the literature suggests that it is OK to do, for instance, dental extractions, dermatologic procedures and routine cataract surgery, so this level may be acceptable for a retrobulbar, assuming the ocular indication warrants it.[8]The point is that you do not want to be doing an emergency lateral cantholysis to decompress an orbital hemorrhage and then find out that the INR was 4.9 but you never checked it. As long as you make a conscientious effort to inform the patient of the risks and make sure the INR is not sky-high, you are doing a good job.

Still—you should never become complacent about blocking patients on Coumadin, and you should recognize that the scales of risks and benefits can shift depending on why you need to do the block and the exact level of the INR.

> **Don't forget** to re-engage some of your atrophic clinical skills in this setting: Talk to and look at the patient. Someone with an INR of 2.1 and no problems with bruising or bleeding is very different from someone with an INR of 2.1 who is covered with bruises and sanguineous Band-Aids.

What about intravitreal injections?

There is more of a consensus that one does not need to worry about stopping anticoagulation at all in this setting—these are tiny needles going through a relatively avascular space, and raising the intraocular pressure with the injection is likely to mitigate any bleeding.[4] Should you check an INR? Most doctors don't—a history of stable anticoagulation seems to be enough. One can't argue against checking it—if you get into trouble you will wish you had checked it, but the logistics of sending every intravitreal injection patient down for a lab test and following up the results would be onerous, if not impossible. The odds are good that you will get away with doing nothing—but once again, don't forget to make sure the patient understands the risk they are taking so no one is surprised if Murphy and his Law appear. They can get more pronounced subconjunctival hemorrhages, though, and they need to be warned about this. Fortunately, the hemorrhages are usually just cosmetic annoyances, although there is at least one case of a severe subconjunctival hemorrhage leading to conjunctival necrosis and the need for surgery.[11]

What about those new oral anticoagulants?

Perhaps the most important thing with the newer drugs is that you have to know their names. It would have been so much easier if they had simply been called "Coumadin Substitute One, Two and Three." But no. It is therefore easy to take a quick look at a patient's med list and—if you don't recognize them—think that the patient is not anticoagulated. And that would be a bad thing to do. Because although the new drugs are convenient for patients, they share one small problem: THERE IS NO WAY TO REVERSE THEM! And you can't use the usual coagulation tests, such as INR, to determine if the drugs are on board and having an effect.

The drugs to watch for are the direct thrombin inhibitor dabigatran (Pradaxa) and the factor Xa inhibitors rivaroxaban (Xarelto) and apixaban (Eliquis). There are plenty of others in the pipeline, so the list will likely grow. A full discussion is well beyond the scope of this book, but there are a few things to be aware of with these meds. First, they have a rapid onset of action—usually within a few hours after taking them. They don't gradually build up like Coumadin, so keep this in mind if you are restarting them after surgery. Also, if they need to be discontinued, the timing of drug cessation depends on the risk of bleeding and the patient's renal function; usually 1-2 days, but sometimes more. The bottom line is to check with someone that knows what they are doing if you need to mess with these drugs.

Preliminary data suggests that there is no increased risk of adverse events with these agents relative to Coumadin, but there is not a lot of data yet on how to proceed as far as ophthalmic procedures.[12] They can probably be considered similar to Coumadin, but all the caveats reviewed above as far as informed consent apply, and it is a good idea to stay on top of the literature as more info is published about the risks of this class of medication.

While we are on the subject of thinned blood, there is one other thing to consider. Don't forget to ask about herbal supplements in patients with ocular hemorrhages. For instance, ginkgo biloba, in particular, has been associated with spontaneous hyphema and retinal hemorrhages.[13] Garlic, ginseng and fish oil may also have anticoagulant properties or interact with anticoagulant medications.[14] It makes sense to be aware of any alternative therapies that patients may be taking.

References

1.   Effects of aspirin treatment on diabetic retinopathy. ETDRS report number 8. Early Treatment Diabetic Retinopathy Study Research Group. *Ophthalmology.* May 1991;98(5 Suppl):757-765.

2.   Mahaffey KW, Granger CB, Toth CA, et al. Diabetic retinopathy should not be a contraindication to thrombolytic therapy for acute myocardial infarction: review of ocular hemorrhage incidence and location in the GUSTO-I trial. Global Utilization of Streptokinase and t-PA for Occluded Coronary Arteries. *J Am Coll Cardiol.* Dec 1997;30(7):1606-1610.

3.   Barequet IS, Sachs D, Priel A, et al. Phacoemulsification of cataract in patients receiving Coumadin therapy: ocular and hematologic risk assessment. *Am J Ophthalmol.* Nov 2007;144(5):719-723.

4.   Charles S, Rosenfeld PJ, Gayer S. Medical consequences of stopping anticoagulant therapy before intraocular surgery or intravitreal injections. *Retina.* Sep 2007;27(7):813-815.

5.   Fu AD, McDonald HR, Williams DF, et al. Anticoagulation with warfarin in vitreoretinal surgery. *Retina.* Mar 2007;27(3):290-295.

6.   Brown JS, Mahmoud TH. Anticoagulation and clinically significant postoperative vitreous hemorrhage in diabetic vitrectomy. *Retina.* Nov 2011;31(10):1983-1987.

7.   Passemard M, Koehrer P, Juniot A, Bron AM, Creuzot-Garcher C. Maintenance of anticoagulant and antiplatelet agents for patients undergoing peribulbar anesthesia and vitreoretinal surgery. *Retina.* Oct 2012;32(9):1868-1873.

8.   Douketis JD, Spyropoulos AC, Spencer FA, et al. Perioperative management of antithrombotic therapy: Antithrombotic Therapy and Prevention of Thrombosis, 9th ed: American College of Chest Physicians Evidence-Based Clinical Practice Guidelines. *Chest.* Feb 2012;141(2 Suppl):e326S-350S.

9.   Law SK, Song BJ, Yu F, Kurbanyan K, Yang TA, Caprioli J. Hemorrhagic complications from glaucoma surgery in patients on anticoagulation therapy or antiplatelet therapy. *Am J Ophthalmol.* Apr 2008;145(4):736-746.

10.   Konstantatos A. Anticoagulation and cataract surgery: a review of the current literature. *Anaesthesia and intensive care.* Feb 2001;29(1):11-18.

11.   Gupta R, Negi A, Vernon SA. Severe sub conjunctival haemorrhage following intravitreal triamcinolone for refractory diabetic oedema. *Eye (Lond).* May 2005;19(5):590-591.

12.   Ing E, Douketis J. New oral anticoagulants and oculoplastic surgery. *Can J Ophthalmol.* Apr 2014;49(2):123-127.

13.   Fraunfelder FW. Ocular side effects from herbal medicines and nutritional supplements. *Am J Ophthalmol.* Oct 2004;138(4):639-647.

14.   Spolarich AE, Andrews L. An examination of the bleeding complications associated with herbal supplements, antiplatelet and anticoagulant medications. *J Dent Hyg.* Summer 2007;81(3):

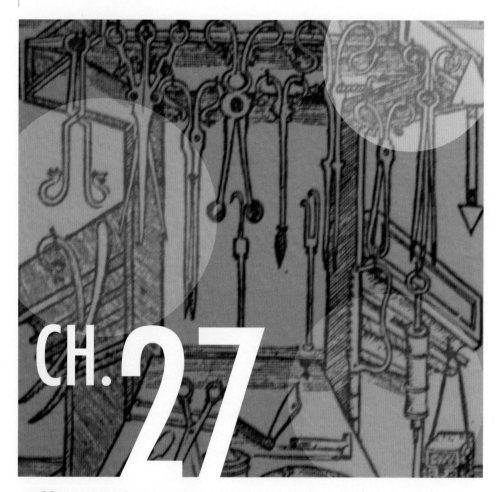

Differential Diagnosis A Rose Is a Rose Is MacTel Type 2

Never trust to general impressions, my boy, but concentrate yourself upon details.
Sir Arthur Conan Doyle, *The Adventures of Sherlock Holmes*

Usually you do not need to use your differential diagnosis powers with diabetic retinopathy, given that the patient already has the systemic diagnosis and the fundus findings are classic. But as this book shows, when it comes to actually treating patients the whole "art of medicine" thing more than makes up for the ease of diagnosis. Still, you should always keep at least a little of your mental bandwidth available to think about the differential diagnosis—it can sometimes make a big difference.

It is easy to come up with an inventory of things that can look like diabetic retinopathy—and the resulting lists are usually divided into: (1) things that can make new blood vessels grow, and (2) things that can make little hemorrhages and swollen capillaries show up all over the place.

Table 1 lists diseases that can make new blood vessels grow and can therefore simulate active proliferative retinopathy. It is based on one of the all-time classic tables from an equally classic paper by Jampol et al.[1], it is a real keeper if you plan on doing a lot of retina. The list is not exhaustive—there are many case reports of neovascularization in various diseases—but it covers most entities.

Table 2 is the standard list for the differential diagnosis of background changes such as hemorrhages and microvascular abnormalities. You can scan it into your smartphone and then you should be good to go for regurgitating facts on rounds, passing boards, impressing chicks and dudes at bars, etc., etc.

Table 1: Differential diagnosis of retinal neovascularization (often peripheral).

Vascular diseases with ischemia:	
Sickling hemoglobinopathies	Other hemoglobinopathies
Small-vessel hyalinosis	Ocular ischemic syndrome
Diabetes mellitus	Retinal embolization (such as talc retinopathy)
Branch retinal vein occlusion	Retinopathy of prematurity
Branch retinal artery occlusion	Familial exudative vitreoretinopathy
Hyperviscosity syndromes	Toxemia of pregnancy
Aortic arch syndromes	Encircling buckle operation
Carotid cavernous fistula	
Inflammatory diseases with possible ischemia:	
Sarcoidosis	Toxoplasmosis
Retinal vasculitis (from any cause including infectious and autoimmune such as lupus)	Acute retinal necrosis
Eales disease	Multiple sclerosis
Any forms of uveitis including pars planitis	Frosted branch angiitis
Behçet's disease	Syphilis
Birdshot uveitis	
Miscellaneous:	
Familial telangiectasia	Longstanding retinal detachment
Cocaine abuse	Retinitis pigmentosa
Choroidal melanoma (and other tumors)	Autosomal-dominant vitreoretinal choroidopathy
Senile retinoschisis	Coagulopathies
Juvenile X-linked retinoschisis	Idiopathic retinal vasculitis, aneurysms and neuroretinitis (IRVAN)

Table 2: Differential diagnosis of background diabetic retinopathy

Radiation retinopathy	Drug toxicity (such as interferon)
Vein occlusions	Preeclampsia
Ocular ischemic syndrome	Inflammatory microvasculitis, such as occurs with lupus
Hypertensive retinopathy	Infectious agents such as HIV (cotton-wool spots) and CMV
Hematologic abnormalities - anemia, leukemia, lymphoma, thrombocytopenia	Certain types of muscular dystrophy
Macular telangiectasias	Valsalva retinopathy
Coats' disease	Purtscher-like retinopathy
Sickle cell retinopathy	Terson syndrome
Age-related microvascular changes	Syphilis

However, if you really want to be able to handle the Giant Smackdown of clinical life, you have to realize that reality tends to be more complex than mere tables. A list of diseases doesn't really give you a good matrix to work with, because you need to worry about different diseases in different situations. Remember that the whole reason to have a differential is to keep yourself and the patient out of trouble. A wise doctor once said that there are really only two diagnoses that you need to think of in any clinical situation: the diagnosis the patient has and the worst possible diagnosis if you are wrong. If want to explore the next level of diabetic differential diagnosis, feel free to read beyond the Land of the Tables...

The diabetic differential diagnosis can be broken down into three situations where you can screw up:

The first situation occurs when you have a patient with known retinopathy and a brand new disease shows up out of the blue. If the disease happens to be something that can look like diabetes, it can remain hidden within the preexisting retinopathy. Diseases such as these may be eminently treatable if you catch them in time, but they can make the patient much worse if you don't.

The second situation occurs in a patient with known diabetes but who, until now, has had no significant retinopathy. If said patient begins to get something funny in their retina, but it is not really diabetic disease, it is easy to call it diabetes and treat it incorrectly because you are blindfolded by the patient's systemic diagnosis.

The third situation is the typical one presented in most texts (and the purpose of tables such as those on the previous page). Namely, what should you think of if you have a patient who does not have known diabetes but has something that looks like diabetic retinopathy? This is fairly easy because you start by ruling out diabetes and then consider everything else covered in the above two situations.

> **Granted,** this categorization is artificial—these things can all overlap—so once you have internalized this knowledge don't go binary and forget that they can be combined in different ways (especially if your patient is unlucky). For instance, if you have a patient with retinopathy of unknown cause, and you skillfully diagnose diabetes, that patient can still get worse from a bunch of things that you are responsible for such as uveitis, a central retinal vein occlusion or, for that matter, sideroblastic anemia. Just don't stop thinking.

In any event, let's look at each one of these scenarios in greater detail. First:

Things that can hide in the signal-to-noise ratio of diabetic retinopathy and can make things worse if you don't think of them.

> **Occam's razor:** the simplest explanation is to be preferred.
>
> **Hickam's dictum:** patients can have as many diseases as they damn well please.

Diabetics are allowed to get other diseases, so if you are totally in the diabetic retinopathy zone you may fail to notice something crucial. Typically the new disease is missed because the superimposed findings are simply attributed to worsening of the underlying diabetic retinopathy. It is a Bad Thing to overlook such problems because if any other disease is added to diabetic retinopathy, the resulting synergy can be far worse than either entity alone.

One problem that can be hard to diagnose in the setting of retinopathy is uveitis. A rip-roaring HLA B-27 flare-up is easy to detect, but smoldering intermediate uveitis or retinal vasculitis can be hidden. For instance, if you think that every floating dot in your slit beam is just a red blood cell, you can miss white blood cells in the vitreous from intermediate uveitis. Or a subtle vasculitis can be mistaken for diabetes-related vascular changes (and there is no doubt that even a little bit of vasculitis can play hell with the retinopathy). You have to be on guard for subtle signs that don't fit in with typical diabetes, like macular edema out of proportion to the microvascular damage, or excessive staining of the vessels and/or nerve on fluorescein angiogram. Recognizing the synergizing presence of uveitis is crucial because the addition of local steroids or systemic immunosuppression can really help control the retinopathy (Figure 1).

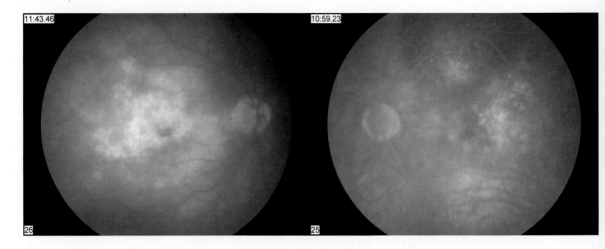

Figure 1: A patient with diabetic retinopathy in both eyes and superimposed mild intermediate uveitis in the right eye. Note the markedly asymmetrical macular edema and the diffuse cystoid changes in the eye with uveitis. Also—and this is subtle—note the slightly increased disc staining in the right eye, especially in the center of the nerve. These findings strongly suggest that something more than diabetes is going on.

Some other examples of things that can rev up the retinopathy include hematologic problems such as anemias, lymphoproliferative disorders or dysproteinemias. If you are following someone for retinopathy and they suddenly have lots of new blot hemorrhages or mild vascular tortuosity, it is easy to think of the changes as just "worsening" retinopathy. If you had seen these patients de novo—without a history of diabetes—you would likely make the connection to a systemic hematologic disease much faster. Try to at least think about these things if a patient's fundus starts to look really bloody—and don't be afraid to check a CBC or serum protein electrophoresis like a real doctor.

Oh, and don't forget that if your patient is on Coumadin, they may have lots of creepy hemorrhages that suggest either hematologic or retinovascular problems, such as a central retinal vein occlusion. You can always check an INR if you are worried, but many times this is just something that goes along with diabetic retinopathy and Coumadin (kind of makes you wonder what their brains look like...).

And finally, never, never, never forget the usual suspects if the retinopathy is acting up with lots of hemorrhages, cotton wool spots and other background changes. These are: poor glucose control, accelerated hypertension, renal failure and hypercholesterolemia. Ironically, rapid glucose control can do this as well (rapid meaning a drop of HbA1c of 3 or more points in a couple of months). All of this is a rehash of Chapter22, but the message merits repetition. If you are sick of reading it, go find another textbook.

What if one eye is a lot worse than the other?

Keep in mind that something strange may be going on in a patient who has very asymmetric disease. Diabetic retinopathy is almost always asymmetric to some extent, but you should worry if there is a big difference between the two eyes. The uveitis patient shown above is one example of this.

However, there are two bad boys you *really* need to keep in mind: central retinal vein occlusion (CRVO) and ocular ischemic syndrome (OIS). Both of these can present with way more hemorrhages and more pronounced macular edema in the worse eye. Both entities can also cause venous dilation that can be quite subtle at first. Sometimes you have to study photos of each eye simultaneously to more easily identify the vascular changes that suggest one of these entities (Figure 2). If the worse eye also has anterior segment neovascularization, then it is practically screaming CRVO or OIS—make sure you listen. (Ocular ischemic syndrome is bad news for diabetics, and diabetics are more likely to get it because they are, well, diabetic. It is important enough that it gets its very own chunk of this chapter later on.)

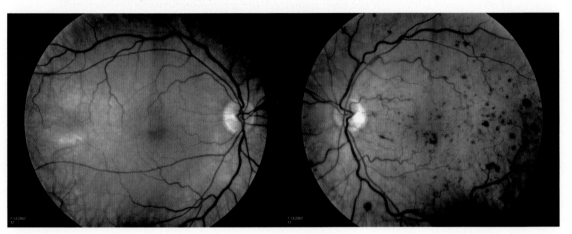

Figure 2: Asymmetric retinopathy due to a mild central retinal vein occlusion. Note the slightly dilated and tortuous veins, which suggest that the left eye has more going on than just accelerated background retinopathy.

If you think you are dealing with venous occlusive disease or ocular ischemia superimposed on diabetes, you have to deal with the ramifications of the diagnosis (e.g., check carotid Dopplers if you are worried about ischemia, consider a systemic work-up if you are worried about a vein occlusion and watch for anterior segment neovascularization for both). You also want to make darn sure the patient is aware of your concerns as you discuss the treatment and prognosis. He or she needs to know that everything you do may not work as well because of the double jeopardy and that the vision may worsen in spite of treatment and, in particular, how the eye may get neovascular glaucoma if the ischemia worsens.

(Remember Chapter 5 and the part about warning the patient that things may get worse, even with perfect treatment? Well, if your patient has diabetes and macular edema from a central retinal vein occlusion that you didn't recognize—and if that patient then gets neovascular glaucoma two weeks after you do a laser for edema—you *know* they will blame your focal for the nightmare they are about to experience. Not good.)*

---

* And they should blame you because you have screwed up twice:
1. By missing the CRVO in the first place.
2. If the macular edema was entirely due to a CRVO, it is a waste of time to do a laser—but that is a tale for a different book.

Other thoughts on asymmetric disease:

As mentioned, diabetic retinopathy can be asymmetric just because it can. Sometimes this is handy because the first eye gives the patient a taste of what is in store for the remaining eye if they don't take care of themselves. Do not hesitate to point this out to them if they don't realize it on their own.

In terms of disease pathology, though, there is one other issue that comes up occasionally in the literature: whether the asymmetric retinopathy is a manifestation of occult carotid disease. It has been suggested that a significant carotid obstruction can lower the blood pressure in the retinal vessels in the ipsilateral eye (unless there is collateral flow around the circle of Willis). The lower blood pressure turns out to be protective—the hydrostatic forces that eat away at blood vessels are lower—so the eye fed by the diseased carotid actually looks healthier.[2]

However, this effect is probably pretty rare, if it exists at all.[3] If carotid disease is going to cause a problem, it is much more likely to result in worsening of retinopathy from ischemia. The real question is whether you need to do carotid Dopplers on all patients with asymmetric disease. This is probably not necessary unless there is a big asymmetry that can't be explained by local eye conditions, or unless one eye develops anterior segment neovascularization. If you do Dopplers on everyone with just a bit of asymmetric disease, you may pick up something interesting on occasion, but it will probably have nothing to do with the retinopathy. Also, the patient may be more likely to end up at the vascular surgeon's office for no good reason. You decide...

Anyway, back to the differential diagnosis of diabetic retinopathy and the second scenario:

Things that can really make you look bad if they show up in a diabetic with no prior retinopathy and you think they are from diabetes.

The first section covered problems that can be "invisible" because they can superimpose themselves on pre-existing diabetic retinopathy, and you can miss them if you are not careful. Now it is time to turn to entities that, in and of themselves, can mimic diabetes. Most of these can be missed if they happen to show up in a diabetic patient—that is, you would be more likely to think of them if the patient wasn't diabetic. (Remember, sometimes Occam's razor can slice you a piece of bad-diagnosis pie.)

Perhaps the most common troublemaker is a branch retinal vein occlusion (BRVO). An acute BRVO can mimic diabetes if it is very mild, but usually the sectoral nature of the hemorrhages and the edema will tip you off. An old, chronic BRVO, however, can be a fooler because the vascular remodeling can spread across the horizontal midline, and the more acute findings that trigger the BRVO pattern-recognition algorithm in your head—like a localized sector of hemorrhage—are no longer present (Figure 3).

Figure 3: An old branch retinal vein occlusion simulating diabetic retinopathy. Note how the vascular changes can look much more like diabetes once the acute changes have resolved. In this case, there are also some hard exudates that have spread to the other side of the fovea, masking the fact that all the microvascular changes are localized above the fovea (something that would normally make you think of a BRVO). The early-phase angiogram clearly shows vascular remodeling in the distribution of a vein above the fovea and the late phase shows the leakage localized to the same area—this is where an angiogram can be very helpful to make the diagnosis. Note that the patient has already had grid laser to the area of leakage, including some grid spots below the fovea (suggesting that someone thought this was diabetes and added grid to non-pathologic retina).

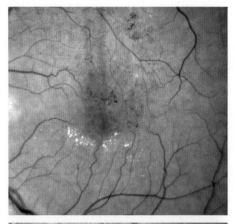

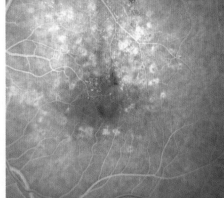

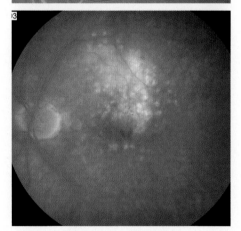

Why is it important to make the distinction?

First of all, the late vascular remodeling that occurs with an old BRVO can simulate easily treatable microaneurysms. Usually these vascular changes are dilated vessels that may provide the only remaining circulation to the fovea. If you decide to laser them like diabetic microaneurysms you could shut down the fovea's blood supply. Bad move. Treating a BRVO with laser tends to involve more of a grid thing rather than a "shoot red" thing. Besides, nowadays most BRVOs with central edema are treated with injections first and laser may be added as an adjuvant. If a patient has a local area of leakage that seems to respect the horizontal midline and does not have much in the way of vascular changes anywhere else, think BRVO and get an FA before you start cooking microaneurysms.

The second problem is that BRVOs can develop screwy-looking collateral vessels over time, and if you haven't realized you are dealing with a BRVO you can mistake them for proliferative disease. If you incorrectly do a PRP on such a patient you will be destroying retina needlessly—and until we figure out how to replace it you will be gaining some serious negative karma. To complicate matters, patients may develop true neovascularization secondary to a BRVO—and not just collateral vessels. These new vessels do need to be treated, but if you mistake them for proliferative diabetic retinopathy you will needlessly treat them with panretinal photocoagulation when they usually just need a sector of photocoagulation to treat the area of ischemia caused by the BRVO.

A central retinal vein occlusion can actually be a bit more problematic than a BRVO when it comes to distinguishing it from diabetic disease, and this is particularly true if the CRVO is mild. Because CRVOs are diffuse, rather than localized like a BRVO, they can simulate both new onset retinopathy or be hidden by preexisting retinopathy (see the prior section). It is a bit easier to sniff out a CRVO if there is no retinopathy to begin with because all the usual CRVO findings stand out as a sudden change, and the unilaterality is telling.

You should keep in the very back of your mind *the possibility of bilateral mild CRVOs in a diabetic who suddenly develops retinopathy. If you have been following diabetics for a while, you know that they usually do not quickly go from zero retinopathy to lots of pathology. The new onset of bilateral disease with features that suggest a CRVO such as venous dilation and tortuosity should make you suspicious. Such a scenario is so unlikely that you will probably never see it, but bilateral CRVOs are almost always a sign of something bad and if you blow them off as diabetes you might miss life-threatening problems like a dysproteinemia.*

Radiation retinopathy is another entity that can closely mimic diabetic retinopathy, but the history of radiation therapy will clue you in (Figure 4). Radiation retinopathy tends to be nastier than diabetes, especially in terms of capillary dropout and ischemia. It also tends to be more refractory to treatment than typical diabetes—and you and your patient need to know that the prognosis may not be as good if radiation damage is part of the problem. Where you need to be on your guard about this is with a known diabetic who didn't tell you—or whom you never asked—about prior radiation treatment. (Remember that stuff in medical school about PMH, ROS, PSH, etc.? This is where it does something more useful than allow you to bill a level-four visit.)

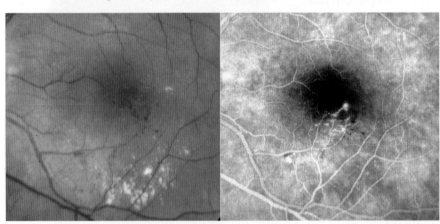

Figure 4: Radiation retinopathy. There is really nothing diagnostic about the appearance, although there is a sense that radiation creates more capillary dropout and ischemia than one would expect from a similar degree of diabetic retinopathy.

Macular telangiectasia type 2 (MacTel type 2—formerly idiopathic juxtafoveal telangiectasia type 2a) is another close mimic (Figure 5). This is the most common of the macular telangiectasias, and it is the one most likely to be confused with diabetic retinopathy. Plus, these patients are more likely to have diabetes—and if they aren't already diabetic, they are prone to becoming so. MacTel type 2 is characterized by tiny microvascular abnormalities around the fovea, especially on the temporal side. The pathology tends to be very symmetrical. (If you think you have a unilateral case, you are most likely looking at an old, small BRVO with late vascular remodeling or, less likely, the type 1 subset of macular telangiectasia related to adult Coats' disease—see the section below.) The appearance on FA is also quite characteristic: There is a very symmetrical doughnut of leakage in the late phases, with more leakage on the temporal side of each fovea.

Texts often refer to the presence of "right-angle venules," a term that makes no sense unless you see a few of these patients. It refers to veins that drain the outer retinal capillaries. (The "right-angle" refers to the fact that, if you look closely, the tip of the venule seems to dive down—directly away from the observer—into the outer capillaries. It does *not* refer to a right-angle turn in the horizontal plane of the retina, which is what one might otherwise think.)

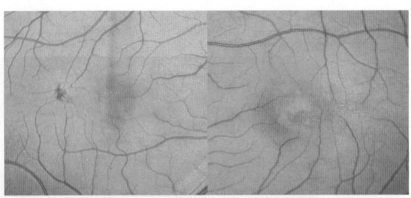

Figure 5-1: MacTel type 2. The right and left eyes of a patient with this entity. The left image shows the typical pigment clustering in the region of the abnormal vessels. This is a great tip-off, but not always present. The right image shows the refractile flecks that can also be seen with this (better seen in the digital version). Finally, you can get a sense that the perifoveal area has a subtle grayish cast in a very symmetric distribution. Note that the blood vessels temporal to both foveas look ratty, and you could easily mistake this for diabetes if you aren't thinking about MacTel.

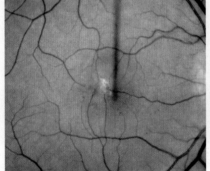

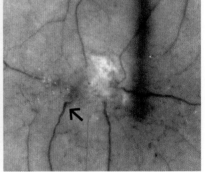

Figure 5-2: (right) MacTel type 2. The dilated veins around the fovea are more obvious in a red free photo (different patient).

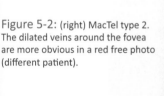

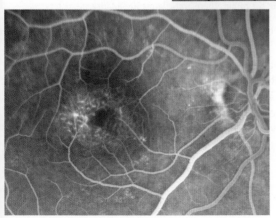

Figure 5-3: (Above right) Close-up of **Figure 5-2**. The arrow shows a "right-angle vein." The view is not stereoscopic, but you can get a sense that the vein is diving down into the outer retina. You can also see some of the refractile deposits seen in MacTel type 2 to the left of the fovea.

Figure 5-4: (Left) Early FA of MacTel type 2. You might call this diabetes, but note how the whole area around the fovea has an odd appearance and there are more abnormalities temporal to the fovea. There would also be a striking symmetry between the two eyes (see next figure).

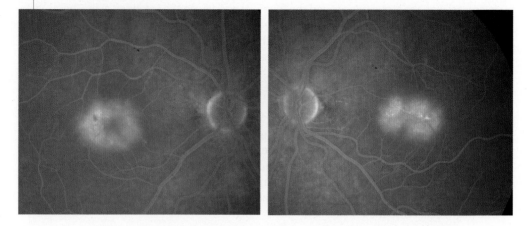

Figure 5-5: (Below) Late FA showing both eyes of a patient with MacTel type 2. Note the symmetric doughnut shape to the edema. If you do not think of this entity when you see this pattern, you may decide to use laser, which can be counterproductive.

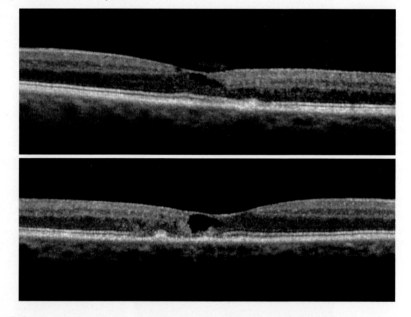

Figure 5-6: Typical MacTel type 2 OCTs. Note the ratty cystic changes, without any obvious retinal thickening—the cysts almost look like someone cut out parts of the retina. There is also some irregularity of the RPE consistent with the associated pigment changes. This is not like diabetic disease at all. (Note that patients can get retinal swelling if they develop a neovascular membrane, but it will look more like macular degeneration than diabetes. See the review mentioned in the text for more details.)

These patients can also get pigment clumping around the vascular abnormalities, as well as tiny golden refractile deposits near the fovea. Both findings are more prominent on the temporal side. OCT testing can show cystic changes, but there is a surprising lack of retinal thickening given the leakage seen on the angiogram. And the cystic changes are kind of weird—they look like chunks of the fovea have been punched out. This is important. Cystic changes on the OCT without any thickening, especially if symmetrical, should make you think of this entity (Figure 5-6).

Although patients tend to get gradual blurring of their vision over time, they do not tend to get severe vision loss. However, a subset of patients can develop very unusual neovascular membranes within and beneath the retina, and these patients can lose a lot of vision if this process is not recognized.

It is very important to consider this entity because laser treatment will not work; in fact, it may make the patient worse. You should be embarrassed if you do consider lasering such patients, because it indicates you have switched off your brain and are going on pattern recognition alone—you are seeing the red spots and leakage on FA, but you are ignoring the fact that the OCT is telling you the retina is not thick and both eyes are very symmetrical. Also, if the patient does get a neovascular membrane, they will then get definite retinal thickening. If you mistake this thickening for worsening diabetic edema, you will be encouraged to do more of the forbidden thing mentioned a few sentences ago. This will again have no useful effect and will now delay effective treatment, allowing your patient to get much worse.

If you think you do have a patient with MacTel type 2, you should congratulate yourself for making a relatively obscure diagnosis. However, there really is not much in the way of proven treatment for the leakage. People are always trying things, ranging from topical nonsteroidals to intravitreal therapy, although nothing seems to make much difference. So if you are considering the diagnosis it is best to get a retina consult to confirm it and to see what the treatment du jour may be. A full discussion is well beyond the scope of this chapter, but Issa, et al. provide a great review on the topic.[4]

The situation with MacTel type 2 is quite different, however, if the patient does develop a neovascular membrane. There is a lot of data suggesting that anti-VEGF agents and/or photodynamic therapy with Visudyne may help prevent severe vision loss. Patients with this problem should be referred quickly and not allowed to languish in your collection of patients who respond poorly to laser.

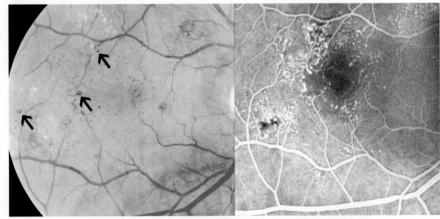

Another entity that can give you weird-looking vessels that may seem diabetic-ish at first is adult-onset Coats' disease (Figure 6). These patients have patches of irregular, bulb-like vessels that tend to leak much later in life relative to the eye-destroying type of Coats' disease that children get (in which the vessels are far more diffuse). This disease is more common in men and is strongly unilateral. There are often far more hard exudates than one

Figure 6: Adult-onset Coats' disease. (The color and the FA are from different points in time.) The arrows in the color photo show how the large, globular vessels will reflect the camera flash—showing up as a white dot on the red surface. The FA highlights the odd-looking bulbous vessels and the fact that the entire capillary bed is enlarged and irregular. This is very different from the more focal damage caused by diabetes. Finally, these photos are of early lesions. There often will be excessive amounts of hard exudates around the vascular lesions if the leakage is allowed to persist.

would see with typical diabetic retinopathy. An FA is very useful because it lights up the offending networks of vessels, which can look quite bizarre. It is important to distinguish this from regular diabetic disease because—unlike diabetic macular edema—you usually need to really treat these vessels aggressively in order to avoid letting the macula fill up with yellow fat. And just to confuse things, this adult-onset Coats' disease is probably part of a spectrum that includes macular telangiectasia type 1 (MacTel type 1). MacTel type 1 has the aneurysmal changes seen in Coats' disease, but it is limited only to the macula (and often just the temporal vasculature around the fovea—Figure 7). Like traditional Coats' disease, MacTel type 1 is usually found in males and is unilateral. It is very different from MacTel type 2, which, as discussed above, is usually bilateral and does not have exudative changes or aneurysmal dilations.

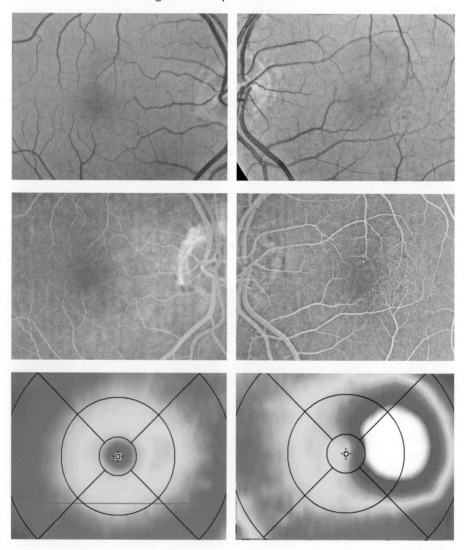

Figure 7: Macular telangiectasia type 1 in the left eye. Note the unilaterality and localized nature of the findings in the upper red free photos and the angiogram in the middle. The marked swelling can be seen in the bottom on the OCT. This patient doesn't have the more diffuse vascular changes seen in the adult-onset Coats' patient in **Figure 6**, nor are there other scattered microvascular changes that one would expect in true diabetic retinopathy. And this doesn't look anything like the weird little bilateral vascular changes seen in MacTel type 2. (Images courtesy of Matthew E. Farber, M.D.)

Most of the above entities have in common the fact that, at least at first, they mimic background diabetic changes. As mentioned at the beginning of the chapter, the differential is very different if you have a patient who is presenting with new vessels growing up off the retina. If you have a patient who presents with typical proliferative retinopathy and does turn out to have diabetes, you can relax and just follow the instructions in the rest of the book. (Well, relax only as far as making the diagnosis. Any patient who walks in the door with proliferative retinopathy is usually in big trouble, both from an ophthalmic standpoint and systemically.)

If the proliferative disease is atypical, then Table 1 can come in handy—as well as a textbook that covers all those diseases. There is, however, one proliferative disease in particular that you should keep in mind: proliferative retinopathy due to hemoglobin SC disease (especially if you have a patient population from the appropriate demographic). The far-peripheral nature of these vessels should make you think of this and prompt you to get a hemoglobin electrophoresis, even if the patient is diabetic. You do not want to mistake this entity for diabetes because treating SC disease requires a little more discretion. Blasting away everything in the periphery is not necessarily a good thing for these patients—they can get ischemic changes from the laser and traction related complications; the full scoop is beyond the scope of this book. (Interestingly, the presence of hemoglobin SC does not seem to increase the risk of diabetic retinopathy.)[5]

But now on to the third scenario:

Patients *without* previously diagnosed diabetes and funny things in their retina that look diabetic.

This is usually the easiest because even an ophthalmologist can diagnose diabetes. (By the way, remember that we are talking about diagnosing Type 2 diabetes here—Type 1 does not show up in your clinic with retinopathy as a presenting sign. Those patients show up in the ER with polydipsia, polyuria and ketoacidosis.)

How do you diagnose diabetes? The pundits argue about this, but Table 3 shows the latest criteria. Just to make things confusing, there are three different sets of criteria: those from the European Diabetes Epidemiology Group, the American Diabetes Association and the World Health Organization. Fortunately, all are similar; the ADA criteria are used here.

There is increasing recognition that glucose intolerance is really more of a spectrum, rather than something that can be specified by a single number. This has led to the definition of prediabetic states such as "impaired glucose tolerance" or "impaired fasting glucose" (Table 4). Such patients are at risk for macrovascular disease, such as heart attack and stroke, and they represent a demographic with significant personal and public health consequences.

Table 3: Criteria for Diagnosing Diabetes

A1C ≥6.5%*† OR
Fasting plasma glucose‡ ≥126 mg/dL (7.0 mmol/L)† **OR**
2-hour plasma glucose ≥200 mg/dL (11.1 mmol/L) during an oral glucose tolerance test; 75-g glucose load should be used† **OR**
Random plasma glucose concentration ≥200 mg/dL (11.1 mmol/L) in persons with symptoms of hyperglycemia or hyperglycemic crisis

*Test should be performed in a lab using a NGSP-certified method and standardized to the Diabetes Control and Complications Trial (DCCT) assay.

†In the absence of unequivocal hyperglycemia results should be confirmed using repeat testing.

‡Fasting defined as no caloric intake for ≥8 hours.

American Diabetes Association. Standards of medical care in diabetes—2013. *Diabetes Care*. 2013;36(suppl 1):S11-S66.

Table 4: Categories of increased risk for diabetes (prediabetes)*

Impaired fasting glucose (IFG): FPG 100 to 125 mg/dL (5.6 to 6.9 mmol/L)
Impaired glucose tolerance (IGT): 2-h PG on the 75-g OGTT 140 to 199 mg/dL (7.8 to 11.0 mmol/L)
HbA1C 5.7 to 6.4 percent

FPG: fasting plasma glucose

* For all three tests, risk is continuous, extending below the lower limit of the range and becoming disproportionately greater at higher ends of the range.

From: American Diabetes Association. Standards of Medical Care in Diabetes 2011.Diabetes Care 2011; 34:S11.

Basically, the diagnosis of diabetes is established when a patient has a fasting blood glucose concentration of 126 mg/dL (7.0 mmol/L) or higher, or a random value of 200 mg/dL (11.1 mmol/L) or higher (confirmed by repeat testing). A hemoglobin A1c can also be helpful now that the test is standardized. A level of ≥6.5 is used to diagnose diabetes. If you think a patient has diabetes based on the eye, but the test results are equivocal, you can get more aggressive with a two-hour glucose tolerance test. This test is a hassle, though, and these patients should really be at their medical doctor getting the full systemic evaluation anyway. The point is that it should be fairly easy to rule in the diagnosis of diabetes if you are seeing worrisome changes in the fundus. Even if you don't diagnose frank diabetes, it is very likely the patient will turn out to have one of the prediabetic states (unless a completely different problem is causing their retinopathy). Note that it was once thought that "prediabetic" patients did not get microvascular changes in their retinas, but it is now recognized that such patients may have mild background findings, although they are unlikely to have any significant retinopathy.[6]

Oh yeah, there is one other simple thing to do if you have a patient with hemorrhages and swellings in the retina, and you may not think of it because you have been too busy learning how to sell your patient a multifocal IOL or something. You can look extremely bad, however, if you don't consider this particular entity and perform the simple test required to detect it. If you can't think of it, you really should go ahead and do that cornea fellowship. (Hint—look at **Table 2.**)

If the patient has a few microvascular abnormalities but does not have any obvious systemic cause, recognize that recent population-based studies have found that perhaps 5 to 10% of patients over 40 to 50 years old can have occasional microaneurysms, retinal hemorrhages, and/or cotton wool spots. This may represent the effect of normal aging on the retinal vasculature, but it turns out that such patients are more likely to have problems such as hypertension, smoking and/or borderline glucose tolerance. Interestingly, these retinal findings can also be a marker for subclinical cerebrovascular and heart disease. In other words, if you have a patient with a few microaneurysms and no diabetes (and none of the other causes outlined in this chapter), don't just scratch your head and go "hrrrm." Inform their doctors and encourage these patients to get a complete physical, because the odds are something will turn up, and finding it may improve their overall health.[7,8]

CHAPTER 27.1

Ocular Ischemic Syndrome—Thermonuclear Retinopathy

Global ocular ischemia may be very difficult to diagnose, particularly if the patient already has lots of diabetic eye disease. You won't see it very often unless you have a practice full of patients with awful disease, but you do not want to miss it if it does show up because it can be treatable if caught early and disastrous if caught late. In the past this syndrome has had a number of confusing names, including retinopathy of carotid insufficiency and venous stasis retinopathy (the latter being most problematic because some people have used the same term to describe a non-ischemic central retinal vein occlusion). Lately, everyone seems to agree that the most useful name is ocular ischemic syndrome (OIS), mostly because that is what the people at Wills Eye Hospital call it, and who's gonna argue with them?

Although OIS can be due to problems such as temporal arteritis or localized ophthalmic artery stenosis, by far the most common cause is atherosclerotic carotid artery obstruction. If it is related to carotid disease there is usually at least a 90% ipsilateral obstruction. Unfortunately, bilateral involvement is common, although it may be sequential. The thing about this entity is that it can show up in very sneaky ways, and you have to keep it in mind because about half of patients with OIS have co-existing diabetes.

Presentation

The actual presentation varies along a multifactorial grid that includes the amount of the obstruction, the rate of obstruction, and the nature of the intraocular response induced by the ischemia. And all of this is can be scrambled up if you are seeing it in the setting of diabetic retinopathy; early signs may be lost amongst the preexisting diabetic damage. This can be a problem. Remember the paragraph above that talked about the need to keep in mind the worst-case scenario when you make a given diagnosis? Well, OIS is usually one of those worst-case scenarios in the setting of aggressive diabetic retinopathy.

Almost all patients have some sort of visual symptoms. They may present with sudden vision loss if there is a relatively acute onset, although many times there is a gradual, variable amount of vision loss, often with episodes of amaurosis fugax that may be atypical. The symptoms can also seem non-specific, for instance, episodic blurring of vision or prolonged vision loss following exposure to bright lights. Patients may complain of colored vision, often reddish or violet in hue. Of course, some of these are the same symptoms that many diabetics routinely complain of once they have significant retinopathy—so you have to be listening for changes in the quality or degree of the complaints and whether they are unilateral. Patients may also complain of vague eye aches, and a very characteristic symptom is a history of facial pain that improves with lying down.

The clinical findings can be quite varied in early, mild disease. Iris neovascularization is common, although it may be very subtle at first. Angle neovascularization leading to frank neovascular glaucoma is not far behind. However, one of the odd things about this entity is that the ischemic ciliary body may not be able to generate enough aqueous to elevate the pressure. Therefore, if the anterior segment neovascularization is subtle you may miss the diagnosis because there will be no elevated pressure to tip you off that something bad is happening. This is especially true if you are running a retina practice where patients are always seen after dilation—you won't see the new blood vessels and you won't have the pressure rise to make you suspicious.

By the way, the above problem means that if the patient ends up having carotid surgery, they may suddenly develop very high pressures as the ciliary body becomes perfused and starts to make aqueous. Both the patient and the vascular surgeon should be warned about this, and you should make arrangements to have someone else be on call to treat the miserable neovascular glaucoma that develops at 3:00 a.m. after their carotid is reopened.

There are some other presentations that need to be kept in mind to appreciate how peculiar this disease can be, even though they don't exactly intersect with the differential diagnosis of diabetes. OIS can result in corneal endothelial dysfunction with corneal edema and folds in Descemet's membrane—in an elderly patient with acute corneal decompensation, you have to think of OIS. OIS can also generate anterior uveitis with some anterior chamber cell and, rarely, even a keratic precipitate or two. Weird.

Posterior segment findings may be superficially similar to background diabetic retinopathy—and this is where you can easily miss the diagnosis. There may be retinal hemorrhages, but they tend to be further away from the posterior pole than typical diabetic hemorrhages, and they also tend to be larger and more blot-shaped (Figure 7). OIS, even without superimposed diabetes, can also cause neovascularization of the nerve, and there may even be microvascular changes such as capillary telangiectasias, microaneurysms, and macular edema.

Let's repeat one point here. *OIS needs to be considered in a patient with unilateral cystoid macular edema and not much diabetic retinopathy to explain it. (Assuming there are no other causes such as uveitis, an early CRVO, traction, etc.)*

OIS patients will often have dilated veins, too, and the combination of the peripheral hemorrhages and venous changes may suggest a mild CRVO in addition to diabetes. Brown and Margargal[8] point out that in OIS, the veins may be dilated but not tortuous, which is different from a CRVO, in which the veins are usually both dilated and tortuous (Figure 8).

Figure 8: Dot and blot hemorrhages in the periphery of a patient with OIS. They are distributed more randomly and are "blotchier" than one would expect from diabetes. (Brown GC, Magargal LE. Int Ophthalmol 1988; 11:239-51. Used with permission).

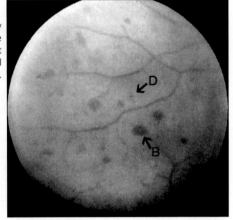

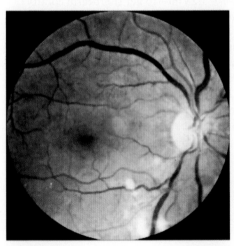

Figure 9: Dilated veins in OIS—without tortuosity. Also scattered cotton wool spots. (Sharma S, Brown GC, Ocular Ischemic Syndrome in Ryan SJ(ed.) Retina 4th Edition. Used with permission.)

Fluorescein angiography may be useful in sorting out the diagnosis. There is often a delay in both choroidal and retinal filling due to global ophthalmic artery hypoperfusion. There may also be late staining of the vessels and disc in early OIS, as well as the aforementioned macular edema. This may make one think of inflammatory disease, but the delayed circulation time should suggest OIS.

Digital ophthalmodynamometry is a classic physical exam maneuver that may allow you to make a very astute diagnosis of OIS, if you can actually remember to do it. Although there are devices to quantitate the pressure required to cause the central retinal artery to pulsate, it is easy to simply view the nerve and push on the eye with your finger. An eye with OIS will often show pulsations of the artery with only mild pressure (be sure you are not mistaking venous pulsations for arterial pulsations). Many times this finding is somewhat subtle and you need to compare one eye to the other to appreciate the difference.

Once you think you are dealing with OIS, the main concern is to make sure that there is no carotid disease that needs to be treated. The patient should have carotid Dopplers and be encouraged to get to their internist to look for other vascular problems such as heart disease.

From an ophthalmic standpoint, if they develop neovascular glaucoma these patients usually need very aggressive panretinal photocoagulation, along with anti-VEGF therapy and whatever is needed to control the pressure. The PRP generally needs to be performed quickly and in high, painful doses, which tend to create symptomatic changes in vision. Also, remember the warning from Chapter 20 on iris neovascularization about how patients with OIS may be at an increased risk for a central retinal artery occlusion after an anti-VEGF injection.[13] This is probably due to the underlying poor perfusion in the eye, but there also may be a direct effect of the drugs on the vasculature. It means that you ought to have a low threshold for doing a paracentesis if you inject patients with OIS. Or use a very low dose of the drug—like .025 ml—to get short-term control of the vessels without raising the pressure to levels that could obstruct the circulation.

Basically, patients with OIS need to understand that you are fighting to save the eye—and they need to have appropriate expectations, because even if the treatment works these eyes don't tend to see well. The brief discussion in this section really does not do justice to this entity, and if you think you are dealing with OIS you should read some of the references that follow.[9-12] The main point is that this is a really bad thing to have happen to a diabetic eye, and it can be very subtle at first. However, you can help save both the patient's eye and their brain if you make the diagnosis.

References

1.   Jampol LM, Ebroon DA, Goldbaum MH. Peripheral proliferative retinopathies: an update on angiogenesis, etiologies and management. *Surv Ophthalmol.* May-Jun 1994;38(6):519-540.

2.   Basu A, Palmer H, Ryder RE, Taylor KG. Uncommon presentation of asymmetrical retinopathy in diabetes type 1. *Acta Ophthalmol Scand.* Jun 2004;82(3 Pt 1):321-323.

3.   Duker JS, Brown GC, Bosley TM, Colt CA, Reber R. Asymmetric proliferative diabetic retinopathy and carotid artery disease. *Ophthalmology.* Jul 1990;97(7):869-874.

4.   Charbel Issa P, Gillies MC, Chew EY, et al. Macular telangiectasia type 2. *Progress in retinal and eye research.* May 2013;34:49-77.

5.   Koduri PR, Patel AR, Bernstein HA. Concurrent sickle cell hemoglobin C disease and diabetes mellitus: no added risk of proliferative retinopathy? *J Natl Med Assoc.* Sep 1994;86(9):682-685.

6.   Tyrberg M, Melander A, Lovestam-Adrian M, Lindblad U. Retinopathy in subjects with impaired fasting glucose: the NANSY-Eye baseline report. *Diabetes Obes Metab.* Aug 2008;10(8):646-651.

7.   Wong TY, Klein R, Amirul Islam FM, et al. Three-year incidence and cumulative prevalence of retinopathy: the atherosclerosis risk in communities study. *Am J Ophthalmol.* Jun 2007;143(6):970-976.

8.   Ojaimi E, Nguyen TT, Klein R, et al. Retinopathy signs in people without diabetes: the multi-ethnic study of atherosclerosis. *Ophthalmology.* Apr 2011;118(4):656-662.

9.   Brown GC, Magargal LE. The ocular ischemic syndrome. Clinical, fluorescein angiographic and carotid angiographic features. *Int Ophthalmol.* Feb 1988;11(4):239-251.

10.   Sivalingam A, Brown GC, Magargal LE. The ocular ischemic syndrome. III. Visual prognosis and the effect of treatment. *Int Ophthalmol.* Jan 1991;15(1):15-20.

11.   Sivalingam A, Brown GC, Magargal LE, Menduke H. The ocular ischemic syndrome. II. Mortality and systemic morbidity. *Int Ophthalmol.* May 1989;13(3):187-191.

12.   Mendrinos E, Machinis TG, Pournaras CJ. Ocular ischemic syndrome. *Surv Ophthalmol.* Jan-Feb 2010;55(1):2-34.

13.   Higashide T, Murotani E, Saito Y, Ohkubo S, Sugiyama K. Adverse events associated with intraocular injections of bevacizumab in eyes with neovascular glaucoma. Graefes Arch Clin Exp Ophthalmol. Apr 2012;250(4):603-610.

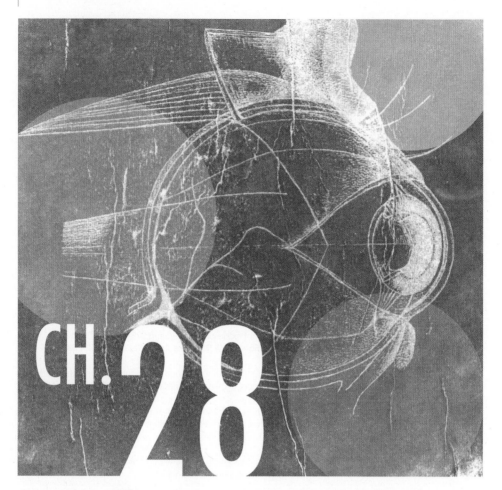

Just How Often Do You Have to Drag Them Back, Anyway?

I haven't had the time to plan returning to the scene because I haven't left it. Mick Jagger

Table 1 is the best overview on how often one should follow up with and consider treating patients with different levels of retinopathy—it is based on guidelines from the American Academy of Ophthalmology.

Table 1: Follow-up interval based on retinopathy findings.

Retinal Abnormality	Suggested Follow-up Interval
Normal or rare microaneurysms	Annually
Mild NPDR	Every 9 months
Moderate NPDR	Every 6 months
Severe NPDR	Every 2-4 months
Clinically significant macular edema	Every 2-4 months*
PDR	Every 2-3 months**
Inactive/Involuted PDR	Every 6-12 months

*This interval will obviously depend on how worried you are and whether the patient needs to be actively treated. If the treatment includes intravitreal injections then this interval may need to be every month at first.

**If this is a patient with active disease that is in the process of being treated they may need to be seen more often to make sure the vessels are regressing and there is no problematic traction. Once things start to stabilize then the visits can be spread out.

Modified from *Diabetic Retinopathy Preferred Practice Pattern* - American Academy of Ophthalmology 2008 and Basic and *Clinical Science Course Section XII* - American Academy of Ophthalmology 2010.

However, some patients do not quite fit into a table, so here are some other things to consider:

First of all, there is some controversy about how often diabetics should be screened if they have no retinopathy. For instance, there is good evidence that suggests that older Type 2 diabetics can be screened every two years until they begin to develop retinopathy.[1] Also, for some reason retinopathy is vanishingly rare before the onset of puberty.[2] As a result, the American Diabetes Association at one point had a more complicated recommendation for pre-pubertal patients with Type 1 diabetes: They should have their first screening examination within three to five years after the diagnosis of diabetes once the patient is age 10 years or older.

Rather than trying to figure out what the preceding sentence means, or trying to remember which older patients are due for their bi-annual examination, it seems much simpler to just insist that all diabetics get examined once a year. Diabetics are understandably not enthusiastic about screening examinations, and human nature is human nature. (When was your last eye exam?) It is all too easy for patients to neglect screening examinations, especially if they are asymptomatic. Then, after a few years go by and they begin to have symptoms from advanced disease, they suddenly remember to get an exam—but it may be too late. It makes sense to have diabetics of all types and ages get used to the idea that an annual eye exam is just part of their life.

The counter-argument is that annual examinations increase overall healthcare costs, which they do. It would certainly be great to spread out the examinations if everyone lived in a perfect world where every patient could be tracked perfectly. However, in the world where most of us live it is probably better to train them to have an annual eye exam than to spread out the visits and risk losing them to follow up—an eventuality that could end up costing everyone a lot more.

> ***Please note*** *that the preceding discussion refers to patients who are known to have diabetes and are known to have no retinopathy. Any older patient with newly diagnosed Type 2 diabetes absolutely needs an examination at the time of diagnosis. Period. There is a significant chance that they may have smoldering retinopathy due to long-standing undiagnosed diabetes, and an eye exam is at the top of their list of things to do.*

There are some other factors to consider when deciding how often to monitor patients once they do have some degree of retinopathy. An extremely important factor is the rate of disease progression. For instance, a patient who quickly goes from minimal background retinopathy to more advanced disease is very worrisome and should be monitored more frequently than the table may suggest. On the other hand, a patient with old, treated proliferative retinopathy that has been stable for years may only need one exam per year or less. Another factor usually related to progression is—once again—the patient's degree of systemic control. And control refers to all the different risk factors such as glucose level, hypertension and elevated lipids. A poorly controlled patient is always at higher risk for getting into trouble (and at higher risk for being lost to follow up), and should be kept on a tighter leash in terms of return-visit frequency.

An additional factor is whether you are seeing the patient for the first time. Unless you have their old records, you have no way of knowing whether such patients have progressive disease. There is nothing wrong with bringing a patient back sooner than their degree of retinopathy would suggest in order to be sure that they are stable. You can reassure yourself about the rate of a patient's progression and reinforce the need to follow up two for one!

Also, remember the effect that pregnancy can have on diabetic retinopathy. Refer to Chapter 24 for the suggested examination schedule for that particular situation—especially the part about encouraging diabetic women to have an eye exam well before they even think about getting pregnant.

Finally, recall the caveats about financial concerns mentioned in Chapter 21. Patients without insurance may simply be unable to afford returning for routine exams, and you should make sure that they are welcome regardless of their ability to pay. Patients with high-deductible plans are often in the same boat. It is a lot easier—and just plain nicer— to do a quick diabetic screening exam for free than to make the patient and society pay for lifelong disability resulting from preventable vision loss.

References

1.   Leese GP. Should diabetes retinal screening intervals change? *Diabet Med*. Jan 2013;30(1):43-45.

2.   Geloneck MM, Forbes BJ, Shaffer J, Ying GS, Binenbaum G. Ocular Complications in Children with Diabetes Mellitus. Ophthalmology. 2015.

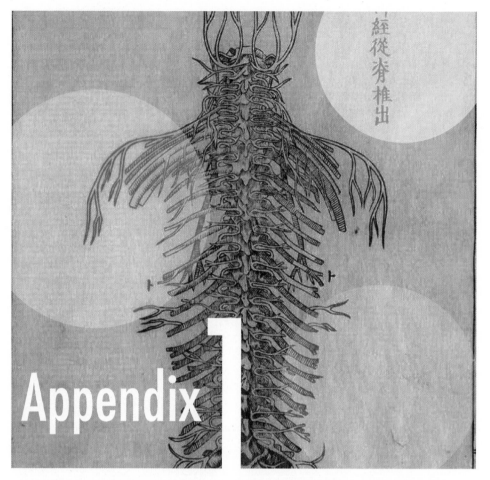

Smile for the Camera: Screening for Diabetic Retinopathy With Lik Thai Lim, MBBCh, FRCOphth

A photograph is usually looked at — seldom looked into. Ansel Adams

As outlined at the beginning of this book, there are an awful lot of diabetics out there, and it takes an awful lot of time to screen them for retinopathy. If you are the only ophthalmologist for a large number of people, you could spend your entire day screening diabetics and never accomplish anything else.

The gold standard for screening is a careful fundus examination, but statistics suggest that 30-50% of patients with diabetes are not screened properly—and the percentages are probably a lot higher in the developing world. The reasons for this are manifold, and include a lack of resources, lack of money, lack of awareness on the part of the patient, and the fact that the examination itself is not fun.

A lot of effort goes to finding ways to screen populations for retinopathy without tying up clinics and staff with complete examinations. Since estimates of the prevalence of sight-threatening eye disease among diabetics ranges from 6 to 14%, there is a good chance that about 1 in 10 screened patients will have something that can be treated to avoid vision loss—again, a number that is likely higher in the developing world.[1,2]

That percentage—one in ten—is worth dwelling on. If you set up a program at the local free clinic, it is like you have granted yourself a superpower that allows you to keep one in ten people seeing. Even better, you don't have to worry about a deluge of uninsured patients. Most clinics don't have a large number of diabetics, and only a subset of those will need to be seen, so you may be adding only a few patients to your schedule each month. Your practice gets major dharma points with little effort!

However, screening can be tricky because there are no "gold standards" for how to identify patients at risk. Most studies have used some sort of retinal photography, and early studies used traditional seven-field stereoscopic fundus photography—a technique called for in the EDTRS. But that method is costly and time consuming. Recently, attention has focused on the use of one, two or three-field photographs as a compromise, often using non-mydriatic cameras (Figure 1).

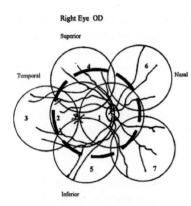

Figure 1: A drawing showing the location of the standard seven-field 30-degree photos as called for in the EDTRS. The dashed circle is approximately what a 45-degree single field photo shows. (From Lin DY, Blumenkranz MS, Brothers RJ, Grosvenor DM. Am J Ophthalmol. Aug 2002;134(2):204-213. Used with permission.)

However, the fewer the fields, the greater the risk of missing something significant. It has been estimated that up to a quarter of significant retinopathy lesions lie outside the area of photograph with a single field 45-degree photograph.[3] Still, doing some degree of screening is far better than doing nothing; when done carefully, the sensitivity and specificity of a single image can be quite high (often into the 80-90% range).[4] And newer wide-field imaging systems can capture a lot of the retina with one image—that may be easier compared to multiple fundus photographs.[5] Even better, OCT testing may soon be available along with photos. That can really increase the specificity and yield.

What about dilation? Although it is easier to take good photos if the patient is dilated, there are issues. First, the non-ophthalmologists at the clinic are going to be concerned about angle closure glaucoma, even though the risk is low. Second, anything that makes it harder for the clinic staff to get their work done will decrease their compliance with getting the patients photographed. That's important. If you tie up the nurses with extra work, they will be less likely to get the photos no matter how interested you are in the system. Finally, there may be liability issues with the use of a mydriatic, especially if patients are driving. Fortunately, newer cameras are able to take good images with an undilated eye. But if you are working in a region where cataracts are also a problem, patients may need to be dilated to increase the number of useful images. And, of course, you have to be sure that whoever is doing the photos can tell the difference between usable and unusable images.

It generally does not take a lot of time to review the images and determine who needs to be seen, at least on a small scale. However, things get more onerous if large numbers need to be screened. Studies have looked at training endocrinologists and even technicians to do the grading with variable success—you can try anything you want but you need to give a nod to any liability issues that might arise.[16] But even if others are doing the reading, there still can be a significant time commitment if hundreds or thousands of photographs need to be evaluated. As a result, efforts are underway to develop computerized screening systems. Look for these to become more and more prevalent, especially in areas where patients wildly outnumber physicians.

You will also need to decide what criteria warrant referral. Different studies use different criteria; you can look at the references at the end of the chapter for more details. But if you are starting to do this on your own, you can decide for yourself. You will probably want to be fairly conservative and bring patients in with even mild-looking disease simply to get them in the system. Of course, another issue is actually getting the patients in once you decide they need to be seen. If they have to travel long distances or give up a day's work you may need to figure out another way to get them evaluated (see Appendix 2). It is amazing how hard it is to get people in—educating the clinic staff about educating the patients about the importance of follow-up is crucial.

A favorite trick is to have the clinic take a $5 deposit to make an appointment, and then give them the $5 back when they actually show up. It gets them in, and until we figure out a way to do brain transplants it helps motivate less motivated patients to take care of themselves.

You may want to check with your malpractice carrier to see what the concerns are, even if you are offering your services gratis to a free-clinic. If you are trying to set up a for-profit entity, that is a completely different can of worms and well beyond the scope of this discussion. You need to assess the feelings of your ophthalmic community and the local medical community, and be very aware of the liability issues.

Another problem has been both the cost of the equipment and the training required to get clinic staff to become proficient at taking photos. Fortunately, efforts are underway to make cheaper cameras that are less user-dependent. An example is the DRS camera by CenterVue (Figure 2). It costs about $18,000 US—well within the range of a grant—and the camera automatically scans the patient's face to hone in on the pupils to take photographs without the need for a trained photographer. A feature like this is really important. As mentioned above, if getting pix becomes a hassle for the clinic staff, they will be much less likely to take them.

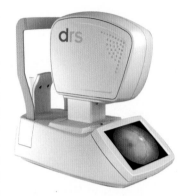

If you can afford it, you will by far see more pathology with a non-mydriatic wide-angle image (Figure 3).[6] The new Optos Daytona camera system is portable and offers a 200-degree view of the fundus.[7] Most importantly, it requires an imager, not a trained photographer. The price is significantly more than the DRS imager above—like a Tesla to a Volt. And with the kind of expansive image obtained, it is likely that non-physician imagers can assess the photos and make referrals as the photos are taken.[8]

Figure 2: DRS automatic camera. Note the lack of any joystick—the camera is designed to find and photograph each eye on its own. Courtesy of CenterVue, San Jose, CA.

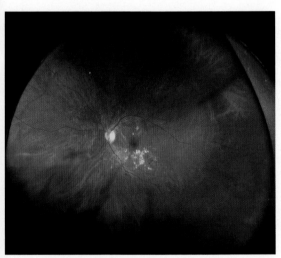

More recently, smartphone adapters have been created that allow fundus photography, including open source designs using 3-D printed parts.[9-11] And a skillful observer can even use the built-in light to do indirect ophthalmoscopy with an unmodified smart phone.[12] Doing this requires some skill, but the images can be evaluated and this approach may have a role, especially in the developing world. But the field of view is limited and it takes some practice to perform imaging this way.

When it comes to photographic screening, this chapter just scratches the surface. There is a lot of information about this subject in the literature, so if you are thinking about doing something along these lines, some good recent reviews are referenced.[13-15]

Figure 3: Wide angle view of the Optos device. You can readily see pathology well outside the area that can be captured by traditional fundus cameras.

References

1. Liesenfeld B, Kohner E, Piehlmeier W, et al. A telemedical approach to the screening of diabetic retinopathy: digital fundus photography. *Diabetes care*. 2000;23(3):345-348.
2. James M, Turner DA, Broadbent DM, Vora J, Harding SP. Cost effectiveness analysis of screening for sight threatening diabetic eye disease. *Bmj*. 2000;320(7250):1627-1631.
3. Lueder GT, Silverstein J, American Academy of Pediatrics Section on O, Section on E. Screening for retinopathy in the pediatric patient with type 1 diabetes mellitus. *Pediatrics*. 2005;116(1):270-273.
4. Browning D. *Diabetic Retinopathy. Evidence-Based Management*. Springer; 2010.
5. Liegl R, Liegl K, Ceklic L, et al. Nonmydriatic ultra-wide-field scanning laser ophthalmoscopy (Optomap) versus two-field fundus photography in diabetic retinopathy. *Ophthalmologica. Journal international d'ophtalmologie. International journal of ophthalmology. Zeitschrift fur Augenheilkunde*. 2014;231(1):31-36.
6. Silva PS, Cavallerano JD, Sun JK, Soliman AZ, Aiello LM, Aiello LP. Peripheral lesions identified by mydriatic ultrawide field imaging: distribution and potential impact on diabetic retinopathy severity. *Ophthalmology*. 2013;120(12):2587-2595.
7. http://www.optos.com/en-US/Products/Retinal-imaging-products/Retinal-imaging-products/Daytona/.
8. Silva PS, Cavallerano JD, Tolson AM, et al. Real-Time Ultrawide Field Image Evaluation of Retinopathy in a Diabetes Telemedicine Program. *Diabetes care*. 2015.
9. Russo A, Morescalchi F, Costagliola C, Delcassi L, Semeraro F. Comparison of smartphone ophthalmoscopy with slit-lamp biomicroscopy for grading diabetic retinopathy. *American journal of ophthalmology*. 2015;159(2):360-364 e361.
10. http://www.ophthnotes.com/smartphone-retinal-camera/.
11. http://www.medgadget.com/2015/05/worlds-first-open-source-smartphone-retinal-camera.html?utm_source=facebook.com&utm_medium=social&utm_campaign=buffer&utm_content=buffer38354.
12. Haddock LJ, Kim DY, Mukai S. Simple, inexpensive technique for high-quality smartphone fundus photography in human and animal eyes. *Journal of ophthalmology*. 2013;2013:518479.
13. Surendran TS, Raman R. Teleophthalmology in Diabetic Retinopathy. *Journal of diabetes science and technology*. 2014;8(2):262-266.
14. Silva PS, Aiello LP. Telemedicine and Eye Examinations for Diabetic Retinopathy: A Time to Maximize Real-World Outcomes. *JAMA ophthalmology*. 2015.
15. Zimmer-Galler IE, Kimura AE, Gupta S. Diabetic retinopathy screening and the use of telemedicine. *Current opinion in ophthalmology*. 2015;26(3):167-172.
16. Silva PS, Cavallerano JD, Tolson AM, et al. Real-Time Ultrawide Field Image Evaluation of Retinopathy in a Diabetes Telemedicine Program. Diabetes care. 2015;38(9):1643-1649.

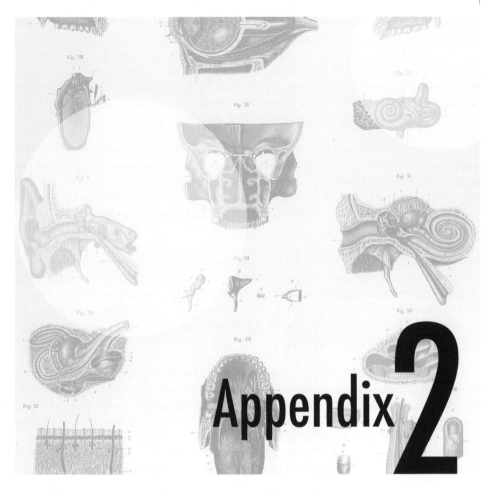

Appendix 2

Building Something Out of Nothing
With Krishna R. Murthy, MRCOphth

The best way to find yourself is to lose yourself in the service of others. Mahatma Gandhi

When it comes to treating retinopathy, there is one problem that is universal: not enough resources to take care of all of the diabetics. It is likely that, wherever you are, you will have patients that are struggling to get care. And it can become a vicious cycle; caring for more indigent patients means fewer resources for everyone. There are a lot of organizations out there that can help you help them, but you have to make the first move.

Whether you are trying to simply get a grant to put a camera in a free clinic, or whether you want to build a regional network to prevent retinopathy, start by learning about who can help you locally. Examples are service clubs such as the Lions Club or Rotary Club. Various religious groups may also be interested, and there are resources available—for instance at public libraries—that can help you identify organizations that might fund the type of project that you are considering.

But remember that most of those resources are not going to start handing you money simply because you are a good person. You need to work to build connections and be willing to put in some sweat equity to demonstrate that your thoughts are pure and what you are doing will provide a good return on their investment.

You might consider working with local diabetic organizations, and even networking with local endocrinologists, podiatrists, and pharmacists. Indeed, for many places one of the biggest obstructions to providing excellent care for diabetic retinopathy is the fact that there are insufficient medical specialists to take care of the entire patient. Figuring out ways to make your location attractive to diabetologists can help your patients a lot more than your injections and lasers.

And don't underestimate the utility of getting to know the regional government administrators. The high-tech nature of our specialty—and the ability to "help the blind to see"—often makes ophthalmology more interesting to bureaucracy types. There are also organizations that specifically help ophthalmology-related initiatives. The American Academy of Ophthalmology maintains a list of organizations on their web site (http://www.aao.org/international/outreach).

You can tap organizations that focus on diabetes in general. Diabetes Monitor has a list of national groups from many countries: http://www.diabetesmonitor.com/resources/international-diabetes-organizations.htm. The World Diabetes Foundation and the International Diabetes Foundation are two additional global entities that can be very helpful. And don't forget the drug companies—both ophthalmic and systemic. It is good for them on a number of levels if you can generate programs that keep diabetics functioning in society. Check with the local reps to see if grants are available.

However, be prepared to hear far more "No's" than "Yes's". It is easy to get frustrated, especially in the developing world. Between lack of resources, unmotivated patients and bureaucratic hassles, you can feel like Sisyphus.

But you can succeed.

A great example of what can be done is the system set up by Dr. Murthy and colleagues in Bangalore.[1] They first went out to the surrounding region to screen diabetics, and then they offered free care to patients with significant disease if they came to their clinic in the main city. It became obvious that although such an approach was altruistic, it was not effective. Transportation was unavailable for many patients; for others the cost of losing a day's wages was so prohibitive that they were unable to get in—even for free care. And for some patients, simply going to the Big City was just too overwhelming.

So the next thought was to bring diagnostic equipment and lasers into the surrounding countryside. Unfortunately, that stuff isn't cheap, and transporting delicate ophthalmic equipment is much easier said than done. And it is really hard to get such a system going when you are trying to care for indigent patients who can't pay enough to cover the cost of the equipment, let alone cover the cost of fixing it when it gets damaged in transit.

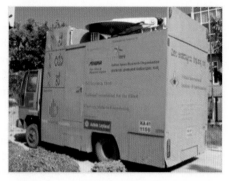

Figure 1: The travelling van filled with retinal equipment.

They applied to local organizations in hopes of getting a grant to cover these start-up costs, but no one would fund the effort. So they went outside their box and applied to the World Diabetes Foundation and were given a grant to obtain equipment. They then worked with volunteer engineers to design a truck that could transport the equipment in specially made shock-absorbing containers (Figures 1 and 2).

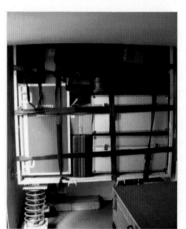

Figure 2: An example of the cases used to protect equipment and the spring shock absorbers used beneath the platforms holding the cases. (Both images courtesy of Krishna Murthy, M.D, Subbakrishna Rao and Prabha Eye Clinic, Bangalore, India.)

One would think that they were all set. But no. New solutions bring new problems. They were worried that they might alienate general ophthalmologists in the countryside by sucking away their patients—even if those ophthalmologists did not do retinal treatments themselves. This is a potential side effect of the "cataract mission" approach to treating patients. Going out and doing as many surgeries as possible in a region isa wonderful endeavor and can improve the quality of many patients' lives—the Aravind model is a classic example of how effective this can be.[2] But treating diabetic retinopathy is an ongoing process; it isn't solved with one surgery. And in some situations, a visiting mission can make it more difficult for locals to invest time and effort into building a self-sustaining clinic. The fact that somebody will show up periodically and do a bunch of treatments for free means that patients are going to wait for missions rather than see the local ophthalmologist.

To address this, Dr. Murthy and colleagues offered to visit each of the regional ophthalmologists, see patients in their office, and teach the regional ophthalmologists how to perform the laser treatments discussed in this book (the logistics of the situation did not allow the use of injections or vitrectomy in the rural areas). At this point, some of the other retinal specialists in Bangalore suggested that this wouldn't work because the general ophthalmologists would then hold onto all their diabetics and keep lasering them without referring them in when needed. But that didn't happen, and it turns out that the new approach worked extremely well. The regional ophthalmologists were able to learn how to evaluate and treat retinopathy, and they didn't need to worry about capital expenditures because they used the equipment brought in once a month on the truck. They were even able to generate revenue because patients didn't have to spend money on transportation or lose time from work. Those ophthalmologists then served as a referral network to get the truly complicated patients into the main retinal office for more advanced care.

Even better, they could implement strategies to expand demand for the program. This included providing educational sessions for community health workers and local general practitioners on diabetes care and screening for complications. Posters were put up at local clinics and pharmacies to increase awareness on the need for eye screening, and the regional ophthalmologists encouraged local physicians to refer patients for screening. The ophthalmologists could even conduct diabetic retinopathy screening camps in more rural areas, and then treat the identified patients on the day the truck comes to their office. And in places where there are no nearby ophthalmologists, a more typical telemedicine screening program can be provided by the truck—like that discussed in Appendix 1— and patients identified as having problems can be treated when the truck returns. The possibilities are limitless.

Soooooo...

There really is no reason why a typical diabetic patient should go blind in the modern era, as long as their disease is caught early enough and they are taking reasonably good care of themselves. As the number of these patients increases, the onus is upon us to do what we can to get them in so that they do not need to suffer. In many situations the only barrier is how willing you are to work on their behalf, and how much help you can get from organizations that are waiting out there to assist you. Like the doctors in Bangalore, you may find that something that seems like a problem at first can actually provide the best solution. Buena suerte.

References

1.   Murthy KR, Murthy PR, Kapur A, Owens DR. Mobile diabetes eye care: experience in developing countries. Diabetes Res Clin Pract. Sep 2012;97(3):343-349.

2.   Natchiar G, Robin AL, Thulasiraj RD, Krishnaswamy S. Attacking the backlog of India's curable blind. The Aravind Eye Hospital model. Archives of ophthalmology. Jul 1994;112(7):987-993

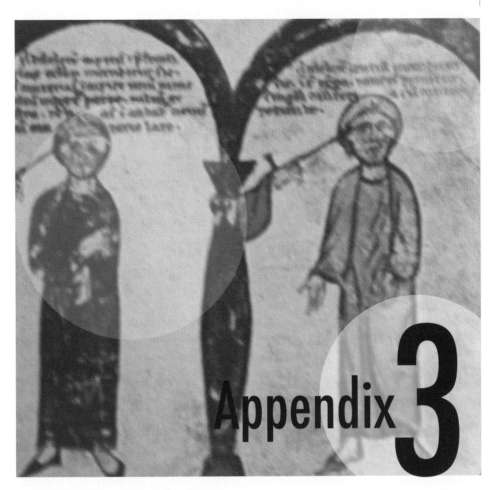

Infrared Techniques

Nothing ever becomes real 'til it is experienced. John Keats

Infrared diode lasers are cheaper yet durable because they are a simpler design. For this reason they may be the laser of choice in situations where financial resources are limited or if the laser can't be pampered and babied like in your nice cushy clinic. There is also data that suggests infrared treatment is as effective as green for diabetic retinopathy, although there are nowhere near as many patients in these studies as in the DRS and ETDRS.[1-3] However, you can't just sit down at an infrared laser and assume you can treat with the same techniques you would use for a green laser. This would be a Very Bad Thing.

Infrared is much trickier to use because the burns can seem unpredictable. They are, in fact, predictable, but it just plain takes a lot of experience and you really need to be aware of the degree of pigment in both the choroid and retinal pigment epithelium as you treat. Green light hits the RPE like a hammer hitting a nail—all the heat you would ever need for a burn is right there. Infrared is not as well absorbed by the RPE and penetrates deeper, so you actually need to heat up both the RPE and inner choroid to get a burn. Don't be surprised if you need to use two to three times more power to do an infrared treatment compared to the powers you would use with a green laser. If there is not much pigment you need to really crank up the power—sometimes it is impossible to get a burn in very pale fundi with an infrared laser.

*Although using an infrared laser can be difficult at first, it does come in handy when the view is hazy. Recall that shorter wavelengths are scattered more than longer wavelengths and that infrared is less absorbed by just about everything in the eye (refer back to **Figure 1 in Chapter 6**). All of this means that it can get through media opacities much better than visible wavelengths.*

Also, the way an infrared burn develops is different from that of a burn using a green laser. With a green laser, the burn intensity gradually increases as you increase the power; there is a nice, gentle linear relationship that has room for error. The retinal response to infrared is more like an "S"-shaped curve, with the steep part starting just when you can see a burn. In other words, a small increase in the power can have a big effect on how hot your burn is once you start getting some uptake.

At first, the infrared burn tends to be elusive; you will see nothing and you will keep turning the power up and up—which can be a creepy feeling. Then, once you start to see some early graying, you have to be very careful because even a tiny increase in power can dramatically increase the intensity of the burn.

This also means that the laser-tissue interaction is much less forgiving. For instance, if you have found a good power, you still have to be very vigilant about the level of pigmentation at the site of treatment. If you move into an area of darker pigmentation you can blow things apart suddenly and unexpectedly—especially if you have fallen into "green-laser mode" and are mechanically stomping away on the foot pedal without paying close attention. Another difference between green and infrared is that the desired end point for a burn is much milder than with a green laser. A grayish-white or whitish burn that might be OK with green will be quite hot with infrared, and you will be treating at the limit of safety. Usually a light graying will do the trick—you can get nasty scars, more pain and maybe even a choroidal hemorrhage if you try to create burns similar to those you would expect with a green laser. Less is definitely more with infrared.

The infrared is also far more demanding of the quality of your focus. Even a slight astigmatic oval or a slight defocusing in the anterior-posterior direction will totally block your ability to create a burn. Conversely, if you choose your power using a spot that is a little out of focus, you can cause a bad burn if you suddenly snap into accurate focus as you are working.

All of this means time and patience. In the beginning you may feel that each spot is taking hours as you fuss with the power and duration settings, and there is no question that each spot does require a lot more finesse. This can be very tedious if you are trying to do a fast and furious PRP, but with experience this becomes much less of a problem.

Perhaps the best way to use an infrared is to use your foot to adjust the power. In other words, pick a duration that is 50 to 100% longer than you might use for green (say .3 second if you normally use .15 for green). Then get the power up to where you are getting the burn you want in lighter areas—remember this may be two to three times the power you would use for green. (Note: You may have to turn the aiming beam way down to be able to watch how the tissue responds to the laser as you apply the power. If the aiming beam is bright, you cannot see subtle changes in the tissue underneath it.)

Once you have a good setting that is giving you reasonable burns, you can then carefully move to more pigmented areas and be prepared to pull your foot off the pedal as soon as you see a burn begin. This way you do not need to be constantly adjusting the power up and down depending on the pigmentation—you can simply change how long you keep the pedal to the metal for each burn. This approach is still fussy, but less time-intensive than resetting the power every five burns or so (which is what will happen with infrared if you are keeping your foot down for the entire duration of every pulse). This technique was discussed in Chapter 10—the difference is that the technique is a luxury with the green but it is more of a necessity with infrared. (Chapter 9 also talked about defocusing the spot to help you control the energy density without having to keep adjusting the laser controls. You can try this with infrared, but usually this wavelength is merciless when it comes to proper focus, so this trick is not as useful as with green.)

There is one other problem with infrared: Because the burns tend to be deeper, patients tend to feel them much more. You can try the usual things—shorter duration, smaller spot, etc., but many times you can't change these settings too much without diminishing your ability to control the safety of the burn. You may need to use more retrobulbar anesthesia than you would with a green laser. One caveat, though. If you block patients you can end up with really deep burns if you aren't paying really close attention to how your spots look, because they can't tell you how much it hurts. There has been at least one case series of patients whose pupils were blown by deep burns after periocular anesthesia.[4] (On the other hand, many patients prefer the infrared without a block, because there is no visible flash of light and they feel the treatment is less intense.)

The infrared laser is not something you should start your laser career with, if at all possible; it is much easier to learn treatment techniques with a green or yellow laser. If you must dive in with infrared, try to do a bunch of PRPs first so that you can get a good sense of how this wavelength behaves before you start treating the macula. This is because you can get nasty burns really fast if you are not careful—something that is not a good idea around the fovea. Also, you usually cannot get microaneurysms to change color with infrared, so don't go crazy turning up the power and trying to whiten microaneurysms.

If you are treating macular edema with infrared, it is much better to get in a very light grid of burns and then wait and see how the patient does. You can do focal treatment as well, but definitely don't try for a color change. Instead, just include the focal treatment as part of the grid. You can always add more treatment overtime if necessary—don't wallpaper the macula with a lot of whitish infrared burns because you will leave a very destructive legacy.

One thing to keep in mind *is that if you are using an infrared laser made by Iridex, you may have the capability of doing micropulse laser. (See Chapter 6 for a description and references.) Your laser representative can help you determine whether this is a possibility. Many of these lasers were purchased with no intention of using the micropulse settings and the original owner may not even know whether this is an option.*

Micropulsing an infrared laser is one technique for creating subthreshold burns, i.e., burns that you cannot detect visually. It is felt that such burns may have a physiologic effect without causing much damage. There are no large controlled trials that prove the efficacy of these approaches, but a lot of docs are adopting the technique as an adjuvant to injections. It may also turn out that micropulse works best with pattern lasers given that there is no identifiable burn to guide treatment location. In any event, the fact that you are reading this appendix suggests that you may be well positioned to take advantage of these techniques if they are proven effective.

Please note that this section is just a brief introduction to the art of lasering in the infrared. If you are learning your trade on this type of laser, hopefully you have a kindly instructor who will take the time to nurture your skills personally. Infrared can be a great wavelength because it can penetrate media opacities and it can be much more affordable, especially in developing countries. It is just that it is a tricky thing to master, so take your time, be careful with your settings, stay very attuned to the amount of pigment in the tissue you are treating and pay close attention to your focus.

References

1. Akduman L, Olk RJ. Diode laser (810 nm) versus argon green (514 nm) modified grid photocoagulation for diffuse diabetic macular edema. *Ophthalmology* 1997;104:1433-41.

2. Bandello F, Brancato R, Trabucchi G, Lattanzio R, Malegori A. Diode versus argon-green laser panretinal photocoagulation in proliferative diabetic retinopathy: a randomized study in 44 eyes with a long follow-up time. *Graefes Arch ClinExp Ophthalmol* 1993;231:491-4.

3. Ulbig MW, Hamilton AM. [Comparative use of diode and argon laser for panretinal photocoagulation in diabetic retinopathy]. *Ophthalmology* 1993;90:457- 62.

4. Patel JI, Jenkins L, Benjamin L, Webber S. Dilated pupils and loss of accommodation following diode panretinal photocoagulation with sub-tenon local anaesthetic in four cases. *Eye (Lond).* Sep 2002;16(5):628-632.

NOTES

NOTES

INDEX